Prostanoids
and Drugs

NATO ASI Series

Advanced Science Institutes Series

A series presenting the results of activities sponsored by the NATO Science Committee, which aims at the dissemination of advanced scientific and technological knowledge, with a view to strengthening links between scientific communities.

The series is published by an international board of publishers in conjunction with the NATO Scientific Affairs Division

A	Life Sciences	Plenum Publishing Corporation
B	Physics	New York and London
C	Mathematical and Physical Sciences	Kluwer Academic Publishers Dordrecht, Boston, and London
D	Behavioral and Social Sciences	
E	Applied Sciences	
F	Computer and Systems Sciences	Springer-Verlag
G	Ecological Sciences	Berlin, Heidelberg, New York, London,
H	Cell Biology	Paris, and Tokyo

Recent Volumes in this Series

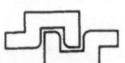

Series A: Life Sciences

Prostanoids and Drugs

Edited by

B. Samuelsson

Karolinska Institute
Stockholm, Sweden

F. Berti

University of Milan
Milan, Italy

G. C. Folco

University of Parma
Parma, Italy

and

G. P. Velo

University of Verona
Verona, Italy

Plenum Press
New York and London
Published in cooperation with NATO Scientific Affairs Division

Proceedings of a NATO Advanced Study Institute on
Prostanoids and Drugs,
held September 5–16, 1988,
in Erice, Italy

Library of Congress Cataloging in Publication Data

NATO Advanced Study Institute on Prostanoids and Drugs (1988: Erice, Italy)
    Prostanoids and drugs / edited by B. Samuelsson . . . [et al.].
        p.   cm.—(NATO ASI series. Series A, Life sciences; v. 177)
    "Proceedings of a NATO Advanced Study Institute on Prostanoids and Drugs,
held September 5–16, 1988, in Erice, Italy"—T.p. verso.
    "Published in cooperation with NATO Scientific Affairs Division."
    Includes bibliographical references.
    ISBN 978-1-4684-7940-9   ISBN 978-1-4684-7938-6 (eBook)
    DOI 10.1007/978-1-4684-7938-6
    1. Prostanoids—Antagonists—Therapeutic use—Testing—Congresses. 2.
Prostanoids—Pathophysiology—Congresses. I. Samuelsson, Bengt. II. North
Atlantic Treaty Organization. Scientific Affairs Division. III. Title. IV. Series.
    [DNLM: 1. Anti-Inflammatory Agents—congresses. 2. Leukotrienes—con-
gresses. 3. Prostaglandins—congresses. QU 90 N779p 1988]
RM666.P858N37   1988
615'.36—dc20
DNLM/DLC   89-22775
for Library of Congress   CIP

© 1989 Plenum Press, New York
Softcover reprint of the hardcover 1st edition 1989

A Division of Plenum Publishing Corporation
233 Spring Street, New York, N.Y. 10013

PREFACE

    This volume, the sixth in the series "The Prostaglandin
System" assembles most of the lecture notes from the
International School of Pharmacology on "Prostanoids and
Drugs" that took place in Erice, Sicily, at the "Ettore
Majorana Center for Scientific Culture" on Sept 5-15, 1989.

    The course, which was a NATO Advanced Study Institute,
comprised detailed discussion of basic metabolic pathways of
arachidonic acid as well as their location in the everyday
practice of clinical medicine. The current status of our
knowledge on drugs affecting prostanoid metabolic pathways,
and/or their functinal effects, together with the use of
prostanoids as drugs, has been reviewed in depth by
distinguished experts. In certain instances a few chapters
might overlap with others to present divergent viewpoints of
authors, for a better assessment of the complexity of
eicosanoid biology.

    It is likely that as our knowledge of prostanoids in
different diseases increases, new diseases may also be
targets for drugs related to these lipid mediators.
We hope that this book will encourage basic scientists and
clinicians to pursue additional biomedical investigations
along these lines of inquiry. Moreover we would like to take
this opportunity to express our gratitude to all the invited
speakers not only for their important contributions before
and during the course but also for their ability in creating
an atmosphere in which all questions were legitimate and all
lines of investigations were encouraged.

                                            B. Samuelsson
                                            F. Berti
                                            G. Folco
                                            G. Velo

ACKNOWLEDGEMENTS

This Advanced Study Institute was sponsored by NATO (ASI no 308/87)). The Course Directors also acknowledge the financial assistance of the following companies:

- Chiesi Farmaceutici S.p.A., Parma, Italy
- Ciba-Geigy S.p.A., Origgio (VA), Italy
- Essex Italia S.p.A., Milano, Italy
- Fidia, Farmaceutici Italiani Derivati Industriali e Affini S.p.A., Abano Terme (PD), Italy
- Glaxo S.p.A., Verona, Italy
- IBI, Istituto Biochimico Italiano S.p.A., Milano, Italy
- ISF S.p.A., Trezzano sul Naviglio (MI), Italy
- Italfarmaco S.p.A., Milano, Italy
- Laboratori Guidotti S.p.A., Pisa, Italy
- Rotta Research Laboratorium S.p.A., Monza (MI), Italy
- Roussel Maestretti S.p.A., Milano, Italy
- S.K.F., Smith Kline & French Laboratories, Philadelphia, USA
- Sclavo S.p.A., Siena, Italy
- Shering, Berlin, W. Germany
- Simes S.p.A., Cormano (MI), Italy

CONTENTS

MOLECULAR BIOLOGY OF LEUKOTRIENE FORMATION

Bengt Samuelsson

Department of Physiological Chemistry
Karolinska Institutet
S-104 01 Stockholm, Sweden

The leukotrienes are oxygenated derivatives of arachidonic acid with biological activities indicating important roles in inflammation and immediate hypersensitivity (1, 2).

The present review summarizes our work on the characterization of the genes and the enzymes involved in leukotrienes formation (3).

Human 5-lipoxygenase

Molecular cloning experiments have been undertaken in order to gain some insights about the structure of 5-lipoxygenase (4). Human leukocyte 5-lipoxygenase was purified and a polyclonal antibody was prepared from immunized rabbits (5). The 5-lipoxygenase antibody was used for immunoscreening of a human lung cDNA library in the expression vector λgt11. Purified intact 5-lipoxygenase, as well as proteolytically and chemically cleaved 5-lipoxygenase peptide fragments were subjected to peptide sequence analyses.

Isolation of fourteen positive phage clones was followed by purification to homogeneity by three successive rounds of antibody screening. One of the clones, λluS1, containing a 397 bp insert, was sequenced and was found to contain a coding sequence for a segment that was known for 17 amino acids from the peptide analyses of the lipoxygenase fragments. This finding established λluS1 as part of the 5-lipoxygenase cDNA.

The λluS1 insert was nick translated and used as a probe for finding clones with longer inserts from the λgt11 human lung cDNA library and a human placenta cDNA library in the λgt11 expression vector. A clone, λpl5BS, containing a cDNA insert long enough (2.6 kbp) to encode 5-lipoxygenase was isolated from the placenta cDNA library. The insert was sequenced and was found to contain 2073 bp from the initiator codon ATG to the stop codon TGA in a continous open reading frame. However, within this insert there were two adjacent exact 51-bp repeating units. This raised the possibility of a cloning artifact within the cDNA insert of λpl5BS. Therefore, two additional independent clone inserts from λpl9AS and λpl6S were sequenced. These clones contained only one copy of the 51-bp unit within their inserts. Consequently, the true 5-lipoxygenase cDNA lacks the repeat (also confirmed by genomic sequence analysis) and the open reading frame would then encode for a mature protein of 673 amino acids with a calculated molecular weight of 77,856.

There are no long segments with noticeably hydrophobic properties in the structure of 5-lipoxygenase. A segment centered around residue 310 and, to some extent, one after position 643 have several consecutive hydrophobic residues but neither segment reveals extreme properties. The protein is fairly rich in tryptophan and aromatic residues. This also and 2 tyrosines, which is highly conserved in all three soybean lipoxygenase isozymes, is a potential iron-binding region (7). Interestingly, a region of 5-lipoxygenase (residues 358-401) possesses 5 of the conserved histidine residues as well as 5 of the conserved acidic and basic residues. This region could possibly comprise the iron-binding domain of 5-lipoxygenase.

The present of a short sequence segment that is related to the interface-binding domain of the human lipoprotein lipase and the rat hepatic lipase has also been reported (12). 5-Lipoxygenase requires calcium and ATP for maximal activity. The amino acid sequence of 5-lipoxygenase was compared to the sequences of calcium- and ATP-binding proteins. Very limited homology was obseved, however.

Human 5-lipoxygenase shows no sequence homology to either bovine cyclooxygenase (13, 14) or to human LTA_4 hydrolase (15, 16).

The human 5-lipoxygenase gene

The 5-lipoxygenase gene has recently been characterized. Three different genomic DNA libraries were screened with several 5-lipoxygenase cDNA probes. Several overlapping clones spanning the gene were isolated and characterized by restriction endonuclease mapping and Southern blot analysis. The human 5-lipoxygenase gene is organized into at least 13 exons (putative exon 3 has not yet been cloned) divided by 12 introns. Exons range in size from 87 bp (exon 8) to 611 bp (exon 13), whereas intron sizes range between 192 bp (intron J) and 10.5 kb (intron F). Exons 1-6, encoding the amino-terminal half of 5-lipoxygenase are spread out over more than 30 kb of DNA, while the carboxy-terminal encoding exons, 7-13 are clustered in a 6 kb segment. The total length of the gene is at least 45 kb. One particular exon (exon 6), which encodes amino acids 278-326, corresponds exactly to one of the most hydrophobic segments of 5-lipoxygenase. It is, therefore, possible that this exon represents an important functional and/or structural domain of 5-lipoxygenase.

A region upstream of the translation initiation site, comprising the putative promoter region of the 5-lipoxygenase gene was sequenced and characterized. The region does not contain typical TATA and CAAT box sequences, however, certain features common to housekeeping gene promoters were found. The region is very GC-rich (80%) and contains 8 potential "GC-box" sites for binding of the transcription factor Sp1. The presence of two 11-bp inverted repeat segments in this region could possibly have some relevance to transcription factor binding and transcriptional regulation. The housekeeping genes are constitutively expressed. Since the 5-lipoxygenase gene shares similar promoter characteristics to the housekeeping genes this raises many intriguing questions about how the 5-lipoxygenase gene is regulated and expressed in a tissue-specific fashion.

LTA_4-hydrolase

Rabbits were injected with LTA_4-hydrolase (purified from human neutrophils) for production of polyclonal antiserum. One clone (λluH6-1) encoded for a β-galactosidase fusion protein carrying epitopes that were recognized by the LTA_4-hydrolase antiserum. The insert from λluH6-1a was nick-translated and used as a probe to find longer clones in the lung cDNA λgt11 library. Twenty strongly positive clones were abtained. These clones were purified and their EcoRI inserts ranged in size from 0.2 to 1.2 kilobases. The insert of the longest clone, λlu209-8A, was sequenced and found to contain 770 bp of cDNA encoding LTA_4 hydrolase, overlapping with 159 bp of the 5' end of the insert of λluH6-1a, and a 405-bp cloning artifact at the 5' end.

Since we were unable to find clones long enough to encode a full-length cDNA with the lung cDNA λgt11 library screening of additional libraries was carried out. Nineteen strongly positive clones were isolated and purified after screening $\approx 4 \times 10^5$ clones from a human placenta λgt11 library. Twelve of these clones contained a 1.1-kb/0.8-kb double-insert pattern. In DNA blot analysis ^{32}P-labeled λluH6-1a insert hybridized to the 0.8-kb insert of the 12 clones (data not shown). The pattern of these clone inserts gave strong reason to believe that an internal EcoRI site is present.

λpl6A contained a 1910-bp insert, excluding EcoRI linkers, with a continous open reading frame of 1830 bp terminated by a TAA stop codon. The open reading frame encodes a protein of 610 amino acids with a calculated molecular weight of 69,140.

LTA_4 hydrolase was analyzed by direct liquid phase sequencer degradation for 34 cycles. Results were in agreement with the deduced sequence and the previously reported 15 N-terminal amino acids (17) CNBr fragments of carboxyl [^{14}C]methylated LTA_4 hydrolase were purified. Five fragments were analyzed. Both total compositions and amino acid sequences of these fragments are in agreement with the structure deduced from the cDNA sequence. Consequently, N-terminal, internal, and near-C-terminal regions of the deduced structure have been directly confirmed by analysis at the protein level.

The cDNA sequence of the λpl6A insert shows no significant sequence homology with the nucleotide sequences in the EMBL data bank (EMBL/GenBank Genetic Sequence Database (1986) EMBL Nucleotide Sequence Data Library (Eur. Mol. Biol. Lab., Heidelberg, Tape Release 10), including those of rabbit and rat liver microsomal epoxide hydrolases (18, 19).

Screening of the protein sequence for internal homologies did not reveal any consistent patterns of long repeats (two 30 residue segments, starting at positions 209 and 393, show some similarities - 10 identities in 29 residues). Secondary structure predictions (20) and calculations of hydropathy (21) reveal mixed patterns, as for many proteins. However, a segment close to position 200 displays some more extreme properties. Thus, the segment 170-185 is the most hydrophilic in the whole protein, 190-205 the one most hydrophobic, and in between is one of two strong predictions for a reverse turn (followed by a prediction of a β-strand). One of the internal repeat segments mentioned above is adjacent to this segment (residues 209-238) and has a prediction for a long α-helix (residues 220-240). Several features therefore center around the segment 165-240, which could be related to the structure and activity of LTA_4 hydrolase. It was previously demonstrated that LTA_4 could be covalently bound to the enzyme (22). The thiol group of Cys-199 within the hydrophobic region, is one of the possible candidates for such an interaction.

Acknowledgements

These studies were supported by the Swedish Medical Research Council (03X-217) and the Knut and Alice Wallenberg Foundation.

RERERENCES

1. Samuelsson, B. (1983) Science.
2. Samuelsson, B., Dahlen, S.-E., Lindgren, J.-Å., Rouzer, C.A. and Serhan, C.N. (1987) Science 237, 1171-1176.
3. Samuelsson, B., Rouzer, C.A. and Matsumoto, T. (1987) In: Adv. in Prostaglandin, Thromboxane and Leukotriene Research (Eds. B. Samuelsson, P. Ramwell and R. Paoletti), Raven Press, N.Y. vol. 17A, pp. 1-11.
4. Matsumoto, T., Funk, C.D., Rådmark, O., Höög, J-O., Jörnvall, H. and Samuelsson, B. (1988) Proc. Natl. Acad. Sci. USA 85, 26-30.

5. Rouzer, C.A. and Samuelsson, B (1985) Proc. Natl. Acad. Sci. USA 82, 6040-6044.

6. Shibata, D., Steczko, J., Dixon, J.E., Hermodson, M., Yazdanparast, R. and Axelrod, B. (1987) J. Biol. Chem. 262, 10080-10085.

7. Shibata, D., Steczko, J., Dixon, J.E., Andrews, P.C., Hermodson, M. and Axelrod, B. (1988) J. Biol. Chem. 262, 6816-6821.

8. Yenofsky, R.L., Fine, M. and Liu, C. (1988) Mol. Gen. Genet. 211, 215-222.

9. Hogaboom, G.K., Cook, M., Newton, J.F., Varrichio, A., Shorr, R.G.L., Sarall, H.M. and Crooke, S.T. (1986) Mol. Pharmacol. 30, 510-519.

10. Sigall, E., Grunberger, D., Craik, C.S., Caughey, G.H., and Nadel, J.A. (1988) J. Biol. Chem. 263, 5328-5332.

11. Thiele, B.J., Black, E., Fleming, J., Nack, B., Rapoport, S.M. and Harrison, P.R. (1987) Biomed. Biochim. Acta 46, 120-123.

12. Dixon, R.A.F., Jones, R.E., Diehl, R.E., Bennett, C.D., Kargman, S., and Rouzer, C.A. (1988) Proc. Natl. Acad. Sci. USA 85, 416-420.

13. Dewitt, D.L. and Smith, W.L. (1988) Proc. Natl. Acad. Sci. USA 85, 1412-1416.

14. Merlie, J.P., Fagan, D., Mudd, J. and Needleman, P. (1988) J. Biol. Chem. 263, 3550-3553.

15. Funk, C.D., Rådmark, O., Fu, J.Y., Matsumoto, T., Jörnvall, H., Shimizu, T. and Samuelsson, B. (1987) Proc. Natl. Acad. Sci. USA 84, 6677-6681.

16. Minami, M., Ohno, S., Kawasaki, H., Rådmark, O., Samuelsson, B., Jörnvall, H., Shimizu, T., Seyama, Y. and Suzuki, K. (1987) J. BIOL. Chem. 262, 13873-13876.

17. Rådmark, P., Shimizu, T., Jörnvall, H. and Samuelsson, B. (1984) J. Biol. Chem. 259, 12339-12345.

18. Heinemann, F.S. and Ozols, J. (1984) J. Biol. Chem. 259, 797-804.

19. Porter, T.D., Beck, T.W. and Kasper, C.B. (1986) Arch. Biochem. Biophys. 248, 121-129.

20. Chou, P.Y. and Fasman, G.D. (1974) Biochemistry 13, 211-221.

21. Hopp, T.P. and Woods, K.R. (1981) Proc. Natl. Acad. Sci. USA, 78, 3824-3828.

22. Evans, J.F., Nathaniel, D.J., Zamboni, R.J. and Ford-Hutchinson, A.W. (1985) J. Biol. Chem. 260, 10966-10970.

FUNDAMENTAL MASS SPECTROMETRY AND EICOSANOIDS RESEARCH

Robert C. Murphy, Keith L. Clay, and Joseph A. Zirrolli

Department of Pharmacology
University of Colorado Health Sciences Center
4200 E. 9th Avenue
Denver, Colorado 80262

INTRODUCTION

Mass spectrometry is an instrument based technique in which the interaction of ions in a vacuum are studied with magnetic and/or electrical fields. The behavior and motion of ions is quite predictable based upon the mass-to-charge ratio (m/z) of the ions and this forms the basis of the mass spectrometric experiment. The first studies in this area were carried out by J.J. Thompson in England close to the turn of the century which lead to his discovery of isotopes of elements. Later experiments by Aston, Dempster as well as many others lead to the development of the fundamental theory of modern instrumentation for mass spectrometry. Mass spectrometry is an exceedingly versatile technique which can provide fundamental information of great value in many disciplines and has been applied directly to virtually all areas of science including biology, chemistry, and physics. Some of the first experiments involving mass spectrometry applied to biology, involved using the quantitative nature of the information which can be obtained. In these studies, Rittenberg used stable isotopes as tracers in order to study the biochemistry of amino acids (1). Fred McLafferty in the mid 1950s illustrated the usefulness of fragmentation of organic ions and was able to deduce the structures of biological substances based upon mass spectrometry (2). These concepts were quickly applied to extremely complex molecules as illustrated by the work of Klaus Biemann in the late 1950s and early 1960s in which he elegantly demonstrated the ability of mass spectrometry to provide data necessary for the structure elucidation of complex natural products (3).

Historically, mass spectrometry has also played an important role in the field of arachidonic acid metabolism. It was used in the 1960s and early 1970s to characterize the primary prostaglandin and thromboxane structures as well as to deduce the structures of their major metabolic degradation products (4). These studies illustrate the qualitative nature of the mass spectrometric data and the use of this technique for structure elucidation. Following the direct interface of the gas chromatograph with a mass spectrometer (3), one of the first application of quantitative mass spectrometry by selected ion monitoring and stable isotope dilution involved the measurement of lipids (5). Mass spectrometry continues to be the method of choice in many laboratories for the quantitative analysis of eicosanoids by stable isotope dilution techniques. Furthermore, there has been a continual close-link between studies of the metabolism of arachidonic acid and advances in mass spectrometry.

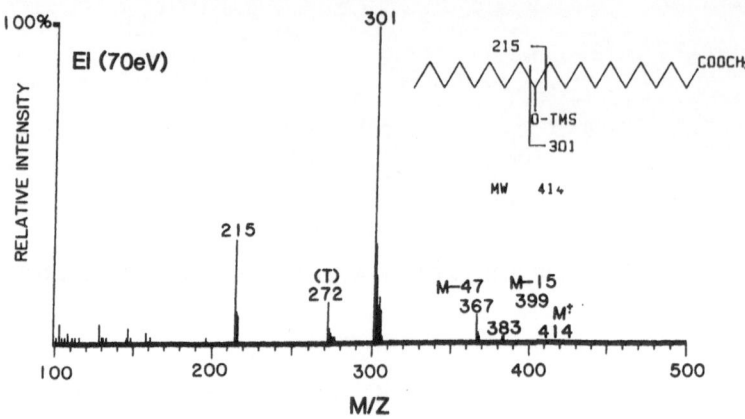

Figure 1 *Electron impact (70 eV) mass spectrum of 12-hydroxyeicosanoic acid derivatized as the trimethylsilyl ether, methyl ester. This derivative was used to facilitate GC/MS anlaysis. The ion at m/z 272 (T) arises from rearrangement of the 12-O-trimethylsilyl group to the carboxyl group prior to fragmentation between c-11 and C-12.*

Qualitative Analysis

There are three general attributes of mass spectrometry which have been responsible for the applicability of this technique to eicosanoid research-specificity, sensitivity, and versatility. Mass spectrometry provides unique information as to the exact masses of ions which originate from a metabolite of arachidonic acid as well as provides information concerning the decomposition of these ions in the gas phase. Furthermore, specificity of the mass spectrometric experiment has been shown to be significantly improved when one directly couples a high resolution separation technique such as capillary gas chromatography or high pressure liquid chromatography directly to the mass spectrometer. These will be discussed later. A second important attribute is the sensitivity of this technique. There is no question that this is a major factor responsible for the application of mass spectrometry to eicosanoid analysis. The basis for the sensitivity enjoyed by mass spectrometry lies with the detection device, the electron multiplier. The electron multiplier is an amplification device which can convert the signal from positive or negative ions into a cascade of electrons typically at a gain in signal from 10^5 and 10^8 fold. While this unique device can be used to detect the presence of one ion (2 x 10^{-24} moles) more routinely the sensitivity is adjusted for ease of operation to values between 10^{-9} to 10^{-12} moles. A third attribute of mass spectrometry is its versatility. Modern techniques of mass spectrometry have now permitted the application of this technique to the analysis of virtually any biochemical substance below a molecular weight of 5 - 7,000 daltons. This means that molecules as large as proteins such as C5A and insulin can be analyzed by mass spectrometry (6) and even this limit has now been extended to the analyses of proteins up to molecular weights above 20,000 (7). Also substances such as inorganic salts can be analyzed and in fact stable isotopes of zinc and calcium have been used in nutritional studies employing mass spectrometric measurements (8). The eicosanoids and their metabolites vary in molecular weight from approximately 200 to 625, the latter being the molecular weight of leukotriene C_4. However, even if one expands the definition of eicosanoids to include those biological substances which contain arachidonic acid such as the glycerophosphatidylcholines then molecular weights close to 1,000 can be encountered. Still, in this mass range, eicosanoid size does not challenge the capability of the modern mass spectrometer.

However, limitations of mass spectrometry should also be mentioned. First of all, the mass spectrometric experiment can be a labor intensive process. It takes extensive training to make an individual proficient in the proper use of the instrument and the preparation of samples prior to analysis. Secondly, the cost of instrumentation can be quite high when compared to other biochemical techniques. However, this cost should be kept in mind with the capability of the instrument to be applied to many areas of biological sciences and its ability to provide fundamental information which might range from protein sequence to quantitative analysis of picomolar amounts of eicosanoids in a biological fluid. A third limitation is that experiments involving gas chromatography/mass spectrometry require that the substance to be analyzed has some vapor pressure so that it can pass into the gas phase at elevated temperature conditions. Not all metabolites of arachidonic acid can satisfy this limiting criterion. For example, the intact sulfidopeptide leukotrienes and in particular LTC_4 and LTD_4 can only be analyzed by special MS techniques which surmount this gas phase requirement. This technique will be discussed briefly later on and is fast atom bombardment mass spectrometry.

Ionization Modes

Several modes of ionization are used to convert a molecule into an ion which can then be handled by the mass spectrometer. Three of these have been most widely used for metabolites of arachidonic acid. They include electron impact ionization, chemical ionization, and fast atom bombardment. Electron impact ionization involves the excitation of the molecule by an energetic electron thermionically emitted from a heated filament with an energy close to 1,600 kcal/mole (70 eV). A portion of this energy is transfered to the molecule in the form of excitation of a ground state electron into an empty, higher energy orbital of the molecule. If the transfer of energy is sufficient to promote an electron completely out of all available orbitals, this leads to the production of a positive ion (since the electron is no longer associated with the molecule). This ion is called the molecular ion and carries the entire weight of the molecule; however, it may rearrange its covalent structure in this state because of excess energy which is often imparted to the molecule during the ionization process. Furthermore, there is typically sufficient energy to break additional carbon-carbon, carbon-hydrogen, and carbon-oxygen bonds in the molecule leading to a host of fragment ions whose abundances make up the classic of spectrum as illustrated in Figure 1 for the 12-hydroxyeicosanoic acid (derivatized for GC/MS analysis).

Chemical ionization mass spectrometry has also had a major impact on eicosanoid research. This technique is similar in some respect to electron impact but differs primarily from the fact that a high pressure of moderating gas is present in the ion source region (9). This moderating gas, such as methane at 1 torr, is ionized by electron impact from a heated filament. However, due to the high pressure of methane, ion molecule reactions and electron capture of secondary electrons can result. For the case of positive ion chemical ionization, one needs to consider the initially formed methane molecular ion (CH_4^+), which can interact with a neutral methane molecule through an ion molecule reaction, generating another species CH_5^+ and $CH_3^{\bullet}$. CH_5^+ is a reactive species which can protonate less acidic species, for example the molecule under study (M), leading to production of MH^+ ions or quasi-molecular ions. This process is energetically less than direct electron ionization and typically a higher population of molecular ions or quasi-molecular ions are observed with chemical ionization mass spectrometry.

If one considers the electron population in the chemical ionization experiment, the initial high energy electrons (70 eV or 1,600 kcal/mole) are step-wise reduced in energy content by multiple interactions with methane molecules due to the high pressure. Furthermore, the electrons which are promoted from the ionized methane molecular ion are also present and these electrons also undergo multiple energy reducing interactions to form an electron plasma (9). This plasma has a population of energies centered around the thermal energy of the ion source. Thus, a plasma of thermal electrons is produced which readily interact with molecules having a high affinity for electrons. Typically one converts an eicosanoid to such an electron capturing compound through derivatization with a polyhalogenated molecule. When such a molecule is present even in trace amounts in the ion source in the presence of a plasma of thermalized electrons, an electron can be captured to form a molecular anion M⁻•. In many cases there is sufficient energy imparted in this electron capture process that some bonds can be broken within the molecule leading to the appearance of fragment anions. However, in general, this fragmentation is substantially less than that observed under electron impact conditions. Figure 2 illustrates the negative ion chemical ionization mass spectrum of a derivatized hydroxy

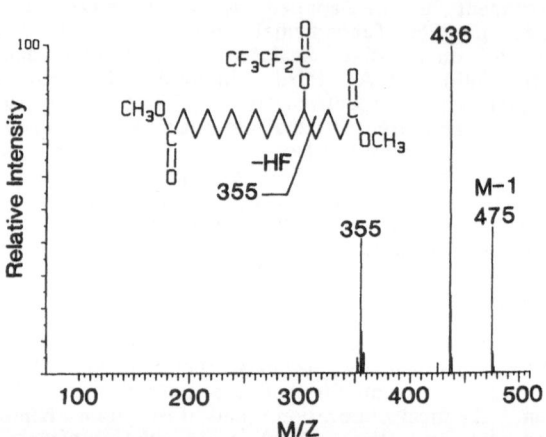

Figure 2 *Negative ion electron capture mass spectrum of 5-hydroxy-1,16-hexadecanedioic acid as the 5-pentafluoropropionyl ester, dimethyl ester. The molecular weight of this derivative is 476.*

dicarboxylic acid derived from a metabolite of leukotriene E_4. This mass spectrum shows a prominent ion at M-1 where a proton is removed from the molecule to form the pseudo molecular anion (M-1) as well as an abundant ion due to the subsequent loss of two moles of HF (m/z 436) as well as a cleavage ion adjacent to the oxygen at carbon-5 derivatized with the pentafluoropropionyl group with loss of HF (m/z 355).

Another important ionization technique is fast atom bombardment which has only been relatively recently described. In 1980 Barber and colleagues (10) found that dissolving a nonvolatile substance in a glycerol matrix and bombarding the matrix with a beam of neutral atoms resulted in the emission of secondary ions which could be analyzed by a mass spectrometer. If the molecule had a sufficient propensity towards the formation of positive or negative ions the biological substance could be observed. A review of the mechanisms involved in the fast atom bombardment experiment have been presented (6). A major application of fast atom bombardment mass spectrometry to eicosanoid research has been in the ability to analyze the sulfidopeptide leukotrienes directly without the need for chemical degradation. This can be illustrated in Figure 3 which illustrates the analysis of negative ions from LTE_4 and N-acetyl-LTE_4 by fast atom bombardment mass spectrometry. In this technique LTE and N-acetyl-LTE were dissolved in glycerol and then bombarded with zenon ions at 6 kv resulting in ions at m/z 438 (M-1)⁻ from LTE_4 (molecular weight 439) and at 42 mass units higher for N-acetyl-LTE_4 at m/z 480 (M-H)⁻ which has a molecular weight of 481. Thus, fast atom bombardment can provide molecular weight information.

Gas Chromatography/Mass Spectrometry

In the early 1960s the gas chromatograph was successfully coupled directly to the mass spectrometer ion source using a separation device to strip off the carrier gas (11). With the advent of improved high vacuum technology and the development of capillary gas chromatography it was found that the gas chromatographic column with relatively low flow rates (1-2 ml/min permitted) could be directly linked to the ion source of the mass spectrometer without the need for a separation device to strip off the carrier gas. Furthermore, the capillary gas chromatographic column offered significant advantages in component resolution capabilities. For example, with capillary columns typically employed from 5-20 meters having internal diameters of 0.2 to 0.5 mm,

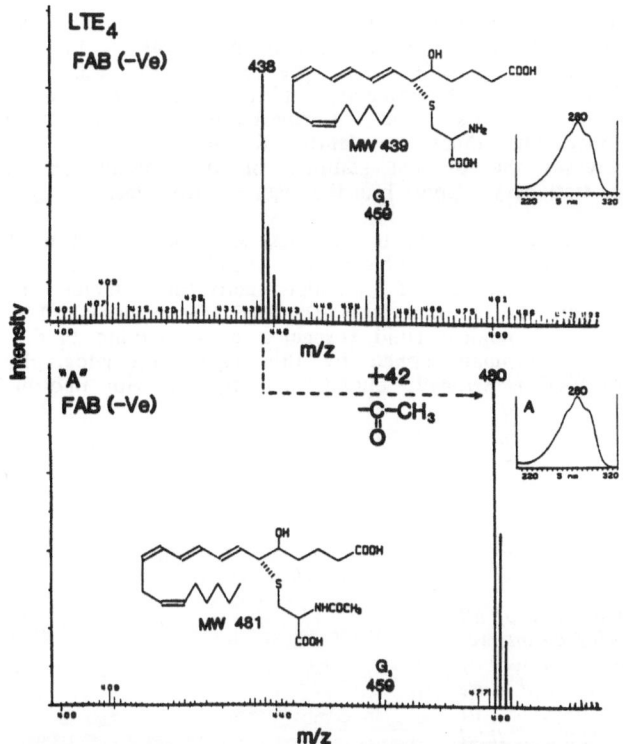

Figure 3 *Fast atom bombardment mass spectra (negation ions) of LTE_4 and N-acetyl-LTE_4 using glycerol as matrix. The inset figures indicate the UV spectra of these two leukotrienes.*

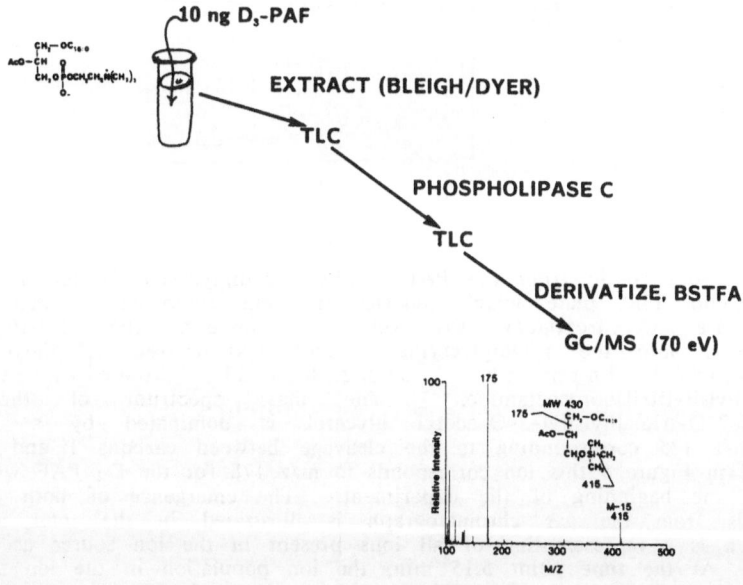

Figure 4 *Flow diagram of a GC/MS-based assay for platelet activating factor (PAF) using D_3-PAF as internal standard. The mass spectrum of the 1,3-diglyceride TMS ether has the most abundant ion at m/z 175.*

one could have total effective plates from 15,000 to 60,000 and still have a capacity of several hundreds of nanograms per peak. For the analysis of eicosanoids one has to consider the type of injector used; there are many available, including a split injector, splitless injector, on-column injector, and falling needle injectors (12). Furthermore, numerous stationary supports are available including those covalently linked to the glass wall. This substantially increases the thermal stability of the column as well as reduces the "bleed" of the stationary support into the mass spectrometer.

Combining gas chromatography to the mass spectrometer led to the development of timed-based experiments to enhance the specificity of the analysis. This is illustrated in the analysis of platelet activating factor from biological fluids seen in Figure 4. In this assay D_3-PAF (for example 10 ng) is added to a known volume of biological fluid suspected of containing PAF. This fluid is then extracted and chromatographed by thin layer chromatography. The band corresponding to PAF is scraped, eluted, and treated with phospholipase C to

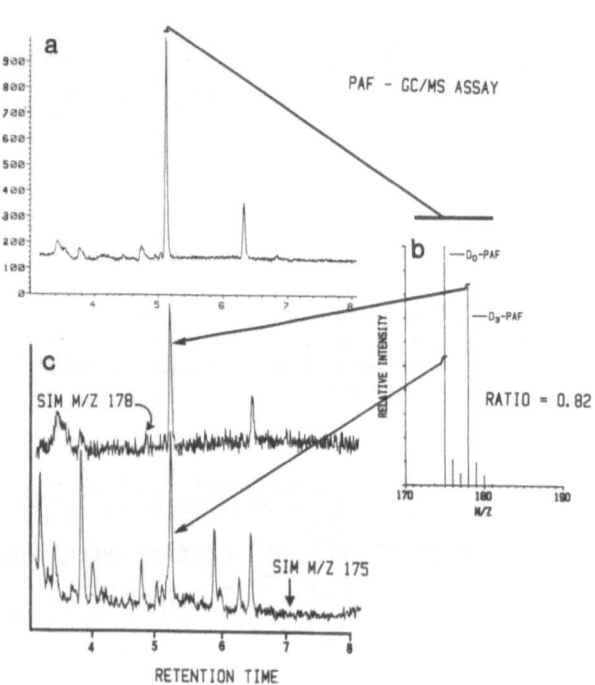

Figure 5 *(a) Summation of all ions recorded during an interval of one scan (typically 1 sec) of a GC/MS experiment are plotted as a function of retention time to obtain the total ionization plot. (b) At any one time ions in the ion source can be observed as illustrated at 5.15 min from m/z 170-190. (c) Presentation of the abundance of a single ion as a function of retention time is the selected ion monitor trace (SIM) as illustrated for m/z 178 and 175.*

form a 1,2-diglyceride from the PAF. This 1,2-diglyceride is chromatographed on a second TLC plate which purifies it from components added by the phospholipase C treatment as well as converts the 1,2-diglyceride quantitatively into the 1,3-diglyceride. This PAF-derived 1,2-diglyceride is derivatized into the trimethylsilyl derivative by bis(trimethylsilyl)trifluoroacetamide. The mass spectrum of the 1-O-hexadecyl-2-O-trimethylsilyl-3-O-acetyl glycerol is dominated by a fragment ion at m/z 175 corresponding to the cleavage between carbons 1 and 2. As illustrated in Figure 5 this ion corresponds to m/z 178 for the D_3 PAF which was added at the beginning of the experiment. The emergence of both of these compounds from the gas chromatograph is illustrated in the total ionization plot which is a representation of all ions present in the ion source as function of time. At the time point 5.15 min, the ion population in the ion source is illustrated in the mass spectrum (Figure 5b) revealing abundant ions at m/z 175 and 178. If one replots the data (which is typically stored in the computer) to the time-based appearance of the specific ions at m/z 175 and m/z 178 (Figure 5c), one obtains selected ion monitoring traces which illustrate the emergence

Figure 6 *A standard curve for a quantitative GC/MS assay of arachidonic acid using D_8-arachidonic acid (MW-492, m/z 311) as internal standard (500 ng) and negative ion electron capture mass spectrometry of the pentafluorobenzyl ester derivative. The ratio of m/z 303 (D_0-arachidonate) to m/z 311 (D_8-arachidonate) relates to the amount of D_0-arachidonate in a linear manner.*

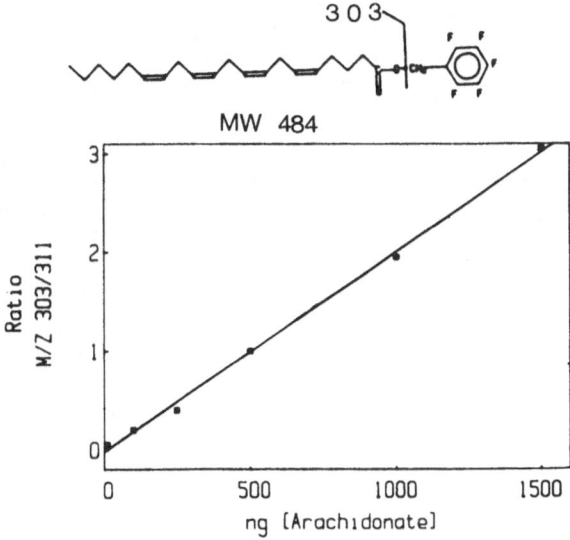

of D_0-PAF and D_3-PAF respectively during the capillary GC/MS experiment. For quantitative analysis, which will be discussed below, one calculates the specific areas for each platelet activating factor species.

Quantitative Analysis

There are many parameters which control the absolute signal strength of ions in the mass spectrometric experiment, for example the gain of the electron multiplier. Therefore, an important question to ask is how can one obtain quantitative data from the mass spectrometer. While there had been several solutions to this problem, the most widely used and accepted approach is to use an isotope labeled internal standard to correct for the variation in ion signal strength and to relate ion abundance to exact quantities of metabolites of arachidonic acid. The basis of this is rather simple. As discussed previously, one adds a known amount of a unique compound, typically a stable isotope derivative of the molecule to be measured to the sample prior to separation and analysis. When carrying out the mass spectrometric experiment, two ions are measured. One characteristic of the desired eicosanoid and the second, the corresponding ion derived from the internal standard. Since the abundance of the internal standard ion is directly related to that amount which was added (which is of course known) this can be used to calibrate the signal strength for the molecule which is endogenous. This correspondence can be seen best by a calibration curve such as that illustrated in Figure 6 for the quantitative analysis of arachidonic acid based upon negative ion electron capture mass spectrometry of the pentafluorobenzyl ester derivative. One routinely sees a straight line relationship over a wide region with standard error of the mean for replicate measurements typically being too small to express in error bars. This technique of isotope dilution mass spectrometry is unsurpassed in precision and accuracy.

A major concern for such an approach is the nature of the internal standard to be employed. A basic problem arises from the fact that stable isotopes do exist in nature at abundances which can cause some effect on the calibration curve. As seen in Table 1, these natural abundances can range from being very high for ^{13}C at M+1, to quite acceptable abundances for those isotopes two mass units higher, for example oxygen-18. Thus, one needs to consider what type of

11

Table I. Natural abundances of isotopes (adapted from Ref. 3) frequently encountered in eicosanoid mass spectrometry

Isotope	% Natural Abundance
^1H	99.985
^2H	0.015
^{12}C	98.9
^{13}C	1.1
^{14}N	99.64
^{15}N	0.36
^{16}O	99.8
^{18}O	0.2
^{19}F	100
^{28}Si	92.2
^{29}Si	4.7
^{20}Si	3.1

stable isotope to be employed and the number of isotopes to be incorporated in order to advance the mass of the internal standard by 1, 2, 3, or perhaps 4 units above that of the native molecule. Furthermore, one must consider the isotopic purity of the internal standard. These can be illustrated in two figures which show the effect of number of isotopes incorporated and the isotopic purity on the standard curve. As seen in Figure 7, the amount of unlabeled material in the isotope internal standard, whether it is 0.1%, 1%, or 5% can effect the lower end of the calibration curve. This is illustrated for LTB_4 by calculating the expected ratio of ions m/z 479/483 from D_{3-} LTB_4 at various isotopic purity. With 5% unlabeled LTB_4 (D_0-LTB_4) present in the $D_{3-}LTB_4$ internal standard, one has a linear range in ion ratios from 0.5 to approximately 10. This should be compared to 0.1% unlabeled D_3-LTB_4 where the linear range is approximately from ratios of .05 to 10.

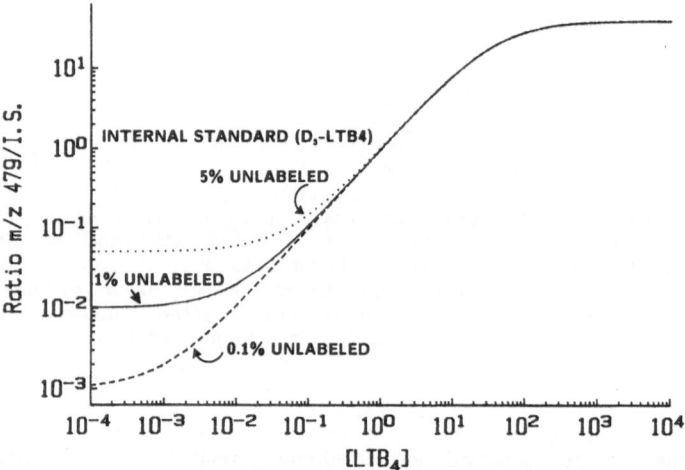

Figure 7 *At high dilution of LTB_4 relative to the internal standard D_3-LTB_4, the standard curve approaches asymptotically a constant value relative to the isotopic purity (5%, 1%, or 0.1% unlabeled material in the internal standard).*

As seen in Figure 8, the number of isotopes incorporated also has a major impact on the range of the calibration curve by advancing the mass above the interference from natural abundance isotopes. For example, if one uses an internal standard which is only one mass unit above that of the native molecule, a severe limitation at the higher end of the calibration curve is realized where a ratio of approximately 1 to 1.5 becomes maximal before no additional change in the ratio is observed for an increase in the amount of unlabeled material (endogenous) present. There is no effect on the lower end of the curve which was illustrated above to correspond to the isotopic purity of the internal standard. However, by using an internal standard which is two mass units above the molecular weight of the native molecule, one can employ ratios which are 10-fold higher before saturation of the measured ratio is observed. As you increase in the number of isotopes to advance the molecular weight above that of the native molecule, you increase the dynamic range of the standard curve.

Figure 8 *At high dilution of the deuterium labeled LTB_4 internal standard (10 to 10^4 more LTB_4 than deuterium labeled LTB_4 in this example), the standard curve approaches asymptotically a constant value related to the natural abundances of all isotopes in the ion (m/z 479) and the number of masses the internal standard is above the nominal mass for LTB_4.*

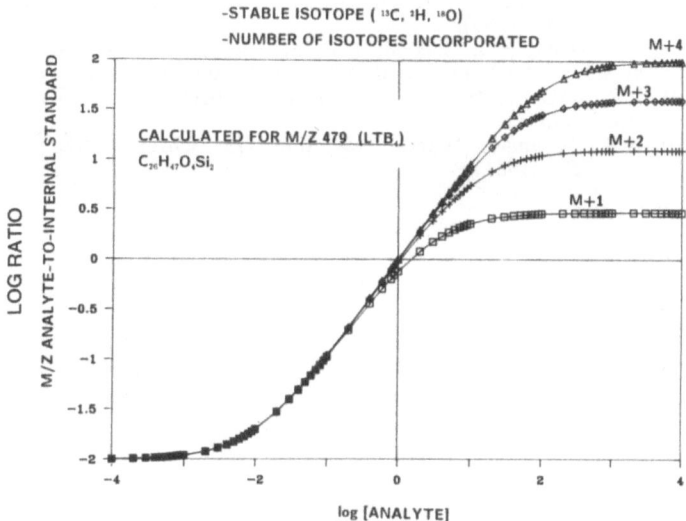

One of the unique aspects of mass spectrometry is that it can be readily optimized for both quantitative and qualitative analysis of numerous molecules including hundreds of different arachidonic acid metabolites which have been structurally characterized. This unique flexibility and sensitivity of the mass spectrometer will ensure its continued application to studies of the metabolism, biosynthesis, and quantitative analysis of metabolites of arachidonic acid in the future.

ACKNOWLEDGEMENTS

This work was supported by a grant from the National Institutes of Health (AI20774).

REFERENCES

1. D. Rittenberg, 1948, Dynamic aspects of the metabolism of amino acids. Harvey Lectures, pp. 200-220 (1948).
2. F.W. McLafferty, Mass spectrometric analysis. Broad applicability to chemical research, *Anal. Chem.* 28:306 (1956).
3. K. Biemann, "Mass Spectrometry: Organic Chemical Applications," McGraw-Hill, New York (1962).
4. B. Samuelsson, M. Goldyne, E. Granstrom, M. Hamberg, S. Hammarstrom, and C. Malmsten, Prostaglandins and thromboxanes, *Ann. Rev. Biochem.*, 47:997 (1978).
5. C.C. Sweeley, W. Elliot, I. Fries, and R. Ryhage, Mass spectrometric determination of unresolved components in gas chromatographic effluents, *Anal. Chem.* 38:1549 (1966).
6. B. Sundquist and R.D. MacFarlane, [252]Cf-Plasma desorption mass spectrometry. Mass Spectrom. Rev. 4:421 (1985).
7. A.G. Craig, A. Engstrom, A. Benick, and P.I. Kamensky, Enhancement of molecule ion yields in plasma desorption mass spectrometry, Proc. Ann. Conf. Mass Spectrom. 35:528 (1987).
8. P.L. Peirce, K.M. Hambidge, C.H. Goss, L.V. Miller, and P.V. Fennessey, Fast atom bombardment mass spectrometry for the determination of zinc stable isotopes in biological samples, *Anal. Chem.*, 59:2034 (1987).

9. A.G. Harrison , "Chemical Ionization Mass Spectrometry," CRC Press, Boca Raton, FL (1983).
10. M. Barber, R.S. Bordeli, R.D. Sedwick, and A.N. Tyler, Fast atom bombardment of solids as an ion source in mass spectrometry, *Nature*, 293:270 (1981).
11. J.T. Watson, "Introduction to Mass Spectrometry," Raven Press, 2nd Ed., New York (1985).
12. R.R. Freeman, "High Resolution Gas Chromatography," Hewlett-Packard, Palo Alto, CA (1981).

QUANTITATIVE ANALYSIS OF EICOSANOIDS BY GAS CHROMATOGRAPHY-

MASS SPECTROMETRY

Francesca Catella, Jana M. Johnson
and Garret A. FitzGerald

Vanderbilt University
Department of Pharmacology
Nashville, TN 37232

INTRODUCTION

Eicosanoids are metabolic products derived from polyunsaturated straight-chain C 20 carboxylic acids. The most abundant substrate in humans is arachidonic acid (AA), a physiological component of the plasma membrane. Following stimulation, AA is released from an ester linkage to phospholipids and oxygenated into an array of compounds whose biological importance has been well established in vitro. On the other hand, the investigation of their potential role in human pathology depends upon assessment of their formation in vivo. Alterations in eicosanoid biosynthesis in pathological conditions and the functional consequences of their pharmacological inhibition or antagonism have indicated their pathophysiological role in vivo[1-5]. Specific and sensitive assays for eicosanoids have been required to address these issues.

The most commonly used methods for the routine measurement of eicosanoids are gas chromatographic (GC) mass spectrometric (MS) techniques and immunoassays (IA) such as radio (RIA) or enzyme immunoassays (EIA). The IAs can usually be performed on a larger scale in a relatively short time and don't require expensive equipment or highly qualified personnel. On the other hand, IA methods may generate misleading results. This is generally due to lack of specificity resulting from inappropriate purification or the use of antisera with high cross-reactivity with different metabolites. For example, RIA measurement of eicosanoids in serum suggested that inhibition of thromboxane synthase resulted in a pronounced increase in prostacyclin formation[6]. A subsequent analysis performed by GC-MS indicated that immunoreactive techniques overestimated the 6-keto-$PGF_{1\alpha}$ concentration, probably due to cross reactivity of the antiserum for 6-keto-$PGF_{1\alpha}$ with other prostaglandins, such as $PGF_{2\alpha}$ and PGD_2 which are formed in greater abundance than prostacyclin in serum[7]. Therefore, any new IA should be validated by characterization of the thin layer chromatography (TLC) pattern of distribution of the extracted eicosanoid-like immunoreactivity, by using multiple antisera and by comparison with GC-MS determinations. RIA results highly comparable with GC-MS results have been indeed attained when the metabolites have been properly purified from biological matrices and a highly specific antiserum has been employed[8,9]. On the other hand, even highly validated IAs have practical limitations. For example, recently, fish oils, rich in the w-3 fatty acid, eicosapentaenoic acid (EPA) have

---

Address correspondence to Dr. FitzGerald

been extensively investigated for their potential antithrombotic properties. Dietary supplementation with fish oil results in decreased formation of TxA_2 (derived from AA), and increased TxA_3[10] (derived from EPA and supposedly less thrombogenic and less pro-inflammatory than TxA_2)[11]. Commonly available IAs cannot discriminate between the eicosanoids derived from AA and those derived from EPA which differ only by one double bond[12]. By contrast, GC-MS techniques can easily discriminate between these two series of compounds.

Another limitation of IA methods overcome by GC-MS is their poor sensitivity. It was suggested that analysis of eicosanoids in plasma could facilitate the investigation of their temporal formation in vivo: this would be desirable when phasic eicosanoid formation might be of interest, such as during ischemic episodes in patients with unstable angina. As far as TxA_2 is concerned, plasma concentrations of its hydration product, TxB_2, are readily confounded by ex vivo platelet activation. However, 11-dehydro-TxB_2 a long lived enzymatic metabolite of TxB_2, has been shown to minimize this problem [13]. Its measurement in plasma requires a detection limit of less than 1 pg/ml. This can be attained by capillary GC- negative ion chemical ionization (NICI)-MS (Fig 1), but it is far below the limit of sensitivity achieved by most commercially available IAs. Combined analysis of 11-dehydro-TxB_2 and 2,3-dinor-TxB_2, indices of the two major pathways of thromboxane metabolism in man, permits one to distinguish altered metabolism from increased biosynthesis of TxA_2[14]. Moreover, combined analysis of metabolites in plasma and urine can be utilized to identify alterations in the volume of distribution and renal clearance of Tx, as might occur due to drug administration or disease.

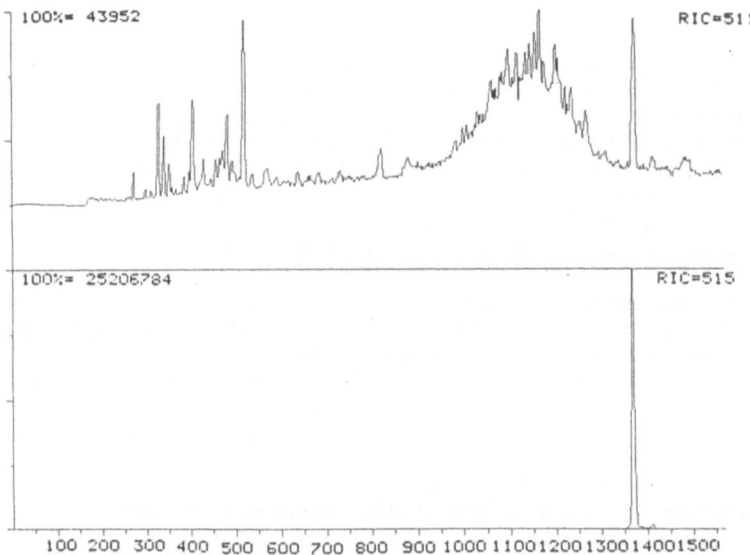

Fig 1)   Selected ion monitoring of 11-dehydro-TxB_2 (m/z 511) and its tetradeuterated internal standard (m/z 515). The plasma concentration of this sample corresponds to 1.4 pg/ml.

The main advantage of GC-MS is that it allows qualitative analysis such as elucidation of structure, and detection of functional groups that are not readily achieved by other techniques.

Although the methods have been refined, GC-MS remains a time consuming approach since samples have to undergo extraction, purification and derivatization prior to injection into the GC-MS.

EXTRACTION AND PURIFICATION

Extraction of sample analytes from the biological matrices (plasma, urine, etc) is usually performed using a reverse-phase cartridge. Samples are retained on these disposable columns and interfering substances can be partly removed by specific solvents. The compound can then be eluted with small amounts of appropriate volatile solvents.

Purification can be attained by TLC before and after derivatization or rely on chemical properties of the different metabolites. The purification of the dinor analogues of 6-keto-PGF$_{1\alpha}$ (the major urinary metabolites of prostacyclin) takes advantage of the fact that these metabolites exist in different forms: the ketone exists in equilibrium with the hemiketal form. In acidic conditions the hydroxyl and carboxyl groups of the hemiketal form react to assume the γ-lactone configuration, allowing extraction with organic solvents. A subsequent wash with a mild aqueous base, not sufficient to hydrolyze the lactone, allows further purification. Finally, hydrolysis to the free acid will permit extraction in organic solvents under acidic conditions[15] (Fig 2).

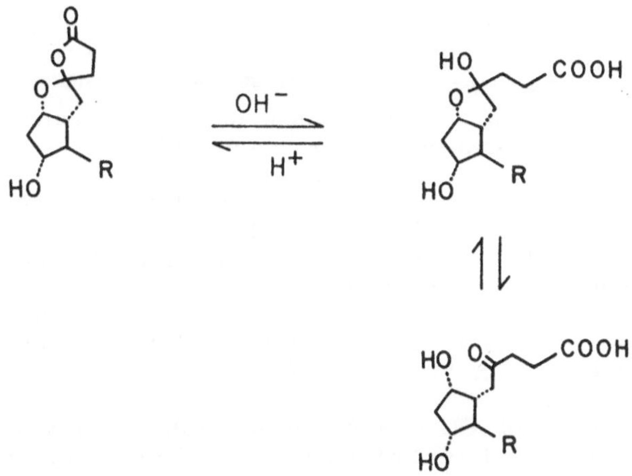

Fig 2)   Dinor metabolites of 6-keto-PGF$_{1\alpha}$ in the free acid and the lactone forms. (By permission, reference 15).

A major urinary metabolite of TxB$_2$, 2,3-dinor-TxB$_2$, is another compound of which the purification has been recently highly simplified and improved. In this case the selective extraction is based on the property of the methoxime derivative of the TxB$_2$ ring to selectively bind to bonded phase phenylboronic acid columns[16] (Fig 3).

More recently immunopurification techniques have been developed. Polyclonal antibodies are immobilized on a stationary phase allowing selective and simultaneous extraction of two or more metabolites[17].

17

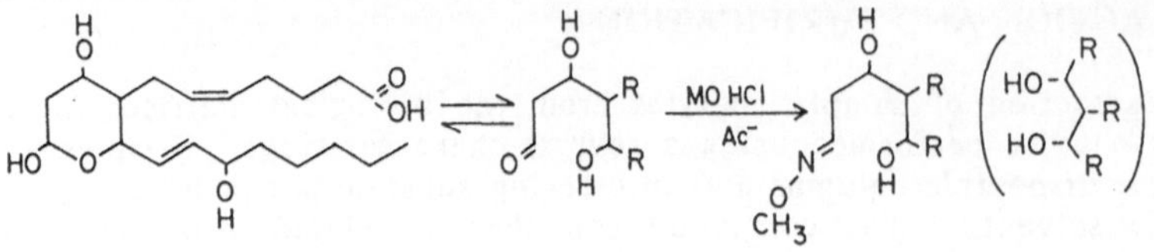

METHOXIME FORMATION IN URINE

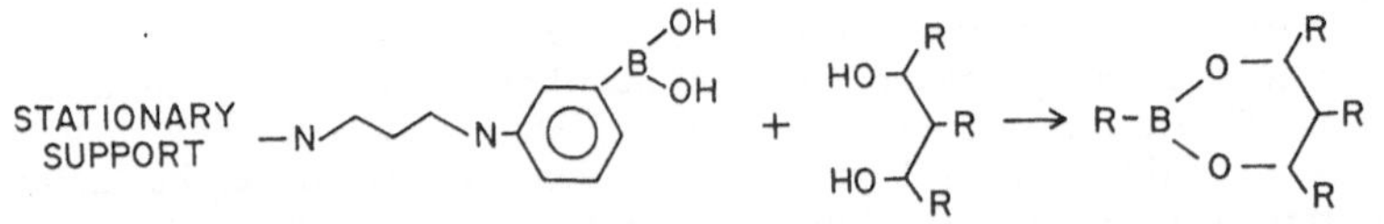

Fig 3)   Dinor-TxB$_2$ exists in equilibrium with an open ring form which is derivatized as the methoxime. Following derivatization, the configuration of the hydroxyls permits condensation with bonded-phase phenylboronic acid to form a stable complex (By permission, reference 16).

DERIVATIZATION

Following extraction and purification, the polar functions of the eicosanoids need to be derivatized in order to improve both their gas chromatographic characteristics and their mass spectrometric fragmentation patterns. Usually the ketone groups are derivatized to methoximes, the hydroxyl groups to the trimethylsilyl (TMS) ethers and the terminal carboxyl groups to the methyl or pentafluorobenzyl (PFB) esters (Fig 4). The latter is an electron capturing group that has the additional advantage of allowing the analysis in the negative ion chemical ionization (NICI) mode. It also directs fragmentation, essentially restricting it to the loss of the PFB group. Taken together, these factors enhance sensitivity by several orders of magnitude.

The substitution of GC packed columns with capillary columns has also facilitated analysis of these compounds. The latter enhance specificity by resolving the metabolites from contaminants originating in biological fluids, and also improve sensitivity by concentrating the compound into a sharp peak.

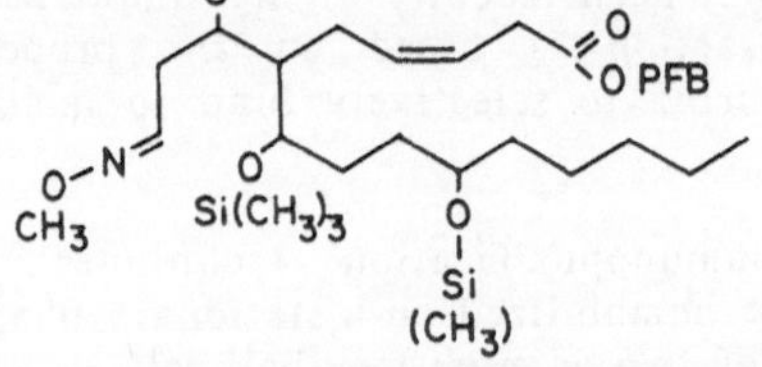

Fig 4)   Derivatization of dinor-TxB$_2$ as the methoxime, TMS ether, PFB ester.

INTERNAL STANDARDS

To achieve precision and accuracy, an internal standard is necessary. The most satisfactory standards are analogues incorporating stable isotopes because they have physicochemical properties almost identical to their natural isomers. This permits accurate quantitation, irrespective of losses during purification or due to incomplete derivatization. The stable isotope dilution technique also permits discrimination between the target compound and other contaminant peaks with different GC retention times.

Quantitation by GC-MS is generally performed in the selected ion monitoring (S.I.M.) mode by measuring the ratio of the integrated areas of the two peaks corresponding to an ion for the endogenous prostaglandin and an ion for the internal standard.

Some, but by no means all, of the stable isotopes are commercially available. The remainder must be chemically or biologically synthesized. For example, deuterium-labeled $PGF_{2\alpha}$ can be obtained from unlabeled PGD_2 by base catalyzed deuteration of C8 and C10 followed by borohydride reduction[18]. The resulting metabolite can be converted to a labeled prostacyclin by chemical means[19]. This analogue has the advantage of being labeled in the cyclopentane ring and therefore it retains the label during metabolic processes that affect the side chains such as the conversion to dinor derivatives. The synthesis of these metabolites can be achieved by incubation of mycobacterium rhodochrous with the primary compounds[20] or by incubation of the hydrolysis product with hepatic cells in culture[21]. Other isotopes such as the tetradeuterated 11-dehydro-TxB_2, can be biologically synthesized by incubation of deuterated TxB_2 with the high speed supernatant of guinea pig liver homogenate in the presence of NAD[22]. Alternatively both the 11-dehydro as well as the dinor metabolites can be labelled by ^{18}O using labeled water as a donor.

CLINICAL APPLICATION

The measurement of eicosanoids by GC-MS has permitted clarification of several controversial issues. Firstly it has established that eicosanoids are not circulating hormones, but autacoids[23]. This implies that prostaglandins and thromboxane act at the site where they are synthesized. By the measurement of the urinary metabolites of PGI_2, it has been possible to calculate the rate of entry of endogenous prostacyclin into the bloodstream as approximately 0.09 ng/kg/min[24]. This corresponds to a value of plasma concentration of less than 3 pg/ml that is not compatible with a role for this compound as a circulating hormone. An analogous approach has indicated that plasma concentration of endogenous TxB_2 are in the range of 2 pg/ml[9]. These data questioned the validity of previous studies based on the measurement of circulating eicosanoids [25].

In contrast to the unreliable assessment of the plasma concentrations of the primary eicosanoids, or their hydration products, the measurement of their major metabolites in plasma and urine offers a reliable index of eicosanoid biosynthesis in vivo. For example, GC-MS measurements of urinary dinor 6-keto-$PGF_{1\alpha}$ and dinor TxB_2 and plasma 11-dehydro-TxB_2 has indicated that unstable coronary syndromes are associated with platelet activation[1].

A limitation of the measurement of the urinary and plasma metabolites is the inability to discriminate their cellular origin precisely. However, different strategies can be applied to imply the source of such compounds. For example, it is possible to assess the contribution of platelets to the urinary excretion of thromboxane metabolites by chronically administering a dose of aspirin that selectively inhibits the platelet cyclooxygenase[26]. The extent of inhibition achieved by this regimen is an index of the proportion of the metabolites derived from platelets. Alternatively, it is possible to analyze whether or not the recovery pattern of these metabolites in urine corresponds to the turnover time of platelets. Using this approach it has been possible to establish that the urinary excretion of 11-dehydro-TxB_2 and dinor-TxB_2 mainly reflects thromboxane biosynthesis by platelets under physiological conditions[14] (Fig 5). This is consistent with their excretion being increased in syndromes associated with platelet activation. By contrast, the urinary excretion of TxB_2 is not affected by acute administration of low doses of aspirin, consistent with the assumption that the primary eicosanoids and their hydration products mainly derive from the kidney under physiological conditions[27].

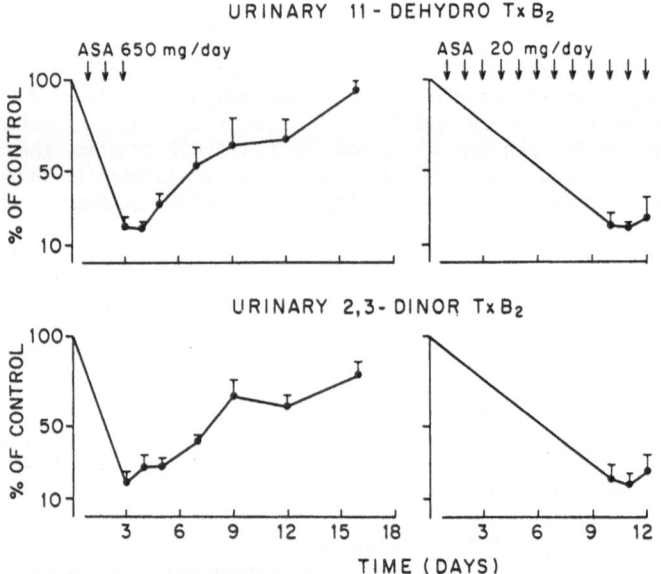

Fig 5)   Left panel: Pattern of recovery of urinary excretion of 11-dehydro-TxB_2 and dinor-TxB_2 following administration of aspirin at a dose inducing complete suppression of platelet thromboxane formation. Right panel: inhibition of the urinary excretion of 11-dehydro-TxB_2 and dinor-TxB_2 induced by aspirin at a dose selectively inhibiting platelet cyclooxygenase (By permission, reference 26).

More recently GC-MS techniques have been applied to measurement of eicosanoids in bleeding time blood and in bronchoalveolar lavage (BAL) fluid to investigate the local formation of these substances at their site of action. Thus, eicosanoid formation in bleeding time blood may reflect the consequences of platelet-vessel wall interactions. Consistent with this hypothesis, the administration of a thromboxane synthase inhibitor results in inhibition of TxB_2 and increased formation of 6-keto-$PGF_{1\alpha}$, probably reflecting utilization of platelet derived endoperoxides by vascular cells[28].

Similarly, pharmacological modulation of the AA metabolism has been shown in sheep BAL fluid after local instillation of ascaris antigen. Following cyclooxygenase inhibition, an approximate 80% reduction in the cyclooxygenase metabolites was accompanied by a concomitant increase in the allergen stimulated release of leukotriene B_4 and C_4[29].

CONCLUSION

In conclusion, GC-MS techniques permit highly specific and sensitive quantitative analyses of eicosanoids; in addition they permit qualitative identification of such compounds. Their application to the measurement of eicosanoids has greatly enhanced our knowledge of the pathophysiological role of these autacoids. More work needs to be done to decrease the degree of purification required and to extend the application of GC/MS to non-volatile samples such as the peptido-lipid leukotrienes. Further development of the combination of MS with liquid chromatography (HPLC-MS) and of tandem mass spectrometry (MS-MS) promises to address both issues.

REFERENCES

1. Fitzgerald, D.J., Roy L., Catella, F., and FitzGerald, G.A. Platelet activation in unstable coronary disease. N. Eng. J. Med.; 315:983-989, (1986).
2. Lewis, H.D., Davis, J.W., Archibald, D.G., et. al. Protective effects of aspirin against acute myocardial infarction and death in men with unstable angina: results of a Veterans Administration cooperative study. N. Eng. J. Med.; 309:396-403, (1983).
3. Cairns, J.A., Gent, M., Singer, J., et al. Aspirin, sulfinpyrazone, or both in unstable angina: results of a Canadian multicenter trial. N. Eng. J. Med. 313:1369-75, (1985).
4. Fitzgerald, D.J., Catella, F., Roy, L. and FitzGerald, G.A. Marked platelet activation in vivo after intravenous streptokinase in patients with acute myocardial infarction. Circulation; 77(1):142-150 (1988).
5. ISIS-2(Second International Study of Infarct Survival) Collaborative Group. Randomised trial of intravenous streptokinase, oral aspirin, both, or neither among 17,187 cases of suspected acute myocardial infarction: ISIS-2. Lancet; i:349-360, (1988).
6. Parry, M.J., Randall, M.J., Tyler, H.M., Myhre, E., Dabe, J. and Thaulow, E. Selective inhibition of thromboxane synthetase by dazoxiben increases prostacyclin production by leukocytes in angina patients and healthy volunteers. Lancet; ii;164, (1982) (letter).
7. Pedersen, A.K., Watson, M.L. and FitzGerald, G.A. Limitations of the measurement of immunoreactive 6-keto-$PGF_{1\alpha}$. Thromb. Res.;33:99-103, (1983).
8. Ciabattoni, G., Maclouf, J., Catella, F., FitzGerald, G.A., and Patrono, C. Radioimmunoassay of 11-dehydrothromboxane B_2 in human plasma and urine. Biochim. Biophys. Acta.; 918:293-7, (1987).
9. Patrono, C., Ciabattoni, G., Pugliese, F., Pierucci, A., Blair, I.A., and FitzGerald, G.A. Estimated rate of thromboxane secretion into the circulation of normal humans. J. Clin. Invest.; 77:590-94, (1986).
10. Knapp, H.R., Reilly, I.A.G., Alessandrini, P. and FitzGerald, G.A. In vivo indexes of platelet and vascular functions during fish-oil administration in patients with atherosclerosis. N. Eng. J. Med., 324:937-942, (1986).
11. Needleman, P., Raz, A., Minkes, M.S., Ferrendelli, J.A., and Sprecher, H. Triene prostaglandins: Prostacyclin and thromboxane biosynthesis and unique biological properties. Proc. Natl. Acad. Sci. USA 76: 944-948, (1979).
12. Braden, G.A., Fitzgerald, D.J., Knapp, H.R. and FitzGerald, G.A. Increased thromboxane $(Tx)A_2$ biosynthesis during coronary thrombosis and thrombolysis with n-3 fatty acid (FA) supplementation. Circulation; 78(4); II-120, (1988).
13. Catella, F., Healy D., Lawson, J.A. and FitzGerald G.A. 11-Dehydrothromboxane B_2: A quantitative index of thromboxane A_2 formation in the human circulation. Proc. Natl. Acad. Sci, USA; 83:5861-65, (1986).
14. Catella, F. and FitzGerald, G.A. Paired analysis of urinary thromboxane B_2 metabolites in humans. Thromb. Res.; 47:647-656, (1987).

15. Falardeau, P., Oates, J.A. and Brash, A.R. Quantitative analysis of two dinor urinary metabolites of prostaglandin I_2. Anal. Biochem.; 115:359-67, (1981).

16. Lawson, J.A., Brash, A.R., Doran, J. and FitzGerald, G.A. Measurement of urinary 2,3-dinor-thromboxane B_2 and thromboxane B_2 using bonded-phase phenylboronic acid columns and capillary gas chromatography-negative-ion chemical ionization mass spectrometry. Anal. Biochem. 150:463-470, (1985).

17. Hubbard, H.L., Eller, T.D., Mais, D.E., Halushka, P.V., Baker, R.H., Blair, I.A., Vrbanac, J.J., and Knapp, D.R. Extraction of thromboxane B_2 from urine using an immobilized antibody column for subsequent analysis by gas chromatography-mass spectometry. Prostaglandins; 33:149, 1987.

18. Brash, A.R., Baillie, T.A., Claire, R.A., and Draffan, G.H. Quantitative determination of the major metabolite of prostaglandins $F_{1\alpha}$ and $F_{2\alpha}$ in human urine by stable isotope dilution and combined gas chromatography-mass spectrometry. Biochem. Med. 16:77-94, (1976).

19. Whittaker, N. Tetrahedron Lett. A synthesis of prostacyclin sodium salt. 32:2805-3808, (1977).

20. Sun, F.F., Taylor, B.M., Lincoln, F.H., and Sebek, O.K. Preparation of two dinor-PGI_2 metabolites from 6-keto-$PGF_{1\alpha}$ by mycobacterium rhodochrous. Prostaglandins 20:729-734, (1980).

21. Balazy, M., Brass, E.P., Gerber, J.G., and Nies, A.S. Facile method for preparation of 2,3-dinor-6-keto $PGF_{1\alpha}$, the major urinary metabolite of prostacyclin. Prostaglandins; 36: 421-430, 1988.

22. Lawson, J.A., Patrono, C., Ciabattoni, G., and FitzGerald, G.A. Long-lived enzymatic metabolites of thromboxane B_2 in the human circulation. Anal. Biochem. 155:198-205, (1986).

23. Blair, I.A., Barrow, S.E., Waddell, K.A., Lewis, P.J., and Dollery, C.T. Prostacyclin is not a circulating hormone in man. Prostaglandins; 23:579-589, (1982).

24. FitzGerald, G.A., Brash, A.R. Falardeau, P., and Oates, J.A. Estimated rate of prostacyclin secretion into the circulation of normal man. J. Clin. Invest. 68:1271-76, (1981).

25. Neri Serneri, G.G., Gensini, F.F., Abbate, R., et al. Abnormal cardio-coronary thromboxane A_2 production in patients with unstable angina. Am. Heart. J.; 109:732-8, (1985).

26. Patrignani, P., Filabozzi P., and Patrono, C. Selective cumulative inhibition of platelet thromboxane production by low-dose aspirin in healthy subjects. J. Clin. Invest. 69:1366-72, (1982).

27. Patrono, C., Ciabattoni, G., Patrignani, P., et al. Evidence for a renal origin of urinary thromboxane B_2 in health and disease. In: Advances in Prostaglandin, Thromboxane, and Leukotriene Research, vol 11, ed. by B. Samuelsson, R., Paoletti, R., and Ramwell, P.W. 493-498, Raven Press, New York, 1983.

28. Nowak, J., and FitzGerald, G.A.: Prostaglandin endoperoxide reorientation at the platelet vascular interface in man. J. Clin. Invest. (in press) 1988.

29. Dworski, R., Sheller, J., Wickersham, N.E., Oates, J.A., Brigham, K.L., Roberts, L.J., II, FitzGerald, G.A. Allergen stimulated release of mediators into sheep bronchoalveolar lavage fluid: Effect of cyclooxygenase inhibition. Am. Rev. Res. Dis. (in press), 1989.

Acknowledgements

Supported by grants (HL30400 and GM15431) from the National Institutes of Health. Dr. Catella holds a Faculty Development Award from the Pharmaceutical Manufacturers' Association Foundation. Dr. FitzGerald is an Established Investigator of the American Heart Association. We are indebted to Ms. E. Stuart for expert editorial assistance.

22

FORMATION AND MECHANISM OF ACTION OF EPOXYEICOSATRIENOIC ACIDS

F.A. Fitzpatrick

Department of Pharmacology
University of Colorado Health Sciences Center
4200 East Ninth Avenue
Denver, CO 80262   USA

INTRODUCTION

Many biologically active eicosanoids originate from cyclooxygenase and lipoxygenase catalyzed metabolism of arachidonic acid (1). These substances include prostaglandins, thromboxanes, and leukotrienes. The enzymological features of their biosynthesis are characterized to a great extent. Their mechanism of action is also well characterized and it appears to involve receptor mediated processes in most instances.

Recently a novel group of eicosanoids has emerged. These are cis-epoxy eicosatrienoic acids (EETs) and certain hydroxyeicosatrienoic acid (HETE) isomers that originate from mixed function oxidase catalyzed metabolism of arachidonic acid (2-11) [Figure 1]. The EETs and HETEs have biosynthetic origins and mechanisms of action that differ substantially from the other eicosanoids. This chapter aims to summarize current information on the formation and mechanism of action of these agents. Presently their role as physiological mediators is uncertain. By comparing and contrasting them with the so called "classical" eicosanoids one may place this issue into focus. Particularly, one may see that conventional paradigms for lipid mediator action may be suboptimal for the EETs.

Biosynthesis. Figure 2 summarizes the biosynthetic properties of dioxygenase enzymes (cyclooxygenase) and monooxygenase enzymes that catalyze EET formation. There are few similarities between these two groups. Notable differences include cofactor requirements; substrate specificity; and details of oxygen insertion into their respective substrates. For example, dioxygenase enzymes have minimal cofactor needs: availability of substrate and oxygen are rate limiting (12). The dioxygenase enzymes have a unique substrate requirement and molecular mechanism. They function on polyunsaturated fatty acids with a 1,4-cis-pentadiene substituent and they insert molecular oxygen antarafacially via abstraction of a proton from an intervening methylene unit (13). The dioxygenases display regiospecificity: the 5-, 12-, and 15-lipoxygenase and the cyclooxygenase are four distinct proteins (13).

In contrast, the monooxygenase requires reduced nicotinamide adenine nucleotides and cytochrome P-450 reductase as cofactors. The monooxygenase displays little substrate specificity: it oxidizes many xenobiotic and endogenous lipid substrates. In doing this, it transfers an activated oxygen atom derived from oxygen-oxygen bond cleavage to the substrate and to water. It should be stressed that the term "epoxygenase" has been applied to the monooxygenase catalyzed oxidation of arachidonic acid. This nomenclature emphasizes chemical features of the products and it differentiates the enzyme from cyclooxygenase and lipoxygenase. There is little evidence for a unique monooxygenase with a substrate specificity for arachidonic acid or related polyunsaturated acids. This warrants attention in view of recent data reporting such an enzyme (8) and the established data indicating that among the many cytochrome P-450 isoenzymes there are some with substrate preferences (14).

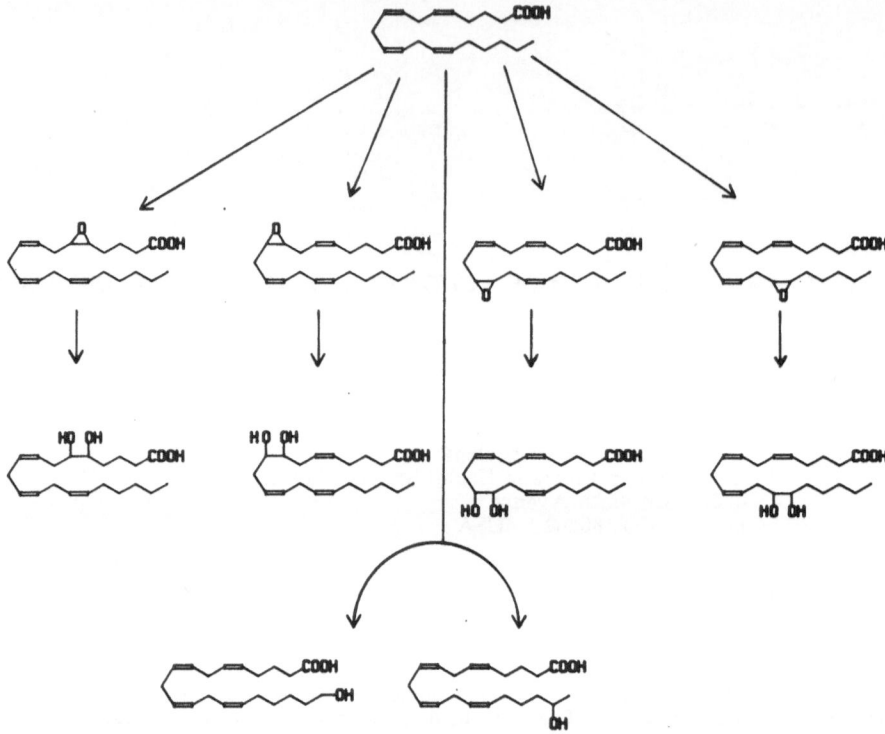

Figure 1 *Structures of epoxyeicosatrienoic acids (EETs) derived from arachidonic acid. Epoxides (left to right): 5,6-EET; 8,9-EET; 11,12-EET; 14,15-EET. Directly below are the vicinal diols derived from hydration of the epoxides. Bottom line shows omega oxidation products.*

Stereoselectivity of product formation represents one of the major differences between the "epoxygenase" pathway and the lipoxygenase pathways. Hydroxyeicosatrienoic acids from either pathway have similar cis-trans diene monohydroxy substituents. The lipoxygenase products are regio- and enantio-specific with an (S) hydroxy configuration at the 5-, 11-, 12-, or 15-position (13). The hepatic epoxygenase produces six regioisomers with no enantioselectivity. It is now advisable to establish the stereochemical configuration of any HETE metabolites, rigorously, in view of the potential for different biosynthetic origins. The significance of this can be appreciated in terms of drug development strategies. For example, drugs that inhibit lipoxygenase enzymes may spare "epoxygenase" enzymes. Consequently, HETEs from the latter could still contribute biological activities.

Occurrence of epoxygenase enzymes and EETs. Hepatic tissue is a rich source of cytochrome P-450 monooxygenase (2-6; 8,10) [Figure 3]. Renal (7,9,11), ocular (15), and pituitary (16) systems also produce detectable amounts of the EETs or HETEs. Renal epoxygenase activity has been characterized at both biochemical and cellular levels. The enzymatic activity predominates within the thick ascending loop of Henle (TALH) cells. Hormonal stimulation of TALH cells activates epoxygenase catalyzed arachidonate metabolism (7).

The EETs occur as endogenous constituents in rat liver (17), kidney (18), lung and urine (19). They may also occur in platelets (20) and endothelial cells (21). Their occurrence as endogenous cellular constituents is not typical of most eicosanoids. Hormonal, neuronal or chemical stimuli initiate their biosynthesis. The prostaglandins, thromboxanes, and leukotrienes have been viewed as autocoid mediators. Cells do not typically incorporate these eicosanoids within membranes or storage vesicles. The occurrence of EETs as "stored" species includes the possibility that these substances have non-autocoid actions. However the formation of these products artifactually, by autooxidation is always a matter of concern [Figure 4].

24

BIOSYNTHESIS

	Cyclooxygenase/Lipoxygenase	Epoxygenase
Enzyme Type:	Dioxygenase	Monooxygenase

Substrate Requirement: 'strict'   'promiscuous'

free PUFA   cis-1,4-pentadiene   xenobiotic or
                                                         endogenous lipids

$=\wedge=$

Co-factor Requirement: minimal   several

- O_2 - O_2
AA   - NADH/NAD$^+$
(except 5-lipoxygenase   - cytochrome P-450
Ca^{++}/ATP/'other')   reductase

Characteristics: - regiospecific   "not regiospecific
                 - stereospecific   (different rates?)
                 - multiple catalytic events   (different enzymes?)
                   (CO/peroxidase)
                   5-Lo/8-Lo)

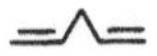

Figure 2

SOURCES OF EPOXYGENASE

Hepatic/Renal/Ocular/Leukocytes Microsomes

Hepatic microsomes best characterized

- high affinity for AA (K_m 40 uM)

- 1:1 stoichiometry for O_2 utilization and NADPH
  NADP

- inhibition by CO, metyrapone (50 uM),
  benzphetamine (500 uM)

- 15-HETE, 12-HETE abundant
  (facilitated oxidation at terminal olefin? greater
  stability?)

- inducer dependent

  i) β-naphthoflavone = ω or ω-1

  ii) pentobarbital = EETs

- rate = 5 - 6 nanomole AA/min/mg

Renal

- TALH cells

- rate approximately 0.1 nanomole AA/min/mg

Figure 3

Biological actions of "epoxygenase" derived EETs and HETEs. Table I summarizes the biological activities reported for various EETs and HETEs derived from the "epoxygenase" pathway. These include stimulation of peptide hormone release from endocrine cells (22-24); inhibition of renal sodium/potassium ATPase (25); mobilization of microsomal Ca^{++} from aortic smooth muscle and anterior pituitary cells (26-27); inhibition of cyclooxygenase activity (28); inhibition of arachidonic acid induced platelet aggregation (28); vasodilation of intestinal microcirculation (29); inhibition of vasopressin

stimulated water transport (30); and angiogenesis and vasodilation of arteries (30). It is uncertain to what extent these are physiological activities. Continued investigations of the pharmacological behavior and the biochemical origins of epoxygenase products may answer that question.

Among the sytems reported, the renal actions of EETs seem most likely to have a physiological role. Renal cortical microsomes produce EETs and also contain them as endogenous species (18). Human urine also contains the 8,9- and 14,15-isomers of epoxyeicosatrienoic acid (19). The levels of these substances appear to vary as a function of renal pathology. Spontaneously hypertensive rats develop an increased capacity for epoxygenase dependent metabolism in parallel with the development of hypertension (32). The mechanism of action and potency of the EETs as inhibitors of renal sodium/potassium ATPase is compatible with a role in maintaining blood pressure. Thus among the systems where EETs display activity the renal system has the most prominent relationships among biosynthesis, action, and mechanism. A caution must be raised about the specificity of renal EET action. Both linoleic and oleic acid are also endogenous sodium/potassium ATPase inhibitors (33). The EETs may be a special case of this precedent, or the activity attributed to oleic and linoleic acid may be due to their autooxidation into corresponding epoxy derivatives.

Rapid and comprehensive metabolism is one of the major factors that has complicated efforts to correlate biosynthesis or occurrence of EETs and HETEs with putative physiological roles. Both enzymatic and non-enzymatic hydration convert EETs into their corresponding vicinal diols (34). Enzymatic conjugation with reduced glutathione (GSH) can also occur (35). Metabolism can "mask" the occurrence of EETs to a great degree.

SUMMARY

The links between epoxygenase metabolites of arachidonic acid and drugs deserve mention in three contexts. First, the EETs originate from the enzymatic system involved in the metabolism of a wide range of pharmaceuticals. Induction, inhibition or modulation of this system could influence formation of EETs and monooxygenase derived HETEs. Second, deliberate inhibition of the cyclooxygenase or lipoxygenase enzymes is a contemporary pharmacological strategy for discovery of antiinflammatory, antiasthmatic, or cardiovascular drugs. Since EETs and HETEs can originate from a different biosynthetic system - one that is not necessarily susceptible to these inhibitors- one must be aware that a shift in the balance of eicosanoid formation is a potential consequence of treatment with such drugs. Finally, the exact mechanism, or mechanisms, of action of the EETs and HETEs is uncertain. They are not necessarily operating at the level of receptor interactions. For instance inhibition of sodium/potassium ATPase best accounts for their action in certain, but not all, circumstances.

TABLE I. Biological Actions of Epoxygense Metabolites

Compound	Concentration	Action
5,6-EET 5,6-DiHETE	.001 - 1 μM	Somatosatin release *in vitro* from hypothalamic median eminence
5,6-EET	.01 - 1 μM	Insulin release *in vitro* from pancreatic islets
14,15-EET; 8,9-EET	.01 - 1 μM	Glucagon release *in vitro* from pancreatic islets
11,12-diHETE	1 μM	Inhibition of Na^+/K^+ ATPase *in vitro*
5,6-EET 8,9-EET 11,12-EET	32 μg/ml 36 μg/ml 25 μg/ml	Vasodilation of intestinal arteriolar blood flow *in vivo*
5,6-EET 11,12-EET 14,15-EET and diHETEs	$\geq$ 1 μM	Inhibition of vasopressin stimulated water flow in toad bladder *in vitro*
5,6-EET 11,12-EET 14,15-EET	$\geq$ 1 μM	Increased $^{45}Ca^{++}$ loss from canine aortic smooth muscle microsomes *in vitro*
5,6-EET	1 μM	Increased $^{45}Ca^{++}$ efflux anterior pituitary; increased cytosolic free Ca^{++}
14,15-cis-EET	10 - 100 μM	Inhibition of cyclooxygenase *in vitro*
14-15-cis-EET, and stereoisomers	1 - 10 μM	Inhibition of platelet aggregation *in vitro*
12(R)-HETE	.01 - 1 μM	Inhibition of Na^+/K^+ ATPase (corneal epithelium) *in vitro*
12(R)-DH-HETE		Vasodilation, angiogenesis

REFERENCES

1. P. Needleman, J. Turk, B. Jakschik, A. Morrison, and J. Lefkowith: Arachidonic acid metabolism. *Ann. Rev. Biochem.* 55:69 (1986).
2. J. Capdevila, N. Chacos, J. Werringloer, R. Prough, and R. Estabrook: Liver microsomal cytochrome P-450 and oxidative metabolism of arachidonic acid. *Proc. Natl. Acad. Sci. USA* 78:5362 (1982).
3. J. Capdevila, Y.Kim, C. Martin-Wixstrom, J.R. Falck, S. Manna, and R. Estabrook: Influence of fibric acid-type of hypolipidemic agent on the oxidative metabolism of arachidonic acid by liver microsomal cytochrome P-450. *Arch. Biochem. Biophys.* 243:8 (1985).
4. J. Capdevila, L. Marnett, N. Chacos, R. Prough, and R. Estabrook: Cytochrome P-450 dependent oxygenation of arachidonic acid to hydroxyeicosatetraenoic acids. *Proc. Natl. Acad. Sci. USA* 79:767 (1982).
5. J. Capdevila, L. Parkhill, N. Chacos, R. Okita, B.S. Masters, and R. Estabrook: The oxidative metabolism of arachidonic acid by purified cytochromes P-450. *Biochem. Biophys. Res. Commun.* 101:1357 (1981).
6. N. Chacos, J.R. Falck, C. Wixstrom, and J. Capdevila: Novel epoxides formed during the liver cytochrome P-450 oxidation of arachidonic acid. *Biochem. Biophys. Res. Commun.* 104:916 (1982).
7. N. Ferreri, M. Schwartzman, N. Abraham, P. Chander, and J. McGiff. Arachidonic acid metabolism in a cell suspension isolated from rabbit renal outer medulla. *J. Pharmacol. Exptl. Therap.* 231:441 (1984).

8. M. Laniado-Schwartzman, M. Davis, J. McGiff, R. Levere, and N. Abraham: Purification and characterization of cytochrome P-450 dependent arachidonic acid epoxygenase from human liver. *J. Biol. Chem.* 263:2536 (1988).

9. A. Morrison and N. Pascoe: Metabolism of arachidonate through NADPH dependent oxygenase of renal cortex. *Proc. Natl. Acad. Sci. USA* 78:7375 (1981).

10. E. Oliw, P.Guengerich, and J. Oates: Oxidation of arachidonic acid by hepatic monooxygenase: Isolation and metabolism of four epoxide intermediates. *J. Biol. Chem.* 257:3771 (1982).

11. E. Oliw, J. Lawson, A. Brash, and J. Oates: Arachidonic acid metabolism in rabbit renal cortex: Formation of two novel dihydroxyeicosatrienoic acids. *Prostaglandins* 22:863 (1981).

12. W.E. M. Lands: Biological consequences of fatty acid oxygenase reactions. *Prostaglandins, Leukotrienes and Medicine* 13:35 (1984).

13. M.Hamberg: Studies on the formation and degradation of unsaturated fatty acid hydroperoxides. *Prostaglandins, Leukotrienes and Med.*, 13:27 (1984).

14. A.Y.H. Lu and S.-B. West: Multiplicity of mammalian microsomal cytochromes P-450. *Pharmacol. Rev.* 31:227 (1980).

15. M. Schwartzman, M. Balazy, J. Masferrer, N. Abraham, J. McGiff, and R. Murphy: 12(R)-Hydroxyeicosatetraenoic acid: A cytochrome P-450 dependent arachidonate metabolite that inhibits Na+/K+ ATPase in the cornea. *Proc. Natl. Acad. Sci. USA* 84:8125 (1987).

16. J. Capdevila, G. Snyder, and J.R. Falck: Epoxygenation of arachidonic acid by rat anterior pituitary microsomal fractions. *FEBS Lett.* 178:319 (1984).

17. J. Capdevila, B. Pramanik, J. Napoli, S. Manna, and J. Falck: Arachidonic acid epoxidation: Epoxyeicosatrienoic acids are endogenous constituents of rat liver. *Arch. Biochem. Biophys.* 231:511 (1984).

18. J.R. Falck, V. Schueler, H. Jacobson, A. Siddhanta, B. Pramanik, and J. Capdevila: Arachidonate epoxygenase: Identification of epoxyeicosatrienoic acids in rabbit kidney. *J. Lipid. Res.* 28: 840 (1987)

19. R. Toto, A. Siddhanta, B. Manna, B. Pramanik, J.R. Falck, and J. Capdevila: Arachidonic acid epoxygenase: Detection of epoxyeicosatrienoic acids in human urine. *Biochim. Biophys. Acta.* 191:132 (1987).

20. L. Ballou, B. Lam, P. Wong and W.Y. Cheung: Formation of 14,15-cis-oxido-5,8,11-icosatrienoic acid from phosphatidylinositol in human platelets. *Proc. Natl. Acad. Sci. USA* 84:6990 (1987).

21. G. Revtyak, A. Johnson, and W. Campbell: Cultured bovine coronary endothelial cells synthesize HETEs and prostacyclin. *Am. J. Physiol.* 254:C8 (1988).

22. J. Capdevila, N. Chacos, J. Falck, S. Manna, A. Negro-Vilar, and S. Ojeda: Novel hypothalamic arachidonate products stimulate somatostatin release from the median eminence. *Endocrinology* 113:421 (1983).

23. R. Cashman, D. Hanks, and R. Weiner: Epoxy derivatives of arachidonic acid are potent stimulators of prolactin secretion. *Neuroendocrinol.* 76:246 (1987).

24. J.R. Falck, S. Manna, J. Moltz, N. Chacos, and J. Capdevila: Epoxyeicosatrienoic acids stimulate glucagon and insulin release from isolated rat pancreatic islets. *Biochem. Biophys. Res. Commun.* 114:734 (1983).

25. M. Schwartzman, N. Ferrer, M. Carroll, E. Songu-Mize, and J. McGiff: Renal cytochrome P-450 related arachidonate metabolite inhibits Na+/K+ ATPase. *Nature* 317:620-622 (1985).

26. G. Snyder, L. Lattanzio, P. Yadagiri, J. Falck, and J. Capdevila: 5,6-Epoxyeicosatrienoic acid mobilizes Ca^{++} in anterior pituitary cells. *Biochem. Biophys. Res. Commun.* 139:1188 (1986).

27. P. Kutsky, J. Falck, G. Weiss, S. Manna, N. Chacos, and J. Capdevila: Effects of newly reported arachidonic acid metabolites on microsomal Ca^{++} binding, uptake and release. *Prostaglandins* 26:13 (1983).

28. F. Fitzpatrick, M.Ennis, M. Baze, M. Wynalda, J. McGee, and W. Liggett: Inhibition of cyclooxygenase activity and platelet aggregation by epoxyeicosatrienoic acids: Influence of stereochemistry. *J. Biol. Chem.* 261:15334 (1986).

29. K.Proctor, J. Falck, and J. Capdevila: Intestinal vasodilation by epoxyeicosatrienoic acids: Arachidonic acid metabolites produced by a cytochrome P-450 monooxygenase. *Circulation. Res.* 60:50 (1987).

30. D. Schlondorff, E. Petty, and J. Oates: Epoxygenase metabolites of arachidonic acid inhibit vasopressin response in toad bladder. *Am. J. Physiol.* 253:F464 (1987).

31. R. Murphy, J. Falck, S. Lumin, P. Yadagiri, J. Zirolli, M. Balazy, J. Masferrer, N. Abraham, and M. Schwartzman: 12(R)-Hydroxyeicosatrienoic acid: a vasodilator cytochrome P-450 dependent arachidonate metabolite from the bovine cornea epithelium. *J. Biol. Chem.* 263:17197-17202 (1988).

32. D. Sacerdoti, N. Abraham, J. McGiff, and M. Schwartzman: Renal cytochrome P-450 dependent metabolism in spontaneously hypertensive rats. *Biochem. Pharmacol.* 37:521 (1988).
33. M. Tamura, H. Kuwano, T. Kinoshita, and T. Inagami: Identification of linoleic and oleic acids as endogenous Na+/K+ ATPase inhibitors from acute volume expanded hog plasma. *J. Biol. Chem.* 260:9672 (1985).
34. N. Chacos, J. Capdevila, J. Falck, S. Manna, C. Martin-Wixstrom, S. Gill, B. Hammock, and R. Estabrook: The reaction of arachidonic acid epoxides (epoxyeicosatrienoic acids) with a cytosolic epoxide hydrolase. *Arch. Biochem. Biophys.* 223:639 (1983).
35. M. Spearman, R. Prough, R. Estabrook, J.Falck, S. Manna, K. Leibman, R. Murphy, and J. Capdevila: Novel glutathione conjugates formed from epoxyeicosatrienoic acids. *Arch. Biochem. Biophys.* 242:225 (1985).

REACTIVE EICOSANOID INTERMEDIATES AND TRANSCELLULAR BIOSYNTHESIS

Jacques Maclouf

Unite 150 INSERM, UA334 CNRS
Hopital Lariboisiere
75475 Paris, France

INTRODUCTION

Most of the studies conducted in the seventies as well as in the early eighties, have been designed to establish the oxidative pathways of arachidonic acid by specific cell types resulting in the determination of the structure of eicosanoids by a given cell. Such an approach has delineated specific enzymatic patterns by certain cells in the blood and vascular system. Such findings are summarized in Table I. Platelets produce mainly 12-hydroxyeicosatetraenoic acid, 12-hydroxy heptadecatrienoic acid and thromboxane A_2. Endothelial cells from human umbilical cord or vascular smooth muscle synthesize mainly prostaglandin I_2 (prostacyclin) and prostaglandins E_2 and $F_{2\alpha}$ whereas this production is different for endothelial cells from the microvasculature. Polymorphonuclear granulocytes synthesize nearly exclusively LTB_4 and eosinophils generate LTC_4. Monocytes, depending upon their origin or their maturation, seem to produce both leukotrienes. In contrast, red blood cells and lymphocytes lack the specific oxygenases to form eicosanoids.

The study of separate biochemical pathways is important at a certain stage of research; it can be observed for instance that enzymes do vary in their requirements for the formation of eicosanoids. Some enzymes such as cyclooxygenase or the 12-lipoxygenase need only arachidonic acid alone where other enzymes (e.g. 5-lipoxygenase) do require cofactors (i.e. Ca^{2+}, ATP, hydroperoxides) to generate leukotrienes.

Historically, the occurrence of unstable intermediates has been a critical concept in understanding the biosynthesis of eicosanoids. The existence of an unstable prostaglandin precursor was suggested as early as 1965 by Samuelsson and co-workers. Yet endoperoxides were only detected and isolated years later (Hamberg and Samuelsson 1973, Nugteren and Hazelhof, 1973) after incubation of sheep vesicular gland microsomes with arachidonic acid. Rearrangement of these endoperoxides lead to the spontaneous formation of prostaglandin $F_{2\alpha}$ and the enzymatic formation of PGD_2. Only $PGF_{2\alpha}$ was produced if a mild chemical reduction of the endoperoxide was employed at an early stage of such incubation experiments. Indeed, trapping experiments showed that upon formation of prostaglandins and thromboxanes, nonenzymatic hydrolysis products of endoperoxides (i.e. $PGF_{2\alpha}$) were released from the platelets (Hamberg *et al.*, 1974).

A similar approach showed that the chemically reactive leukotriene A_4 was a common intermediate in the production of leukotriene B_4 and leukotriene C_4 (Borgeat and Samuelsson, 1979; Murphy, Hammarström, and Samuelsson, 1979): formation of the unstable allylic epoxide was detected in the transformation of arachidonic acid into 5,6-dihydroxy-eicosatetraenoic acid (2 isomers) and 5,12-dihydroxy- eicosatetraenoic acid (3 isomers) in rabbit polymorphonuclear leukocytes). Trapping experiments with 10 volumes of methanol, ethanol or ethylene glycol showed that short term incubations of human polymorphonuclear leukocytes with the calcium ionophore A23187, lead to the formation of corresponding 12-O-alkyl derivatives of the 5,12-dihydroxy acids together with the formation of the leukotriene B_4.

Table I *Eicosanoid metabolism by specific human blood or vascular cells*

<u>Red Blood Cells</u>:	No oxidative metabolism
<u>Platelets</u>:	Cyclooxygenase, thromboxane synthase ($\underline{PGH_2}$, $\underline{TXA_2}$, PGE_2, $F_{2\alpha}$, D_2)
	12-lipoxygenase, peroxidase ($\underline{12\text{-HETE}}$)
<u>Neutrophils</u>:	5-lipoxygenase, leukotriene hydrolase ($\underline{LTA_4}$, $\underline{LTA_4}$, 5-HETE)
	15-lipoxygenase, peroxidase (15-HETE)
<u>Eosinophils</u>:	5-lipoxygenase, leukotriene C_4 synthase (LTA_4, $\underline{LTC_4}$)
	15-lipoxygenase, peroxidase ($\underline{15\text{-HETE}}$)
<u>Monocytes</u>*:	5-lipoxygenase, leukotriene hydrolase, leukotriene C_4 synthase (LTA_4, LTC_4, LTB_4)
	Cyclooxygenase, isomerases, thromboxane synthase, prostacyclin synthase (PGE_2, TXB_2, 6-keto-$PGF_{1\alpha}$
<u>Lymphocytes</u>:	No oxidative metabolism
<u>Endothelial Cells</u>:	
-Umbilical vein	Cyclooxygenase, prostacyclin synthase, isomerases ($\underline{PGI_2}$ $\underline{PGF_{2\alpha}}$ PGD_2, PGE_2)
-Capillaries	Cyclooxygenase ($\underline{PGE_2}$ or $\underline{PGD_2}$ or $\underline{PGF_{2\alpha}} \geq PGI_2$
<u>Smooth Muscle Cells</u>:	Cyclooxygenase ($\underline{PGI_2}$)

* Monocyte/macrophage

All these studies revealed that although chemically unstable, metabolic intermediates could be formed within the cell. Availability of these substances was crucial to study the regulation of specific enzymes such as thromboxane synthase, prostacyclin synthase, the various isomerases, glutathione peroxidase, leukotriene A_4 hydrolase, or leukotriene C_4 synthase. Additional work using these reactive intermediates of the arachidonic acid cascade has lead to the discovery of what is now known as the transcellular metabolism of arachidonic acid (McGee and Fitzpatrick, 1986).

Transcellular metabolism of arachidonic acid metabolism: A complex biochemical reality

It has been observed that the production of eicosanoids by mixed cell populations differs from that expected from each individual cell. Although the concept of transcellular metabolism has been extended to a variety of other situations (Table II), we will limit ourselves to examples concerning reactive eicosanoid intermediates. *In vitro* evidence for this phenomenon typically involves two steps: 1) Incubation of the reactive intermediate (generated by cell A) with cell B results in the formation of another product-X and 2) co-incubation of the two cell populations should also be accompanied by the formation of X.

<u>1) Transcellular metabolism of the reactive intermediates in various *in vitro* systems</u>

In 1977 it was demonstrated that incubation of sodium arachidonate or prostaglandin endoperoxides with human umbilical vein endothelial cells or with bovine aortic endothelial cells resulted into the formation of prostacyclin (Weksler *et al*.). These studies suggested that endothelial cells possessed the capacity to generate prostaglandin I_2 directly from arachidonate via cyclooxygenase and the capacity to convert externally formed prostaglandin endoperoxides into prostaglandin I_2. The first transcellular metabolism experiment was carried out by Marcus *et al*. (1980) with platelet-derived, ^{3}H-labeled endoperoxides that was transformed into ^{3}H-prostacyclin by vicinal aspirin-treated

Table II *Metabolism of lipidic mediators in various cell-cell cooperations*

DONOR CELL	COMPOUND	ACCEPTOR CELL	EFFECT
	Intermediate		
Platelet	PGH_2	Endothelial cell	Increased PGI_2
Neutrophil	LTA_4	Red Blood Cell	Increased LTB_4
		Platelets	Synthesis LTC_4
		EC, SMC	Synthesis LTC_4
	Inactive metabolite		
Platelet	12-HETE	Neutrophil	Synthesis 5,12- or 12,20-diHETE[1]
	Active metabolite		
Eosinophil	LTC_4, LTD_4	EC, Parenchyma	Production of PGI_2 and TXB_2[2]
Neutrophil	PAF	Lung cell(s)	Synthesis of LTC_4 and LTD_4[3]
		Kidney	Synthesis of TXA_2

[1] Borgeat *et al.* (1981), Lindgren *et al.* (1981), Maclouf *et al.* (1982), Marcus *et al.* (1982, 1984, 1988)
[2] Benjamin *et al.* (1983), Cramer *et al.* 1983
[3] Voelkel *et al.* (1982)

endothelial cells. Coincubation of both cell types resulted in an increased production of prostacyclin as compared to that produced by endothelial cells alone. Further evidence for the existence of transcellular metabolism was provided from experiments focused on the metabolism of leukotriene A_4 by cells which do not possess 5-lipoxygenase. In 1984, Fitzpatrick *et al.* demonstrated that LTA_4, at physiologic concentrations, could be transformed into LTB_4 by human red blood cells. Indeed these cells were found to contain LTA_4 hydrolase (McGee and Fitzpatrick, 1985). Further experiments using mixed incubations of neutrophils and red blood cells showed that activated neutrophils generate less LTB_4, when compared to that obtained when neutrophils were incubated in the presence of red blood cells (McGee and Fitzpatrick, 1986). More recently, Feinmark and Cannon (1986) and Claesson and Haeggström (1988) reported that endothelial cells from porcine aorta or human umbilical cord, respectively, could metabolize leukotriene A_4 into the peptido LTC_4. Both groups also demonstrated that cellular coincubations of vascular cells with neutrophils (which normally do not produce LTC_4), resulted in a substantial synthesis of peptido leukotrienes. Similar observations were recently extended to smooth muscle cells which exhibited nearly identical properties as endothelial cells (Feinmark and Cannon, 1987). Yet it is still unclear whether endothelial cells have a higher capacity to generate LTC_4 from LTA_4 as compared to smooth muscle cells. In recent studies (Maclouf and Murphy, 1988), we reported that human platelets possess a very efficient capacity to metabolize LTA_4 into LTC_4 whether LTA_4 was added exogenously or was derived from activated human neutrophils.

2) Transcellular metabolism of an unstable intermediate during cellular coincubations

Several strategies have been used to support the concept of *in vitro* transcellular metabolism involving two separate cell types. 2) During coincubations of red blood cells with neutrophils, the increased production of leukotriene B_4 paralleled the decrease in the formation of the nonenzymatic breakdown products of LTA_4 as compared to that obtained with neutrophils alone (McGee and Fitzpatrick, 1986). This result was consistent with an uptake of leukotriene A_4 (released from neutrophils) by vicinal acceptor erythrocytes to generate leukotriene B_4. 2) Challenge of human neutrophils with the calcium ionophore

A23187 was accompanied by the release into the cell supernatant of an unstable intermediate that could be converted into leukotriene C_4 when added to platelets (Maclouf and Murphy, 1988). The stability of this substance was dependent upon time and pH, both criteria being consistent with the presence of leukotriene A_4 in the supernatant of activated neutrophils. 3) Finally, evidence for the participation of the two cell types in transcellular metabolism was supported by experiments that labeled the acceptor (platelet or endothelial cell) glutathione by the addition of $[^{35}S]$-Cysteine. Coincubation of neutrophils with labeled endothelial cells (Feinmark and Cannon, 1986, Claesson and Haeggström, 1988) or platelets (Maclouf and Murphy, 1988) resulted in the formation of $[^{35}S]$-leukotriene C_4 as the direct result of substrates being provided from each cell.

As mentioned above, transcellular metabolism imparts to mixed cells, a metabolic capability distinct from what would have been predicted from Table I. As seen from the above described examples, such events *in vivo* could result either in an increased production of an eicosanoid (i.e. production of LTB_4 by mixtures of neutrophils and erythrocytes) or to the production of an eicosanoid that cannot be accomplished without coincubation of the two cells (e.g. LTC_4 production by neutrophil/endothelial cells or neutrophils/platelets).

In vitro transcellular metabolism of an unstable intermediates from activated cells

Until now, all studies dealing with cellular activation either from isolated blood cells or cells in culture use end-product eicosanoids as an index of cell activation. These studies measure the product resulting from the specific terminal enzyme as a marker of a specific cell type. From these considerations, the urinary measurement of either dinor-thromboxane B_2 or dinor-6-keto prostaglandin $F_{1\alpha}$ has been currently ascribed to reflect *in vivo* platelet or endothelial cell activation, respectively, in thrombotic or cardiovascular disorders (FitzGerald *et al.* 1986).

The putative existence of transcellular metabolism *in vivo* through multi cellular cooperations raises a serious objection to these latter assumptions. In nearly all examples of this metabolism described so far, only the donor cell (i.e. producing the unstable intermediate) needs to be activated. Biosynthesis of a given metabolite formed by transcellular reactions as a consequence of cell activation will only be secondary to the primary activation of the donor cell. Strictly speaking, the contribution of the acceptor cell which may be of crucial importance for the generation of the biologically active metabolite would be very difficult to demonstrate *in vivo*. In addition, this last point also raises an interesting question concerning the quantitative evaluation of eicosanoids as a reflection of a single cell type (see above). In the case of leukotrienes for instance, red blood cells as well as platelets and endothelial cells have a higher capacity to transform leukotriene A_4 into leukotrienes B_4 and C_4 respectively, than do the neutrophils to generate the unstable intermediate LTA_4. One would thus predict that the overall production of leukotrienes would be limited by the capacity of the human neutrophils to generate significant amounts of leukotriene A_4 in response to "physio-pathological" stimuli.

Release of unstable metabolic intermediates outside the cells have been demonstrated with the concomitant formation of their end-products, thus lending support to the concept of transcellular metabolism. The amount of intact endoperoxides present in platelet suspensions after 1 min incubation with thrombin was evaluated from the difference between the amounts of $PGF_{2\alpha}$ present in samples treated with ethanol with or without the additive stannous chloride (Hamberg *et al.*, 1974). Dahinden *et al.* (1985) have shown that mast cells can convert exogenously added LTA_4 to LTC_4 and have hypothesized that such event may occur during neutrophil/mast cell interactions because activated neutrophils can release LTA_4. Moreover, cellular coincubations have established a relationship between decrease of non enzymatic breakdown products of LTA_4 vs increase of LTB_4 (McGee and Fitzpatrick, 1986). One could still argue that the rather drastic conditions employed during which these cells were challenged resulted in a saturation of the specific enzymes from the donor cell (i.e. thromboxane synthase and leukotriene hydrolase) in their capacity to metabolize PGG_2/PGH_2 or LTA_4 generated, respectively. The lower level of production of leukotriene A_4 under milder conditions would render questionable the reality of a transcellular metabolism aside the artifactual conditions of the calcium ionophore A 23187. However, it was reported that a much weaker agonist of neutrophil activation (e.g. formyl peptides) generated an enhanced production of leukotriene B_4 in neutrophil/red blood cells as compared to neutrophil incubations alone (McGee and Fitzpatrick, 1986). These experiments strongly suggested that even at low level of stimulation, neutrophils release sufficient leukotriene A_4 into the external medium to support transcellular metabolism. We have also found that mild stimulation of neutrophils in the presence or absence of platelets (i.e. 100 fold lower production of peptido leukotrienes than with the calcium ionophore) resulted in the production of LTC_4 only when platelets were present. These findings strongly imply that release of a metabolic intermediate into the external medium by the donor cell or in the very close vicinity of the acceptor cell, occurs during various degrees of stimulation. As a corollary, the neutrophil 5-lipoxygenase releases only part of its products (e.g. leukotriene A_4) to the inside of the cell for conversion by the LTA_4 hydrolase. Only a few studies have been carried out to quantitatively assess the proportion of unstable intermediate released outside the cell. In this respect, studies dealing with the subcellular localization of these critical enzymes are of great interest. Such studies have revealed that cyclooxygenase is located mainly on the reticulum endoplasmic and that it is oriented towards its cytosolic surface (Rollins and Smith, 1980, DeWitt et al., 1981). This finding is consistent with the fact that approximately 80 % of the synthesized endoperoxides have been shown to be transformed into thromboxane A_2 (Hamberg et al., 1974) with a low proportion being released in the outside milieu (Marcus et al 1980). The interface of transfer from one cell to another and the mechanisms of uptake by the acceptor cell must be remarkably efficient in order to trap these highly reactive metabolic intermediates. Until now, acceptor enzymes such as prostacyclin synthase or leukotriene C_4 synthase have been found in the membrane pellet of the cell (Jakschik et al., 1982, Yoshimoto et al., 1988). However, the cytosolic localization of leukotriene hydrolase (McGee and Fitzpatrick, 1985) raises serious questions concerning the mechanisms of substrate transfer to the inner compartment of the cell.

The study of transcellular metabolism using cells found in blood may have little relevance to pathological situations involving adhering cells. However, it may provide a useful model to study mechanisms that are very likely to occur at the organ level. Altering the ratio of cells would mimic what could be expected under pathological conditions in which the vicinity of the donor cell exposed to its neighbor acceptor cells could be dramatically altered. It can also be speculated that incubation of cells in suspensions have the lowest efficiency in transcellular biosynthesis. The close vicinity of cells in in vivo situations such as after adhesion or in the context of a tissue may permit more efficient reactive substrate uptake via gap junctions between adjacent cells rather than via the extracellular matrix or fluid phase.

The concept of transcellular metabolism focuses attention on the use of selective inhibitors or antagonists, rather than fairly non specific compounds acting at the oxygenase(s) level. In this context, the use of thromboxane synthase inhibitors has been shown to lead in vitro and in vivo to a decrease in thromboxane synthesis with a concomitant rise of the prostacyclin synthesis by endoperoxide shunting (Oates et al., 1988). Pharmacological strategies based on inhibiting acceptor cell biosynthesis rather than the donor cell biosynthesis thus become of interest.

ACKNOWLEDGEMENTS

This research was supported by Centre National de la Recherche Scientifique (CNRS).

REFERENCES

Benjamin C.W., Hopkins N.K., Oglesby T.D. and Gorman R.R. Agonist specific desensitization of leukotriene C_4-stimulated PGI_2 biosynthesis in human endothelial cells. Biochem. Biophys. Res. Commun. 117:780-787, 1983.

Borgeat P., Picard S., Vallerand P. and Sirois P. Prostaglandins Med. 6:557- 570, 1981.

Borgeat B. and Samuelsson B. Arachidonic acid metabolism in polymorphonuclear leukocytes: Unstable intermediate in the formation of di-hydroxy acids. Proc. Natl. Acad. Sci. USA 76:3213-3217, 1979.

Braquet P., Touqui L., Shen T.Y. and Vargaftig B.B. Perspectives in platelet-activating factor research. Pharmacol. Rev. 39:97-145, 1987.

Cramer E.B., Pologe L., Pawlowski N.A., Cohn Z.A. and Scott W.A. Leukotriene C promotes prostacyclin synthesis by human endothelial cells. Proc. Natl. Acad. Sci. USA 80:4109-4113, 1983.

Claesson H.E. and Haeggström J. Human endothelial cells stimulate leukotriene synthesis and convert granulocyte-released leukotriene A_4 into leukotrienes B_4, C_4, D_4 and E_4. Eur. J. Biochem. 173: 93-100, 1988.

Dahinden C. A., Clancy R.M., Gross M., Chiller J.M. and Hugly T.E. Leukotriene C_4 production by murine mast cells: Evidence of a role for extracellular leukotriene A_4. Proc. Natl. Acad. Sci. USA 82:6632-6636, 1985.

DeWitt D., Rollins T.E., Day J.S., Gauger J.A. and Smith W.L. Orientation of the active site and antigenic determinants of prostaglandin endoperoxide synthase in the endoplasmic reticulum. J. Biol. Chem. 256: 10375-10382, 1981.

Feinmark S.J. and Cannon P.J. Endothelial cells leukotriene C_4 synthesis results from intercellular transfer of leukotriene A_4 synthesized by polymorphonuclear leukocytes. J. Biol. Chem. 261: 16466-16472, 1986.

Feinmark S.J. and Cannon P.J. Vascular smooth muscle cells leukotriene C_4 synthesis: requirement for transcellular leukotriene A_4 metabolism. Biochim. Biophys. Acta, 922:125-135, 1987.

Fitzgerald D.J., Roy L., Catella F. and FitzGerald G.A. Platelet activation in unstable coronary disease. N. Engl. J. Med. 315:983-989, 1986.

Fitzpatrick F.A., Liggett W., McGee J., Bunting S., Morton D. and Samuelsson B. Metabolism of leukotriene A_4 by human erythrocyte: A novel cellular source of leukotriene B_4. J. Biol. Chem. 259:11403-11407, 1984.

Hamberg M. and Samuelsson B. Detection and isolation of an endoperoxide intermediate in prostaglandin biosynthesis. Proc. Natl. Acad. Sci. USA 70:899-903, 1973.

Hamberg M., Svensson J. and Samuelsson B. Prostaglandin endoperoxides. A new concept concerning the mode of action and release of prostaglandins. Proc. Natl. acad. Sci. USA 71:3824-3828, 1974.

Jakschik B.A., Harper T. and Murphy R.C. Leukotriene C_4 and D_4 formation by particulate enzymes. J. Biol. Chem. 257:5346-5349, 1982.

Lindgren J.A., Hansson G. and Samuelsson B. FEBS Lett. 128:329-335, 1981.

Maclouf J., Fruteau de Laclos B. and Borgeat P. Stimulation of leukotriene biosynthesis by platelet-derived 12-hydroperoxy-icosatetraenoic acid. Proc. Natl. Acad. Sci. USA 79:6042-6046, 1982.

Maclouf J. and Murphy R.C. Transcellular metabolism of neutrophil-derived leukotriene A_4 by human platelets. J. Biol. Chem. 263:174-181, 1988.

McGee J.E. and Fitzpatrick F.A. Enzymatic hydration of leukotriene A_4 hydrolase: Purification and characterization of a novel epoxide hydrolase from human erythrocytes. J. Biol. Chem. 260:12832-12837, 1985.

McGee J.E. and Fitzpatrick F.A. Erythrocyte-neutrophil interactions: Formation of leukotriene B_4 via transcellular biosynthesis. Proc. Natl. Acad. Sci. USA, 83:149-1353, 1986.

Marcus A.J., Weksler B.B., Jaffe E.A. and Broekman M.J. Synthesis of prostacyclin from platelet-derived endoperoxides by cultured human endothelial cells. J. Clin. Invest. 66:979-986, 1980.

Marcus A.J., Broekman, M.J., Safier L.B., Ullman H.L., Islam N., Serhan C.N., Rutherford L.E., Korchak H.M. and Weissman G. Formation of leukotrienes and other hydroxy acids during platelet-neutrophil interactions in vivo. Biochem. Biophys. Res. Commun. 109:130-137, 1982.

Marcus A.J., Safier L.B., Ullman H.L., Broekman M.J., Islam N., Oglesby T.D. and Gorman R.R. 12S,20-dihydroxyicosatetraenoic acid: A new icosanoid produced by thrombin- or collagen-stimulated platelets. Proc. Natl. Acad. Sci. USA 81:903-907, 1984.

Marcus A.J., Safier L.B., Ullman H.L., Islam N., Broekman M.J., Falck J.R., Fischer S., Von Schacky C. Platelet-neutrophil interactions: 12S-hydroxyeicosatetraen-1,20-dioic acid: A new eicosanoid synthesized by unstimulated neutrophils from 12S-20-dihydroxyeicosatetraenoic acid J. Biol. Chem. 263:2223-2229, 1988.

Nugteren D.H. and Hazelhof E. Isolation and properties of intermediates in prostaglandin biosynthesis Biochim. Biophys. Acta 326:448-461, 1973.

Oates J.A., FitzGerald G., Branch R.A., Jackson E.K., Knapp H.R. and Roberts II, J. Clinical implications of prostaglandin and thromboxane A_2 formation. N. Engl. J. Med.319:689-698, 1988.

Rollins T.E. and Smith W.L. Subcellular localization of prostaglandin-forming cyclooxygenase in Swiss mouse 3T3 fibroblasts by electron microscopic immunocytochemistry. J. Biol. Chem. 255: 4872-4875, 1980.

Samuelsson B. J. Am. Chem. Soc. 87:3011-3013, 1965.

Voelkel N.F., Worthen S., Reeves J.T., Henson P.M. and Murphy R.C. Nonimmunological production of leukotrienes induced by platelet-activating factor. Science 218:286-288, 1982.

Weksler B.B., Marcus A.J. and Jaffe E.A. Synthesis of prostaglandin I_2 (prostacyclin) by cultured human and bovine endothelial cells. Proc. Natl. Acad. Sci. USA 74: 3922-3926, 1977.

Yoshimoto T., Soberman R.J., Spur B. and Austen K.F. Properties of highly purified leukotriene C_4 synthase of guinea pig lung. J. Clin. Invest. 81:866-871, 1988.

METABOLISM OF SULFIDOPEPTIDE LEUKOTRIENES

Danny O. Stene and Robert C. Murphy

Department of Pharmacology
University of Colorado Health Sciences Center
4200 E. 9th Avenue
Denver, Colorado 80262

INTRODUCTION

Until recently there has been very little known about the ultimate metabolite fate of the sulfidopeptide leukotrienes. A basic principle of the pharmacology of mediator substances requires that mechanisms exist for biological inactivation of these very potent molecules. One such mechanism might be simple uptake of leukotrienes by the cells which make or respond to them. Studies showing that LTC_4, produced in the isolated perfused lung in response to the calcium ionophore A23187, was largely retained by the lung over a span of 10 minutes, and that very little conversion to LTD_4/LTE_4 took place, suggesting the possibility that a reuptake mechanism for LTC_4 in the lung existed (1). Other eicosanoids (LTB_4, 6-keto-PGF_1, thromboxane B_2 and PGE_2) were largely released into the perfusate. It is also possible that LTC_4 was retained through binding to tissue proteins with high affinity and not taken up into cells. Since direct experiments have now shown that leukotrienes are not stored in cells from which they are released, and, while the retention of LTC_4 by the isolated perfused rat lung has not been fully explained, simple reuptake of LTC_4 in the lung seems unlikely. At present it is thought that metabolic biotransformation is the primary mechanism of inactivation of the leukotrienes.

A mechanism for the local inactivation of the sulfidopeptide leukotrienes through metabolism has been described. When neutrophils or other phagocytic leukocytes are activated to ingest particles or bacteria, the phagocytes respond with a respiratory burst. This reaction produces the reactive oxygen species hydrogen peroxide, superoxide, and hydroxyl radical (2). It has been shown that activated human neutrophils metabolize various peptide chemotactic factors (C5a and N-formyl peptides) by myeloperoxidase-catalyzed oxidation of thioethers (3). This reaction is dependent on H_2O_2 and halide ion and is inhibited by adding methionine or non-specific reducing agents. Studies of neutrophil inactivation of LTC_4 have shown that this myeloperoxidase-catalyzed reaction can convert LTC_4 into sulfoxides and into 6-trans-LTB_4 (4). The same oxidation products can be obtained by incubation of LTC_4 with hypochlorous acid which is the product formed by myeloperoxidase, H_2O_2 and Cl^-. Soluble human eosinophil peroxidase has been shown to catalyze the H_2O_2/Cl^- dependant transformation of LTC_4 to 6-trans-LTB_4 (5). Also, hydroxyl radical generated in the presence of ferrous iron destroys the biological activities of LTC_4, D_4, E_4, and B_4 (6).

In spite of these observations, it seems unlikely that local, oxidative inactivation of leukotrienes by reactive oxygen species is the primary mechanism of inactivation for these molecules. It is not obvious *a priori* that the *in vitro* conditions employed in the experiments noted above would be representative of the microenvironment in which leukotrienes function. The omission of protein from the incubations, the high concentrations of leukocytes (10^7 PMN/ml), the omission of other cell types, and the extended incubation times (30 minutes) might provide conditions which would favor the reactions described and not reflect the microenvironment experienced by leukotrienes synthesized *in vivo* (7). Significant amounts of LTC_4-sulfoxide or 6-trans-LTB_4 have not been reported in studies of leukotriene metabolism in the isolated perfused rat lung (8). Also, as will be discussed below, these metabolites have not been reported in studies where leukotriene synthesis has been stimulated *in vivo*. It seems most likely that the primary mechanism for leukotriene bioinactivation was through hepatic extraction of leukotrienes that escape into the circulation, followed by enzymatic oxidation of the fatty acid backbone of the molecule.

ω-Oxidation of LTB_4 by neutrophils has been described (9). 20-Hydroxy-LTB_4 and 20-carboxy-LTB_4 have been characterized as major metabolites of LTB_4. These metabolites were shown to be substantially inactive as chemoattractants (10). Thus, it appears as if LTB_4 could be inactivated locally by cells which also synthesize this molecule. It has also been shown that isolated rat hepatocytes can extract LTB_4 and metabolize it by way of ω-oxidation (11). Recently, a rat hepatic microsomal monooxygenase was partially purified which converts LTB_4 to 20-hydroxy-LTB_4 (12). The enzyme was oxygen and NADPH dependent and appeared to be physiochemically different from the enzymes which catalyze similar oxidations of laurate and prostaglandins. Interestingly, this enzyme catalyzes three successive ω-oxidations of LTB_4 to from 20-carboxy-LTB_4 (13).

The question as to whether or not LTB_4 is primarily metabolized in the tissue in which it is synthesized or in the liver, has not been resolved. Some of the same objections which were raised against the reactive oxygen mechanisms discussed above might also be applied to local inactivation of LTB_4 by neutrophil ω-oxidation. Metabolites of $[^3H]$-LTB_4 injected into monkeys have been found in urine (14). Of the radioactive material recovered, 40% was found to be volatile, indicating perhaps that β-oxidation of the LTB_4 had occurred. It may be then that LTB_4 was oxidized by those cells which released this mediator, and that the liver also oxidized any LTB_4 which escaped unchanged into the circulation. Further metabolism by β-oxidation might then have followed in the liver. This speculation was supported by the observation that isolated rat hepatocytes metabolized LTB_4 to 18-carboxy-20,19,-dinor-LTB_4 (11).

Over the last six years an important role for the liver has been demonstrated for the metabolic inactivation of the sulfidopeptide leukotrienes. When $[^3H]$-LTC_3 was injected into mice, whole body autoradiography showed major concentrations of the radiolabel in the liver and bile (15). Reverse phase HPLC analysis (RP-HPLC) of radioactive material extracted from these tissues revealed peaks identified as LTC_3, D_3, and E_3, as well as unidentified metabolites in the HPLC solvent front. $[^3H]$-LTC_3 was also taken up by the isolated rat liver, and by isolated rat hepatocytes (16). Metabolism of the LTC_3 was again apparent from radiolabeled materials eluting in the solvent front of a RP-HPLC system. These metabolites were also found in the bile from the isolated rat liver. Specific uptake of LTC_4, D_4, and E_4 by isolated rat hepatocytes was shown to be temperature, and ATP dependant with a high affinity Km of about 1 μM (17). Again, these leukotrienes were transformed to unidentified polar metabolites. A transplantable ascites tumor cell line, AS-30D hepatoma cells, was found to be unable to take up LTC_4 (18). These cells converted LTC_4 to D_4 and E_4 but not to any other metabolites. Thus, it appeared that metabolism of sulfidopeptide leukotrienes by liver may follow uptake of the leukotrienes into the hepatocyte.

One of the rat liver metabolites of LTC_4 has been identified as N-acetyl-LTE_4. After subcutaneous injection of $[^3H]$-LTC_4 into rats, N-acetyl-LTE_4 was found in the feces (19). This metabolite was purified by RP-HPLC and characterized by fast atom bombardment mass spectrometry, and the fatty acid backbone by gas chromatography-mass spectrometry following catalytic reduction/desulfuration. N-acetyl-LTE_4 had bioactivity similar to that of LTE_4 in the guinea pig ileum bioassay. When LTC_4 synthesis was stimulated in the rat by injection with endotoxin or platelet activating factor (50 nmole/kg body weight), N-acetyl-LTE$_4$ was found in the collected bile (20). N-acetyl-LTE$_4$ was identified by co-migration with chemically synthesized N-acetyl-LTE$_4$ in several HPLC systems. It was also shown that pretreatment of rats with D-penicillamine prevented the metabolism of intravenous [^{3}H]-LTC$_4$ to N-acetyl-LTE$_4$. In these experiments D-penicillamine, which inhibited dipeptidase, caused an accumulation of [^{3}H]-LTD$_4$ in the bile, whereas in the controls, N-acetyl-LTE$_4$ and other biliary metabolites more polar that LTC$_4$ were predominant (21). These polar metabolites, as in all of the studies noted so far, accounted for most of the radiolabeled metabolites (up to 45% of the total radiolabel used), indicating that metabolism beyond N-acetyl-LTE$_4$ had occurred.

Several investigators have noted the similarity between the glutathione S-conjugate/mercapturic acid pathway of drug detoxication, and the synthesis of LTC$_4$ (a glutathione S-conjugate of LTA$_4$), and the subsequent biotransformation of LTC$_4$ to N-acetyl-LTE$_4$ (a mercapturic acid) (22). The enzyme LTC$_4$ synthase has been clearly distinguished from those enzymes responsible for glutathione conjugation of xenobiotics (23). It has not been determined whether or not the other enzymes, γ-glutamyl transferase, dipeptidase, and N-acetyl-transferase, were the same for both pathways. N-acetyl-transferases which acetiylate LTE$_4$ at its amino group have been isolated from microsomal fractions of kidney and liver; they have also been found in the cytosol of many tissues, and both forms used acetyl-CoA as the acetate donor (24). An LTE$_4$ specific N-acetyl-transferase has not been thoroughly characterized; however, N-acetyl-LTE$_4$ was formed when LTE$_4$ and acetyl-CoA were incubated with subcellular particulate fractions from rat liver, spleen, lung, and skin (25). These subcellular fractions were characterized only by the centrifugal force used to prepare them, but the particulate nature of the preparations suggested that the N-acetyl-transferase involved was a membrane bound enzyme.

The importance of biliary excretion of LTC$_4$ metabolites has been demonstrated in studies of leukotriene enterohepatic circulation (26). After intraduodenal administration of tritium labeled leukotrienes in rats or in monkeys, polar metabolites were recovered from bile and urine. In mutant rats defective in hepatobiliary excretion of conjugated bilirubin, dibromosulfophthalein, and ouabain, intravenous administration of [^{3}H]-LTC$_4$ resulted in 5-fold higher radiolabel accumulation in the liver compared with controls (27). Also, radiolabel which appeared in bile of the mutants was only 1.8% of that found in controls. Intraduodenal administration of [^{3}H]-N-acetyl-LTE$_4$ was found to undergo enterohepatic circulation. In mutants, labeled material which appeared in bile was only 5% of controls. Also, the proportion of N-acetyl-LTE$_4$ relative to polar leukotriene metabolites was higher in the bile of transport mutants as compared to controls. These observations suggested that after hepatic elimination, a major route of excretion of leukotriene metabolites was via biliary secretion. They also pointed out that enterohepatic circulation would complicate the interpretations of biliary or urinary metabolite measurements.

As mentioned above, a major metabolite in the rat of LTC$_4$ is N-acetyl-LTE$_4$. The liver appears to be the major site for this biotransformation, although rat lung has recently been shown to make this metabolite (28). This metabolic transformation does not appear to occur in primates. In monkeys injected with [^{3}H]-LTC$_4$ only [^{3}H]-LTE$_4$ and polar metabolites were detected, 40% in bile, and 20% in urine by five hours (29). As in the other studies, polar metabolites were unidentified and amounted in this case to as much as ten times more than the LTE$_4$ detected. Similar results were obtained when [^{3}H]-LTC$_4$ was injected into human subjects (30). Of the dose administered, 48% was recovered in urine over 72 hours. Only 13% of the administered dose was identified in urine as LTE$_4$. N-acetyl-LTE$_4$ was not detected.

The biotransformation of the sulfidopeptide leukotrienes by hepatic tissues or *in vivo* has in all cases resulted in appearance of metabolites which were more polar than LTC$_4$ in RP-HPLC systems. The goal of the present work was to develop a model in which these polar metabolites could be structurally characterized. Because LTC$_4$ was rapidly converted to LTE$_4$ *in vivo*, the metabolism of LTE$_4$ was studied. Further, because the liver appeared to be the major site of biotransformation of LTE$_4$ *in vivo*, a model of hepatic leukotriene metabolism was

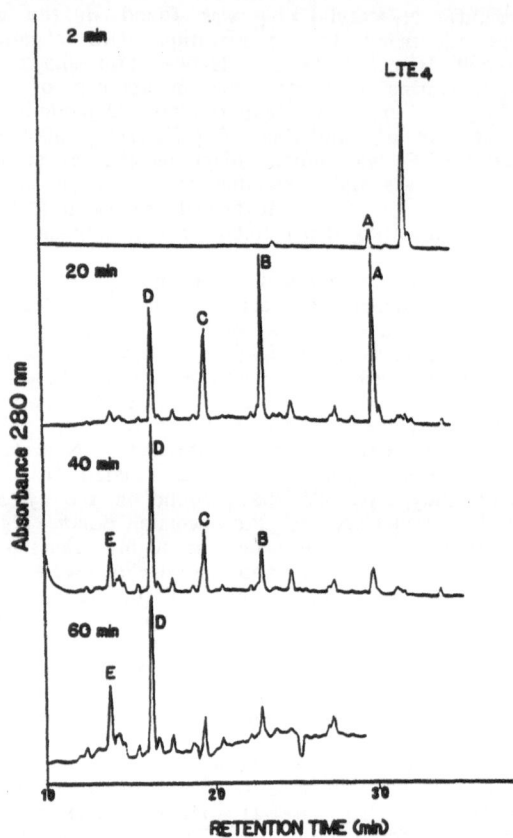

Figure 1 *Separation of metabolites obtained following incubation of* LTE_4 *with isolated rat hepatocytes (32). Incubations were carried out at 2, 20, 40, 60 min. Metabolites A, B, C, D, and E were structurally characterized using mass spectrometric techniques.*

desired. The isolated rat hepatocyte has been extensively characterized biochemically and widely accepted as a model of hepatic function in general, and so was chosen as a model of hepatic metabolism (31).

Quite polar metabolites of LTE_4 resulted from incubation of this substance with isolated rat hepatocytes (32,33). When a gradient RP-HPLC suited to the separation of highly polar substances was used (Figure 1), six different metabolites of LTE_4 were isolated and their abundance varied with the time of incubation. The UV absorption spectra of the isolated metabolites A - D, and F had λ_{max} 280 nm with 10 nm vibronic shoulders suggesting intact conjugated trienes with an allylic thioether (34). Metabolite E contained a conjugated tetraene allylic to a thioether as suggested by its λ_{max} 310. These observations indicated that the major portion of LTE_4's chemical skeleton remained in the isolated metabolites and suggested that, as with prostaglandins and LTB_4, ω-oxidation of LTE_4 might explain the increased polarity of the metabolites. Furthermore, the observation that a substantial amount of volatile radioactivity was also generated during this incubation suggested that metabolism might involve loss of carbons 14 and 15 which were the sites of tritium incorporation in the tracer employed. Metabolites E and F did not contain the tritium label, and so these metabolites must have been altered in some way at carbons 14 and 15 and might have been the source of some of the volatile radioactivity.

The RP-HPLC retention time of Metabolite A suggested that it was N-acetyl-LTE_4, and this was confirmed by RP-HPLC of synthetic N-acetyl-LTE_4. When isolated rat hepatocytes were incubated with Metabolite A, this compound was found to be metabolized to products with RP-HPLC retention times and UV spectra which were the same as those derived from LTE_4 (Figure 2). This experiment

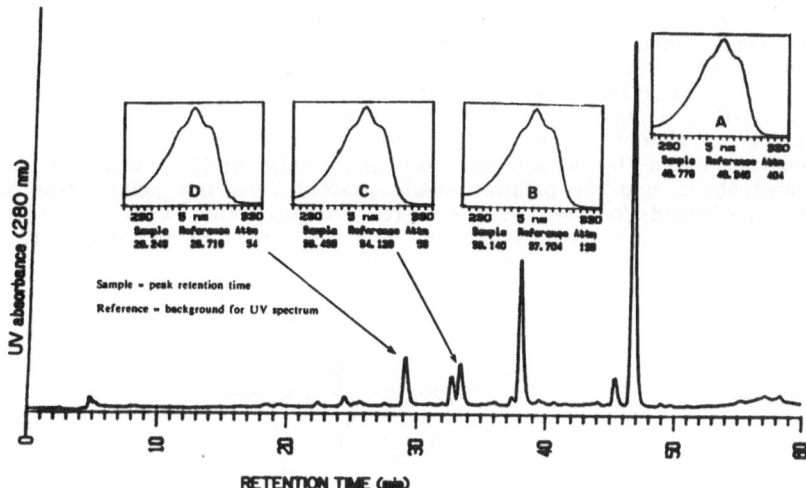

Figure 2 *HPLC separation (conditions different from Figure 1) of metabolites obtained following incubation of N-acetyl-LTE₄ with isolated rat hepatocytes. Metabolites D, C, and B have UV spectra illustrated in the insets at retention times of 29.2, 33.4, and 38.1, respectively. These metabolites were identical to those obtained by LTE₄ metabolism.*

indicated that N-acetyl-LTE$_4$ might be the immediate precursor for the other metabolites.

The structures of LTE$_4$ metabolites A-F (Figure 1) were identified by ultraviolet spectroscopy, mass spectrometry, and ancillary techniques (32). These structures, shown in Figure 3, suggested a single major pathway for the metabolism of LTE$_4$ by isolated rat hepatocytes. Initial acetylation of the cysteine nitrogen was followed by oxidation of the terminal methyl group, presumably by initial NADPH-dependent ω-hydroxylation followed by oxidation to a carboxylic acid as has been described for other eicosanoids (12). Once the ω-terminal methyl group has been oxidized to a carboxylic acid, sequential β-oxidation from the ω-terminus would account for the chain shortened metabolites.

The formation of Metabolite D was interesting in that it served to demonstrate some of the enzymatic details involved in the β-oxidation of unsaturated fatty acids. When β-oxidation reaches a position of unsaturation along a carbon chain, alternative enzymatic steps become necessary to continue chain-shortening. Enzymes have been identified which catalyze isomerization of the double bonds in order to produce the traditionally expected intermediates in β-oxidation. Such double bonds may be encountered in an odd or an even number of carbons from the initial carboxylic acid, and there have been separate enzymes characterized which isomerize these double bonds (35). If the double bond is found in an odd position, such as in arachidonic acid (the first double bond is at C-5), the enzyme cis(3)-trans(2) enoyl-CoA isomerase (after one round of β-oxidation) would shift the double bond at Δ^3 to the Δ^2 position, which would then be an appropriate isomer for the enoyl-CoA hydratase of β-oxidation. Although the name cis(3)-trans(2) enoyl-CoA indicates a definite substrate preference, a Δ^3 trans double bond can be a substrate for this enzyme (36). If the double bond is at an even number position, as in the ω-oxidized LTE$_4$ metabolites, then a somewhat more complex set of reactions are

41

observed. After the formation of the CoA thioester of Metabolite C, acyl-CoA dehydrogenase (mitochondrial) or acyl-CoA oxidase (peroxisomal) would catalyze the formation of the 2,4-dienoyl-CoA ester. This conjugated diene intermediate would not be an efficient substrate for enoyl-CoA hydratase; rather, the enzyme 2,4-dienoyl-CoA reductase would catalyze the hydrogenation of carbons-2 and -5, leading to a trans double bond between carbons-3 and -4. This Δ^3-CoA intermediate would be a substrate for the cis(3)-trans(2) enoyl-CoA isomerase mentioned above, and the pathway would proceed from this point. The activities of the 2,4-dienoyl-CoA reductase and (cis)3-trans(2) enoyl-CoA isomerase would result in the saturation of the double bond at carbon-15 of Metabolite C, and so account for the structure found for Metabolite D (33).

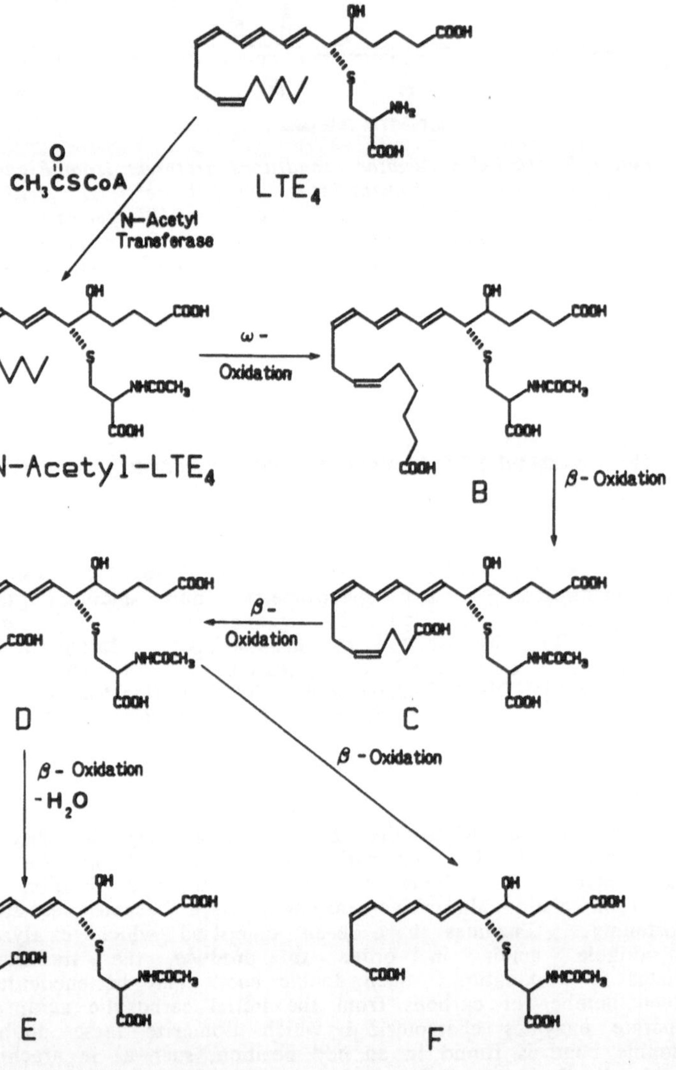

Figure 3 *LTE$_4$ Metabolites from Isolated Rat Hepatocytes.*
A. N-acetyl-LTE$_4$
B. 20-carboxy-N-acetyl-LTE$_4$
C. 18-carboxy-19,20-dinor-N-acetyl-LTE$_4$
D. 16-carboxy-17,18,19,20-tetranor-14,15-dihydro-N-acetyl-LTE$_4$
E. 16-carboxy-17,18,19,20-tetranor-Δ^{13}-N-acetyl-LTE$_4$
F. 14-carboxy-15,16,17,18,19,20-hexanor-N-acetyl-LTE$_4$

The identification of a conjugated tetraene (Metabolite E) was somewhat surprising. It was possible that during β-oxidation of Metabolite D and formation of the 14-hydroxyacyl-CoA thioester intermediate, dehydration to a thermodynamically more stable conjugated tetraene thioester could have produced Metabolite E (Figure 4). Another possible path for the formation of this metabolite would be the initial reduction of carbons-14 and -15 followed by double bond isomerization of this Δ^2 double bond to the Δ^3 isomer through the reverse action of cis(3)-trans(2)-enoyl-CoA isomerase. Experiments to test these two possible mechanisms have yet to be conducted, but the loss of the tritium label from this metabolite must be related to its formation.

While a complete understanding of the metabolic fate of endogenous sulfidopeptide leukotrienes is unknown, it is clear that ω-oxidation followed by β-oxidation is a primary route of LTE_4 metabolism in the rat. It is of interest to note that no evidence of β-oxidation from the C-1 carboxyl has been found. Prostaglandin metabolism is known to occur by β-oxidation from both the C-1 and C-20 positions following ω-oxidation of the C-20 carbon atom. One important structural feature of leukotrienes which might account for this difference in metabolism is the occurrence of a C-5 hydroxyl group. From molecular models it is obvious that strong interactions may take place between the C-1 carboxyl and the C-5 hydroxyl groups which could prevent the C-1 hydroxyl from serving as an adequate substrate for acyl-CoA synthetase. These interactions would involve hydrogen bonding between the C-5 hydroxyl proton and the C-1 acidic oxygen. Under acidic conditions, a lactone may be formed by this interaction, and lactonization has been used as part of an LTB_4 assay (37).

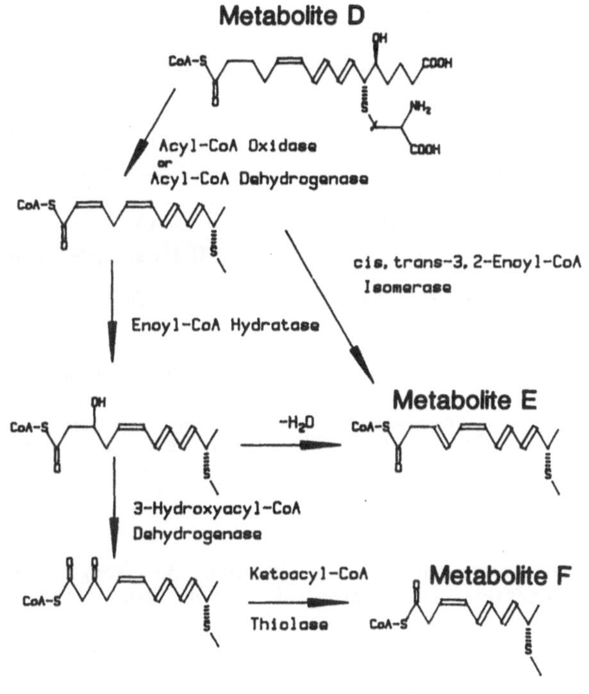

Another question of interest with LTE_4 metabolism by isolated rat hepatocytes concerns the subcellular location of the metabolic events. The initial N-acetylation of LTE_4 appears to occur preferentially in the cytosol from studies

Figure 4 *Proposed pathways for the formation of LTE_4 metabolites E and F from metabolite D by β-oxidation.*

conducted by Orning (25). Subsequent metabolism occurs by way of NADPH-dependant microsomal ω-oxidations (12). Chain shortening by β-oxidation might occur in peroxisomes and/or mitochondria. The preference of peroxisomes for long chain fatty acids and the chain shortening of $PGF_{2\alpha}$ by peroxisomal β-oxidation suggests that these organelles are involved in LTE_4 metabolism (38).

Most recently, the structures of several urinary LTE_4 metabolites have been reported (39). [^{3}H]-LTE_4 was injected into the peritoneal cavity of rats and urine collected over an 8 hour period. Approximately 10-15% of the injected LTE_4 appeared in the urine during the collection period. The radioactive metabolites were extracted and purified by HPLC. The major metabolite was mixed with synthetic 16-carboxy-17,18,19,20-tetranor-14,15-dihydro-N-acetyl-LTE_4

43

(Metabolite D) and the two materials co-eluted upon RP-HPLC (Figure 5). These experiments suggest that LTE_4 undergoes β-oxidation *in vivo* as it did in isolated hepatocytes. Furthermore, these experiments establish that β-oxidation products are eliminated in urine. Studies in primates have also identified 20-hydroxy-LTE_4 and 20-carboxy-LTE_4 as urinary metabolites (40). Therefore, oxidative metabolites of LTE_4 are known to be eliminated in the urine of primates.

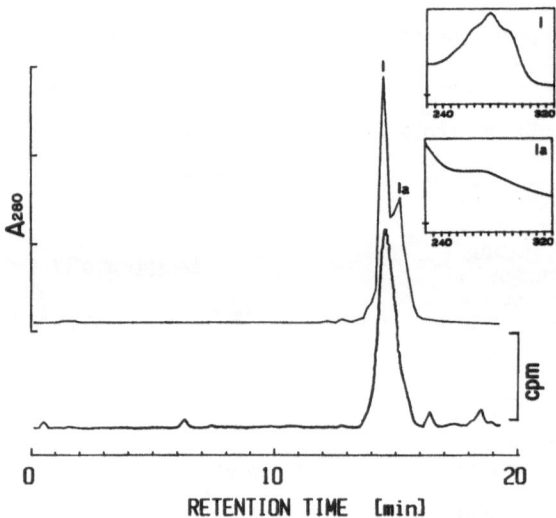

Figure 5 *Co-injection of synthetic 16-COOH-DH-N-acetyl-LTE$_4$ with a major metabolite of LTE$_4$ appearing in the urine of a rat injected with [^{3}H]-LTE$_4$. The absorbance at 280 nm corresponds to the elution of the synthetic material with the UV spectrum indicated in the inset (I). Other urinary components eluted at a slightly different retention time with ultraviolet spectra indicated in the inset (Ia). The radioactive metabolite of LTE$_4$ eluted at the retention time indicated by the scale CPM.*

We are now in a position to suggest that specific metabolites of sulfidopeptide leukotrienes of known structure occur in the urine of rodents and primates which might reflect whole body production of this important class of inflammatory mediators. This may open new possibilities in basic and clinical research to probe the role that 5-lipoxygenase products play in health and disease.

ACKNOWLEDGEMENTS

This work was supported, in part, by a grant from the National Institutes of Health (HL25785). Mass spectrometry was supported by grant RR01152.

REFERENCES

1. J.Y. Westcott, T.J. McDonnell, P. Bostwick, and N.F. Voelkel, Eicosanoid production in isolated perfused lungs stimulated with calcium ionophore A23187. *Am. Rev. Respir. Dis.*, in press.
2. R.K. Root, J. Metcalf, N. Oshino, and B. Chance, 1975, H_2O_2 release from human granulocytes during phagocytosis I. Documentation, quantitation, and some regulating factors. *J. Clin. Invest.*, 55:945.

3. R.A. Clark and S. Szot, 1982, Chemotactic factor inactivation by stimulated human eosinophils mediated by myeloperoxidase-catalyzed methionine oxidation. *J. Immunol.*, 128:1507.

4. C.W. Lee, R.A. Lewis, E.J. Corey, A. Barton, H. Oh, A.I. Tauber, K.F. Austen, 1982, Oxidative inactivation of leukotriene C_4 by stimulated human polymorphonuclear leukocytes. *Proc. Natl. Acad. Sci. USA*, 79:4166.

5. E.J. Goetzl, 1982, The conversion of leukotriene C_4 to isomers of leukotriene B_4 by human eosinophil peroxidase. *Biochem. Biophys. Res. Commun.*, 106:270.

6. W.R. Henderson and S.J. Klebanoff, 1983, Leukotriene B_4, C_4, D_4, and E_4 inactivation by hydroxyl radicals. *Biochem. Biophys. Res. Commun.*, 110:266.

7. M.A. Veill, W.R. Henderson, and S.J. Klebanoff, 1985, Oxidative degredation of leukotriene C_4 by human monocytes and monocyte-derived macrophage. *J. Exp. Med.*, 162:1634.

8. T.W. Harper, J.Y. Westcott, N.F. Voelkel, and R.C. Murphy, 1984, Metabolism of LTB_4 and LTC_4 in the isolated perfused rat lung. *J. Biol. Chem.*, 259:14437.

9. G. Hansson, J.A. Lindgren, S.E. Dahlen, P. Hedqvist, and B. Samuelsson, 1981, Identification and biological activity of novel ω -oxidized metabolites of leukotriene B_4 from human leukocytes. *FEBS Lett.*, 130:107.

10. S.J., Feinmark, J.A. Lindgren, H.E. Claesson, C. Malmsten, B. Samuelsson, 1981, Stimulation of human leukocyte degranulation by leukotriene B_4 and its ω-oxidized metabolites. *FEBS Lett.*, 136:141.

11. T.W. Harper, M.J. Garrity, and R.C. Murphy, 1986, Metabolism of leukotriene B_4 in isolated rat hepatocytes. Identification of a novel 18-carboxy-dinor-LTB_4 metabolite. *J. Biol. Chem.*, 261:5414.

12. M.C. Ramano, R.D. Eckardt, P.E. Bender, T.B. Leonard, K.M. Straub, and J.F. Newton, 1987, Biochemical characterization of hepatic microsomal leukotriene B_4 hydroxylases. *J. Biol. Chem.*, 262:1590.

13. R.J. Soberman, J.P. Sutyak, R.T. Okita, D.F. Wendelborn, L.J. Roberts, and K.F. Austen, 1988, The identification and formation of 20-aldehyde leukotriene B_4. *J. Biol. Chem.*, 263:7996.

14. W.E. Serafin, J.A. Oates, W.C. Hubbard, 1984, Metabolism of leukotriene B_4 in the monkey. Identification of the principal nonvolatile metabolite in urine. *Prostaglandins*, 27:899.

15. L.-E. Appelgren and S. Hammarstrom, 1982, Distribution and metabolism of ^{3}H-labeled leukotriene C_3 in the mouse. *J. Biol. Chem.*, 257:531.

16. K. Ormstad, N. Uehara, S. Orrenius, L. Orning, and S. Hammarstrom, 1982, Uptake and metabolism of leukotriene C_3 by isolated rat organs and cells. *Biochem. Biophys. REs. Commun.* 104:1434.

17. N. Uehara, K. Ormstad, L. Orning, and S. Hammarstrom, 1983, Characteristics of the uptake of cysteine-containing leukotrienes by isolated hepatocytes. *Biochim. Biophys. Acta*, 732:69.

18. G. Weckbecker and D.O.R. Keppler, 1986, Leukotriene C_4 metabolism by hepatoma cells deficient in the uptake of cysteinyl leukotrienes. *Eur. J. Biochem.*, 154:559.

19. L. Orning, E. Norin, B. Gustafsson, and S. Hammarstrom, 1986, *In vivo* metabolism of leukotriene C_4 in germ-free and conventional rats. *J. Biol. Chem.*, 261:766.

20. W. Hagmann, C. Denzlinger, S. Rapp, G. Weckbecker, and D. Keppler, 1986, Identification of the major engoenous leukotriene metabolite in the bile of rats as N-acetyl leukotriene E_4. *Prostaglandins*, 31:239.

21. M. Huber and D. Keppler, 1987, Inhibition of leukotriene D_4 catabolism by D-penicillamine. *Eur. J. Biochem.*, 167:73.

22. R.C. Murphy, R. Mathews, and W. Pickett, W., Leukotrienes and thromboxanes: Metabolites of essential fatty acids with significant untoward pharmacological properties, *in:* "Nutritional Factors: Modulating Effects of Metabolic Processes," E.G. Bassett, ed., Raven Press, N.Y. (1981).

23. M. Soderstrom, S. Hammarstrom, and B. Mannervick, 1988, Leukotriene C synthase in mouse mastocytoma cells. An enzyme distinct from cytosolic and microsomal glutathione transferases. *Biochem. J.*, 250:713.

24. J. Caldwell, Conjugation reactions of nitrogen centers, *in:* "Metabolic Basis of Detoxication," W.B. Jakoby, J.R. Bend, and J. Caldwell, eds., Academic Press, New York (1982).

25. K. Bernstrom and S. Hammarstrom, 1986, Metabolism of leukotriene E_4 by rat tissues: Formation of N-acetyl leukotriene E_4. *Arch. Biochem. Biophys.*, 244:486.

26. C. Denzlinger, A. Guhlmann, W. Hagmann, P.H. Scheuber, F. Scheyer, D. Wilker, D.K. Hammer, and D. Keppler, 1986, Cysteinyl leukotrienes undergo enterohepatic circulation. *Prostag. Leukotr. Med.*, 21:321.
27. M. Humber, A. Guhlmann, P.L.M. Jansen, and D. Keppler, 1987, Hereditory defect of hepatobiliary cysteinyl leukotriene elimination in mutant rats with defective hepatic anion excretion. *Hepatology*, 7:224.
28. J.Y. Westcott, T.J. McDonnel, and N.F. Voelkel, 1988, Alveolar transfer and metabolism of eicosaniods in the rat. In press.
29. C. Denzlinger, A. Guhlmann, P.H. Scheuber, D. Wilker, D.K. Hammer, and D. Keppler, 1986, Metabolism and analysis of cysteinyl leukotrienes in the monkey. *J. Biol. Chem.*, 261:15601.
30. L. Orning, L. Kaijser, and S. Hammarstrom, 1985, *In vivo* metabolism of leukotriene C_4 in man: Urinary excretion of leukotriene E_4. *Biochem. Biophys. Res. Commun.*, 130:214.
31. S.R. Wagle and W.R. Ingebretsen, Isolation, purification, and metabolic characteristics of rat liver hepatocytes, *in*: "Methods in Enzymology," J.M. Lowenstein, ed., Academic Press, New York (1975).
32. D.O. Stene and R.C. Murphy, 1988, Metabolism of leukotriene E_4 in isolated rat hepatocytes: Identification of beta-oxidation products of sulfidopeptide leukotrienes. *J. Biol. Chem.* 263:2773.
33. R.C. Murphy and D.O. Stene, 1988, Oxidative metabolism of leukotriene E_4 by rat hepatocytes. *Ann. NY Acad. Sci.*, 524:35.
34. H.P. Koch, 1949, Absorption spectra and structure of organic sulfur compounds. Part I. Unsaturated sulphides. *J. Chem. Soc.*, 387.
35. W.-H. Kunau and P. Dommes, 1978, Degradation of unsaturated fatty acids. Identification of intemediates in the degradation of cis-4-decenoyl-CoA by extracts of beff liver mitochondria. *Eur. J. Biochem.*, 91:533.
36. C.-H. Chu, L. Kushner, D. Cuebas, and H. Schulz, 1984, The activity of 3-hydroxyacyl-CoA epemerase is insufficient to account for the rate of linoleate oxidation in rat heart mitochondria. Evidence for a modified pathway of linoleate degradation. *Biochem. Biophys. Res. Commun.*, 118:162.
37. J.A. Zirrolli, A. Fradin, J. Maclouf, and R.C. Murphy, 1988, Analysis of LTB_4 and 20-hydroxy-LTB_4 in whole blood challenged with zymosan. Proc. Ann. Conf. Mass Spectrom. 36:, in press.
38. V. Diczfalusy, S.E.H. Alerson, and J.I. Pedersen, 1987, Chain-shortening of prostaglandin $F_{2\alpha}$ by rat liver peroxisomes. *Biochem. Biophys. Res. Commun.*, 144:1206.
39. P. Perrin, J. Zirrolli, D. Stene, J.P. Lellouche, J.P. Beaucourt, and R.C. Murphy, *In vivo* formation of β-oxidized metabolites of leukotriene E_4 in the rat. *Prostaglandins*, submitted.
40. H.A. Ball and D. Keppler, 1987, ω-oxidation products of leukotriene E_4 in bile and urine of the monkey. *Biochem. Biophys. Res. Commun.*, 148:664.

LIPOXINS: BIOSYNTHESIS, METABOLISM AND PHYSIOLOGICAL FUNCTIONS

Carol F. Ng, Hsioa-Yung Ho* and Patrick Y-K Wong

Department of Pharmacology, New York Medical College
Valhalla, NY, USA and *Institute of Biomedical Science
Division of Eicosanoid and Lipid Mediators Research
Academic Sinica, Taipei, Taiwan, R.O.C.

Lipoxygenase products of arachidonic acid are important lipid mediators in inflammatory responses, immunity, and other physiological and pathophysiological processes (1). Recently, a new class of conjugated trihyroxytetraenes derived from oxygenation of arachidonic acid (AA) and eicosapentatenoic acid (EPA) via interactions between the 5- and 15 lipoxygenase pathways have been reported by Serhan et al. (2) and Wong et al. (3). This novel group of compounds are denoted as "Lipoxin" (LX) A_4/B_4 and A_5/B_5, respectively.

Lipoxins possess a number of biological activites. When added to human neutrophils it stimulated the release of superoxide anion without inducing its aggregation (1). Lipoxin A_4 has also been shown to contract guinea pig parenchymal strips and dilate arterioles in hamster cheek pouch (8). Other activities of LXA_4 include activation of protein kinase C and inhibition of natural killer cell cytotoxicity (7) (9). It has been suggested that these conjugated tetraene compounds can be formed during cell-cell interactions, utilizing 15-HPETE or 15-HETE (15-hydroxyeicosatetraenoic acid) from lung alveolar macrophages, endothelial cells, eosinophils and neutrophils (4). In addition, rat basophilic leukemic cells (RBL-1), which contains the 5-lipoxygenase, have been shown to produce lipoxin A_4 and B_4 when stimulated by calcium ionophore A23187 and FMLP (5). Serhan and co-workers suggested that oxygenation of AA at the C-15 position, leading to the formation of 15-HPETE, is the initial step in the formation of lipoxins (2). Ueda et al.(6) reported that LXA_4 and LXB_4 can also be synthesized by purified 12-lipoxygenase from 15-HPETE. In this report 5-lipoxygenase, which is enriched in RBL-1 cells and potato tubers, were used to study the mechanism involved in the generation of lipoxins. In this study we also report the existence of a 6,7-dihydro-reductase activity in partially purified potato enzyme fraction that metabolized lipoxin B_4 to 6,7-dihyro-lipoxin B_4.

MATERIAL AND METHODS

Calcium ionophore A23187 and fMLP (formyl-methionyl-leucyl-phenylalanine) were purchased from Sigma Co. (St. Louis, Mo.) . 15-HPETE was prepared by incubating $[1-^{14}C]$ -arachidonic acid with soybean lipoxygenase as described (3).   Lipoxin A_4 and B_4 standards were generously supplied by Dr. J. Rokach of Merck Frosst Canada.   RBL-1 cells (American Type Tissue Culture) were grown in supsension cultures in MEM supplemented with 20% fetal bovine serum (Sigma) . After harvest, the cells were washed and suspended in Dulbecco's phosphate-buffered saline, pH 7.4.   The cell suspension $(2-3 \times 10^8)$ was added to an incubation vessel containing 15-HPETE (16 μM) dissolved in a minimum volume of ethanol.   Either calcium ionophore A23187 (5 μM) or fMLP (22 μM) was added to the suspension and incubated for 30 min at 37°C and stopped by the addition of two volumes of ethanol.   The residues were analyzed by RP-HPLC as described (3).   After HPLC, the samples with lipoxin UV spectrum were collected, methylated with diazomethane and reinjected onto the same column and eluted with methanol/water (65:35) (2).   The identity of lipoxins were determined by the criteria of their ultra-violet spectrum (UV), co-elution with synthetic standards and by GC/MS (2,3).

Partially purified 5-lipoxygenase was obtained from potato homogenate by brief homogenizaton of potato tubers (Russet Burbank) in acetate buffer (pH 4.5) followed by filtration through gauze and precipitation with ammonium sulfate (50% saturation after a prior precipitation at 25% saturation).   The protein obtained was dialyzed as described by Galliard et al. (10).   The partially purified potato enzyme (15mg of protein) was added to incubation vessels containing 15-HPETE in ethanol (the amount of ethanol was less than 1%) and 1.0 ml of 50 mM phosphate buffer (pH 6.8).   The suspension were incubated for 30 min in a shaking water bath at 37°C and stopped by the addition of two to three volumes of ethanol.   The incubation precipitate was filtered and the ethanolic filtrate was evaporated to dryness.   The residue was dissolved in 2 ml of sodium borohydride in distilled water, followed by incubation on ice for 10 min.   RP-HPLC analysis was run on a dual pump system equipped with a Vercopack C18 column (3.9 mm x 30 cm, 10u), a Rheodyne Model 7125 sample injector and a 700 max variable wavelength detector (Shimadzu SPD-6AV).   The products were eluted with a linear gradient of methanol/water/acetic acid (50:50:0.01 v/v) (solvent A) to methanol (solvent B) for 40 min at a flow rate of 1 ml/min.   UV detector was set as 301 nm for the detection of LXs.   The methyl ester of the LX and dihydro LXs was converted to trimethylsilyl ester as described by Wong et al. (3).   The sample was dissolved in hexane (25 μl) and injected into the gas chromatography mass spectrometer (Hewlett-Packard 5988) equipped with a cross methyl silicone capillary column (0.3 mm x 12m).   Helium flow was set at 16 ml/min and oven temperature was programmed from 130°C to 300°C at 5°C/min, injector temperature at 250°C, ion source at 200°C.   Electron energy was set at 70 ev.

RESULTS AND DISCUSSION

Incubation of RBL-1 cells with 15-HPETE and challenged with either A23187, or fMLP generated products with a UV spectrum indicative of conjugated tetraene compounds.   Following incubation and extraction, the lipid soluble materials were purified by RP-HPLC, which revealed 3 major and 1 minor peaks (Fig. 1) showing typical UV spectrum of lipoxin (11). These fractions were collected and processed as described above.   Four peaks showing the same lipoxin UV spectra were obtained.   The major peak (R.T. 22 min) which co-eluted with LXB_4ME standard was converted to trimethylsilyl derivative and analyzed by GC/MS.   The C-value was 24.0 and the mass spectrum showed ions of high intensity at m/z: 173 (base peak), 203.   Ions of lower intensities were observed at 582(M), 409,394 and 379.   These ions are similar to those reported for LXB_4 (11).

Other components having similar UV data were tentatively assigned as isomers of LXB$_4$. Peaks II and III (Fig. 1) were collected, methylated and reinjected onto a second RP-HPLC. Five peaks displaying the same UV spectra was obtained. The major fraction (R.T. 25 min), which co-eluted with LXA$_4$ME standard was converted to the trimethylsilyl derivative and further analyzed by GC/MS. The C-value was 24.1 and the prominent ions were at m/z 203 (base peak), 173, 582(M), 482 and 379. These ions and C-value were identical to those reported for LXA$_4$ (2).

In comparing the two agonists used to stimulate the production of lipoxins, particulary LXA$_4$, the greatest amount was generated with A23187 (4.8±1.0 µg). This was followed by the chemotactic peptide fMLP (2.0±0.74 µg), which was 58% less than that produced by A23187 (Fig. 2). In addition both A23187 and fMLP stimulated the formation of LXB$_4$ (1.2±0.57 µg and 0.55±0.07 µg, respectively). To further investigate the biotransformation of 15-HPETE, we used partially purified 5-lipoxygenase from potato tubers. The incubation generated products with a UV spectrum indicative of both conjugated tetraene (λmax at 301 mn and shoulders at 287 and 315 mn) and conjugated triene (λmax at 268 and shoulders at 258 nm and 279 nm) compounds (Fig. 3A and 4B). The lipid materials obtained were further purified by RP-HPLC. The conjugated triene compounds which co-eluted with the tetraene compounds were collected, methylated and converted to trimethylsilyl derivatives for GC/MS analysis. The mass spectra showed ions of high intensity at m/z 73 (base peak) and ions of lower intensity at m/z 582, 492 and 409 with M$^+$ of 582. There were eight isomers with C-values of 24.0, 24.2, 24.25, 24.3, 24.35, 24.4, 24.55 and 24.6, all containing m/z 582. Their mass-spectra were similar to those reported for LXB$_4$ and its isomers (4). (Fig. 3B). A new conjugated triene component was observed on GC/MS analysis. It produced a C-Value of 23.5 with a mass spectrum displaying ions at m/z 584(M) , 569(M-15), 494(M-90), 484(M-100), 411(M-173), 303, 203 and 173 (Fig. 4B). Molecular ion of this new compound was found to be 584 with two mass units higher than that of LXB$_4$. Together with the U.V.data, C-value and the mass-spectrum of this compound, we suggest that this is a dihydro-metabolite of LXB$_4$ in which the C$_{6,7}$ double bonds has been reduced. The assignment of 6,7-dihydro - LXB$_4$ correlates with its UV absorption which indicate the presence of a conjugated triene rather than a tetraene system. In this study, 5-lipoxygenase partially purified from potato tubers was used to synthesize lipoxins which generated various isomers with LXB$_4$ as the major product. The results suggest the presence of a 6,7-dihydroreductase activity in the potato enzyme fraction.

Biological activity of LXA$_4$ generated from RBL-1 cells was examined in an isolated preparation of rat tail artery. The preparation was suspended in a 6 ml organ bath filled with oxygenated Krebs solution and kept at 37°C. The tissue was precontracted with 0.125 µM of phenylephrine (PE). Following relaxation of the tissue, administration of 3nM LXA$_4$ from RBL-1-fractions display 12% of the maximum contraction induced by PE, whereas a known LXA$_4$ standard (3nM) elicited 17.6% of the maximum contraction. Since some isomers of LXA$_4$ do not possess biological activity (12), this would account for the difference in the musculotropic response observed with the standard as compared to the biological sample containing isomers of LXA$_4$. The existence of several LXA$_4$ isomers was confirmed by the second RP-HPLC chromatography analysis.

The results obtained in this study suggest that RBL-1 cells can utilize exogenous 15-HPETE to generate lipoxins. Agonists such as

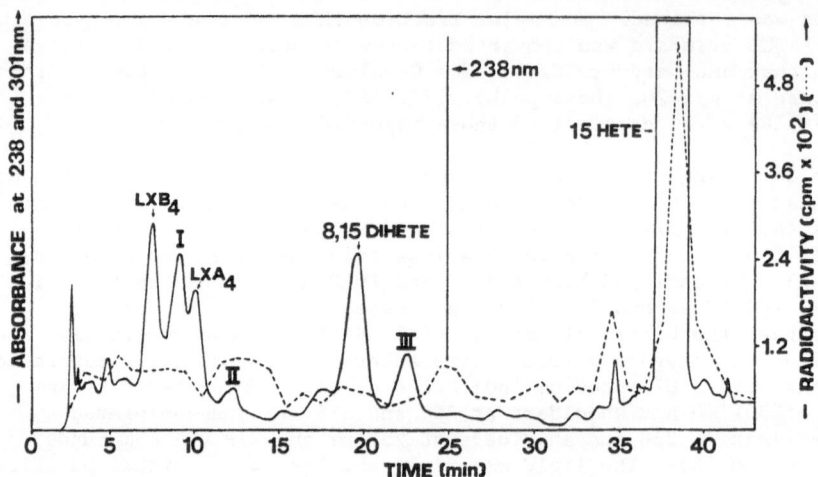

Fig. 1. RP-HPLC chromatogram of 15-HPETE metabolites isolated after incubation of RBL-1 cells with 15-[1-^{14}C]-HPETE.

Fig. 2. LXA$_4$ generation after incubation of 15-[1-^{14}C]-HPETE with RBL-1 cells under different agonists stimulation.

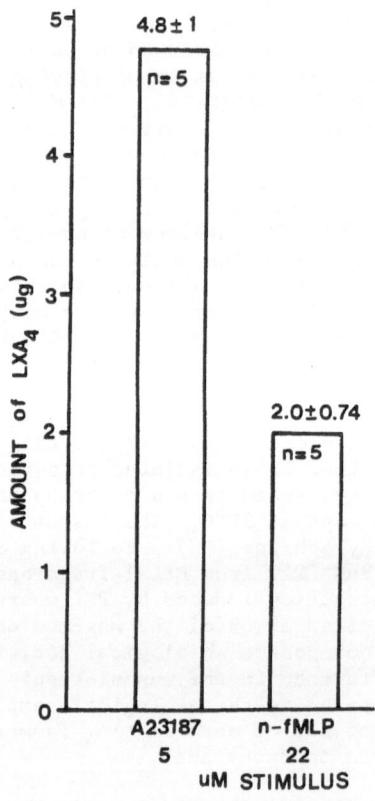

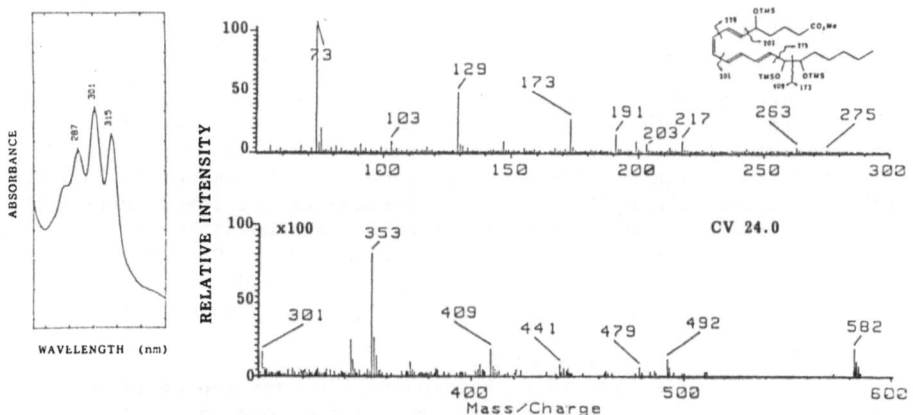

Fig. 3. U.V. spectrum of Lipoxin fractions after incubation of partially purified potato 5-lipoxygenase with 15-HPETE (A). Mass spectrum
of the methylester trimethylsilyl derivative of LXB$_4$ isolated and
purified from RP-HPLC (B).

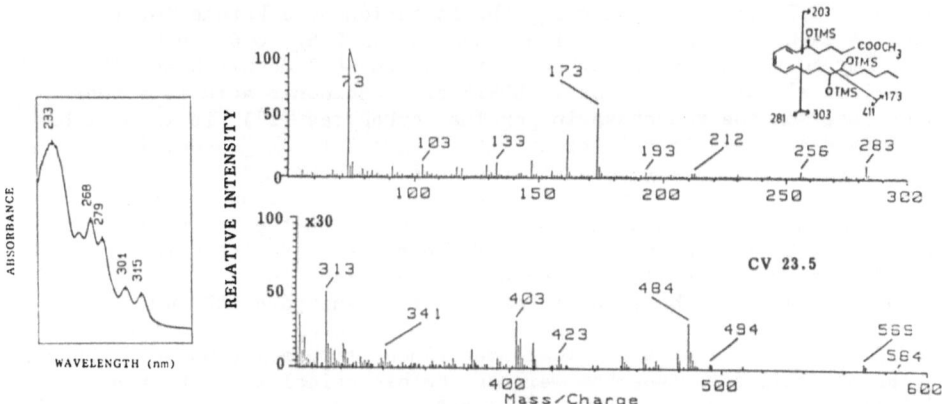

Fig. 4. U.V. Spectrum of a dihydro-lipoxin fraction after incubation
of partially purified potato reductase with 15-HPETE (A). Mass spectrum of the methylester trimethylsilyl derivative of 6,7-dihydro-LXB$_4$
isolated and purified from RP-HPLC (B).

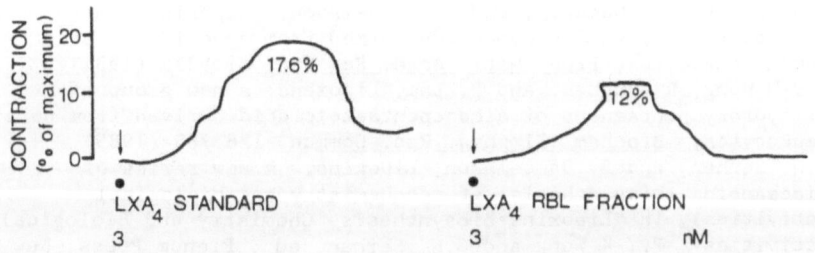

Fig. 5. Biological activity of LXA$_4$ fraction eluted from RP-HPLC (Ref
Fig. 1) as compared with LXA$_4$ synthetic standard on perfused rat tail
arteries.

A23187 and fMLP may mobilize calcium to activate the 5-lipoxygenase pathway for oxygenation of exogenous 15-HPETE. This is followed by the generation of 5,15-diHPETE, epoxytetraene intermediates, and finally the formation of lipoxins. Thus these results suggest that RBL-1 cells can use 15-HPETE or 15-HETE donated by neighboring cells to make lipoxins when concurrently the 5-lipoxygenase pathway is activated by stimuli that induce an influx of calcium. The fact that the amount of lipoxins generated varies with different agonists suggests the involvement of different receptors mediating cellular events and possibly the induction of different cellular sites for the oxidative burst. Once the cell has generated and released these biologically active products, they can further attenuate or amplified the physiological response of neighboring cells.

The metabolism of lipoxin B_4 to dihydro-LXB_4 may represent a major metabolic pathway of lipoxins. Powell and coworkers recently reported the formation of dihydro-LTB_4 in porcine leukocytes via a mechanism that involves the generation of 12-oxo-LTB_4 intermediate by a dehydrogenase step and the formation of dihydro-LTB_4 by a reductase (13). This mechanism is applicable for the formation of dihydro-prostaglandins. They are not generated by a direct reduction of prostaglandins but rather via 15-oxo-prostaglandin, which serves as a substrate for the reductase to form 13,14-dihydro-15-oxo-prosta-glandins. In view of the chemical structure of the final reduced product, 6,7-dihydro lipoxin B_4, the formation of a ketone inter-mediate is highly unlikely. The reduction of LXB_4 to 6,7-dihydro LXB_4 may go through a direct reduction of the 6-7 double bond. Since Powell et al. had found that 15-HPETE of arachidonic acid is a poor substrate for the reductase in porcine leukocytes (13), it is possible that 15-HPETE used in this study with potato 5-lipoxygenase, is converted first to LXB_4 then reduced to 6,7-dihdro-LXB_4. The specificity of this reductase may only reduce $C_{6,7}$ double bond of LXB_4 because 6,7-dihydro-LXA_4 was not detected in the incubation extract by GC/MS. Since Lipoxins of the series A resisted reduction by 6,7-dihydro reductase, other routes of biological inactivation remains to be discovered. Thus, the formation of 6,7-dihydro-LXB_4 may represent a unique metabolic pathway for the metabolism of lipoxin of the B series. The physiological importance of this metabolic pathway in human or other cell types as well as the biological activities of 6,7-lipoxin B_4 remains to be elucidated.

REFERENCES

1. B. Samuelsson, S.E. Dahlen, J. Lindren, C.A. Rouzer, and C.N. Serhan, Leukotrienes and lipoxins: structure, biosynthesis, and biological effects, Science 237:1171 (1987).
2. C.N. Serhan, M. Hamberg, and B. Samuelsson, Lipoxins: novel series of biologically active compounds formed from arachidonic acid in human leukocytes, Proc. Natl. Acad. Sci USA. 81:5335 (1984).
3. P.Y-W Wong, R. Hughes, and B. Lam, Lipoxene: a new group of trihydroxy pentaenens of eicosapentaenoic acid derived from porcine leukocytes, Biochem. Biophys. Res. Commun. 126:763 (1985).
4. C.N. Serhan, and B. Samuelsson, Lipoxins: a new series of eicosanoids (biosynthesis, stereochemistry and biological activities), in "Lipoxins Biosynthesis, Chemistry and Biological Activities", P.Y-K Wong and C.N. Serhan, ed., Plenum Press, New York (1988).

5. C.F. Ng, B.K. Lam, K. Pritchard, M. Stemerman, and P.Y-K Wong, Formation of lipoxins by rat basophilic leukemic cells, Fed. Proc. 5:5634 (1988).
6. N. Ueda, C. Yokoyama, S. Yamamoto, B.J. Fitzsimmons, J. Rokach, J. Oates, and A.R. Brash, Lipoxin synthesis by arachidonate 12-lipoxygenase purified from porcine leuokcytes, Biochem. Biophys. Res. Commun. 149:1063 (1987).
7. A. Hansson, C.N. Serhan, J. Haeggstrom, M. Ingelman-Sundberg, and B. Samuelsson, Activation of protein kinase C by lipoxin A and other eicosanoids. Intracellular action of oxygenation produces arachidonic acid, Biochem Biophys Res. Commun 134:1215 (1986).
8. S.E. Dahlen, J. Raud, C.N. Serhan, J. Bjork, and B. Samuelsson, Biological activities of lipoxin A include lung strip contraction and dilation of arterioles in vivo, Acta Physiol Scand. 130:643 (1987).
9. U. Ramstedt, J. Ng, H. Wigzell, C.N. Serhan, and B. Samuelsson, Action of novel eicosanoids. Lipoxin A and B on human natural killer cell cytotoxicity: effects on intracellular cAMP and target cell binding, J. Immunol. 135:3434 (1985).
10. T. Galliard, and J.A. Matthew, Enzymic reactions of fatty acid hydroperoxides in extracts of potato tuber, Bio. Biophys. Acta. 398:1 (1975).
11. C.N. Serhan, M. Hamberg, B. Samuelsson, J. Morris, and D.G. Wishka, On the stereochemistry and biosynthesis of lipoxin B, Proc. Natl. Acad. Sci. USA, 83:1983 (1986).
12. S.E. Dahlen, L. Franzen, J. Raud, C.N. Serhan, P. Westlund, E. Wikstrom, T. Bjorck, H. Matsuda, SE. Webber, C.A. Veale, T. Puustinen, J. Haeggstrom, K.C. Nicolaou, and B. Samuelsson, Actions of lipoxin A_4 and related compounds in smooth muscle preparations and on the microcirculation in vivo, in "Lipoxins Biosynthesis Chemistry and Biological Activities", P.Y-K Wong, and C.N. Serhan, ed., Plenum Press, New York (1988).
13. W.S. Powell, and F. Gravelle, Metabolism of 6-trans isomers of leukotriene B_4 to dihydro products by human polymorphonuclear leukocytes, J. Biol. Chem. 263:2170 (1987).

LEUKOTRIENES IN THE LUNG AND CARDIOVASCULAR SYSTEM

Priscilla J. Piper, Marwa N. Samhoun, Dolores M. Conroy, H.B. Yaacob, N.C. Barnes*, Jane M. Evans* and J.F. Costello*

Department of Pharmacology, Royal College of Surgeons of England, London WC2A 3PN and *Department of Thoracic Medicine Kings College School of Medicine and Dentistry, London SE5, U.K.

The formation of leukotrienes (LTs) from arachidonic acid derived from phospholipids of the cell membrane is initially catalysed by 5-lipoxygenase[1]. Metabolism of the unstable epoxide LTA_4 leads to the formation of LTB_4 and the cysteinyl-containing LTs C_4, D_4 and E_4. All these LTs have potent, although different, biological activities. LTB_4 is a powerful chemotactic agent for leukocytes whereas LTs C_4, D_4 and E_4 have potent smooth muscle stimulating actions and account for the biological activity of the allergic mediator previously known as slow-reacting substance of anaphylaxis (SRS-A)[2]. Leukotriene B_4 has pro-inflammatory actions but little smooth muscle stimulating activity of its own whereas cysteinyl-containing LTs have potent actions in the cardiovascular system and in the airways in vitro and in vivo (see[3,4]).

GENERATION OF LEUKOTRIENES

Leukotrienes are released by both immunological and non-immunological challenge of human lung in vitro but the exact cellular origin of LTs in unclear. The LTs generated from lung vary both with the stimulus used and between the parenchyma (small airways and blood vessels) and bronchi. Dahlén et al[5] showed the formation of LTs C_4, D_4 and E_4 during antigen challenge of asthmatic lung tissue but did not detect LTB_4. In our studies, when chopped parenchyma from normal human lung was stimulated with anti-IgE, generation of LTB_4 was detected (Table 1). Challenge of parenchyma with the calcium ionophore A23187 results in formation of larger quantities of both LTB_4 and LTD_4, LTB_4 being the predominant LT formed. In this study, levels of LTE_4 were not determined. When human chopped bronchial tissue was challenged with A23187, LTB_4 was generated but no cysteinyl-containing LTs were detected[6].

A 5-lipoxygenase system is also present in vascular tissue[7]. Brocklehurst[2] showed that SRS-A was released by antigen challenge of blood vessels from sensitized guinea pigs. Subsequently, Piper, Letts & Galton[7] demonstrated that the calcium ionophore A23187 released LTB_4 and cysteinyl-containing LTs from porcine blood vessels. However, the quantity of LTs generated varied between blood vessels and the highest concentration of LTs detected was generated by pig cerebral arteries, although renal, coronary and pulmonary vessels released sufficient LTB_4, LTC_4, LTD_4 and LTE_4[8] to have significant biological activity. Human arteries can also be

Table 1. Generation of leukotrienes from human lung parenchyma stimulated with A23187 or anti-IgE.

Stimulus:	A23187 5 ug ml^{-1} (n = 5)		Anti-IgE 1:160 (n = 4)	
	LTB$_4$	LTD$_4$	LTB$_4$	LTD$_4$ pmol g^{-1}
Normal	664	472	20	16
	976	441	12	20
	764	250	10	64
	429	233	-	-
	310	27	11	N.D.
Mean ± sem	629±119	285±81	13±2	25±14
asthmatic	130	205	9	32
asthmatic	220	1308	N.D.	N.D.

N.D. = None detected

stimulated to release LTs. Generation of LTs from umbilical and coronary arteries by A23187 has been demonstrated[9] and intralobar pulmonary arteries challenged immunologically with anti-IgE or with A23187 produced LTB$_4$ and cysteinyl-containing LTs[10]. The amounts released by anti-IgE and determined by radioimmunoassay were: LTB$_4$ 6.71±1.55, LTC$_4$ 7.37±2.48 and LTD$_4$ 11.98±5.49 pmol g^{-1} (n=5). Non-immunological stimulation released higher quantities of LTs[10]. Since the lung contains a large quantity of small blood vessels in addition to large and small airways, vascular tissue may be an important source of LTs released from lung contains a large quantity of small blood vessels in addition to large and small airways, vascular tissue may be an important source of LTs released from lung tissue.

ACTIONS OF LEUKOTRIENES IN THE LUNG

a) In vitro

The fact that cysteinyl-containing LTs have very potent actions on airway smooth muscle has been well documented (see[3,4,5]). On the other hand, LTB$_4$ has little direct smooth muscle stimulating activity on human bronchus (HBr) and any initial contraction rapidly develops tachyphylaxis. There are specific receptors for cysteinyl-containing LTs on airway smooth muscle. In guinea-pig trachea, there are distinct receptors for LTC$_4$ and LTD$_4$; LTE$_4$ appears to occupy the LTD$_4$ receptor[11]. However, in HBr, there seems to be one receptor which is acted on by LTs C4 or D$_4$[12]. LTC$_4$ and LTD$_4$ contract isolated HBr at the picomolar level and are more potent than LTE$_4$. However, whilst being less active than LTs C$_4$ or D$_4$, LTE$_4$ causes contractions of HBr which are longer lasting than those induced by its parent LTs[13].

Leukotriene E$_4$ is a metabolite of LTC$_4$ and is itself further degraded. In rodents, LTE$_4$ undergoes N-acetylation[14]. The N-acetyl derivative of LTE$_4$ (N-AcLTE$_4$) retained considerable biological activity and is about equiactive with LTE$_4$ in contracting guinea-pig trachea (GPT) and lung parenchymal strip (GPP)[15]. N-AcLTE$_4$ contracts isolated HBr, is less active than LTD$_4$ but, like LTE$_4$, causes protracted responses. However, the oxidative metabolites of LTE$_4$, 20-COOH LTE$_4$, 18-COOH 19,20 dinor LTE$_4$, 16-COOH 17,18,19,20 tetranor LTE$_4$ and 20-COOH-NaLTE$_4$ have no spasmogenic activity on HBr in vitro[16]. This shows that biological activity of the cysteinyl LTs is destroyed by shortening and oxidation of the fatty acid backbone but not by metabolism of the peptide side chain.

Challenge of superfused strips of HBr and lung parenchyma (HP) from an asthmatic patient with anti-IgE, in the presence of antihistamine, anticholinergic and adrenoceptor blocking drugs, caused long-lasting contractions which closely resembled those induced by LTE_4[8]. The LT antagonist FPL 55712 (1.9 μM) inhibited the immunologically-induced contractions, strongly suggesting that LTs were generated within the bronchial strip. In another similar experiment, LTs in the effluent were quantitated by radioimmunoassay. LTB_4, LTC_4 and LTD_4 were present but in levels of less than picomols per ml[8].

b) In vivo

Leukotrienes are active in causing narrowing of both large and small airways in normal man when given by inhalation. As predicted by studies on isolated HBr in vitro, LTs C_4 and D_4 are more active than histamine by about 3 orders of magnitude[17]. Although less active than LTC_4 or LTD_4, LTE_4 is still 2 orders of magnitude more active than histamine. As previously shown in studies in vitro, bronchoconstriction induced by LTE_4 is also longer lasting than that of the other LTs[18]. Leukotrienes given by inhalation cause wheezing in normal subjects[17] but were reported to induce cough in only one study[19]. Actions of LT metabolites have not been investigated in man.

Asthmatic subjects also bronchoconstrict to inhaled LTC_4 or LTD_4 and show hyperreactivity to these agonists (see[18]). However, the sensitivity to LTs is increased 4-fold whereas the sensitivity to histamine is increased by a factor of 11. There is some evidence that cysteinyl-containing LTs may induce hyperreactivity of the airways. A non-bronchoconstrictor dose of LTD_4 increased the sensitivity of normals to inhaled prostaglandin (PG) $F_{2\alpha}$ (see[18]) and inhaled LTE_4 increased the sensitivity of asthmatics to methacholine[20].

Leukotriene B_4 is present in sputum of patients with inflammatory diseases of the airways[21,22] and might be expected to contribute to hyperreactivity of the respiratory tract. However, LTB_4 inhaled alone or in conjunction with PGD_2 failed to increase bronchial reactivity to histamine in normal subjects[23].

LEUKOTRIENE ANTAGONISTS

In order to investigate whether LTs play a significant role in asthma, it will be necessary to find whether a potent LT antagonist substantially improves the condition of asthmatics. Recently, a number of antagonists of cysteinyl-containing LTs, which are most active against LTD_4, have been synthesised and shown to be potent antagonists of LTs in various animal models in vitro and in vivo. The structures of some of these antagonists are based on that of FPL 55712. Inhaled FPL 55712 or a related compound, FPL 59257, partially inhibited bronchoconstriction to inhaled LTC_4 or LTD_4 in normal subjects[19] and improved FEV_1 in asthmatic patients[24].

Some of the new LT antagonists have been investigated in man. L-649,923 is structurally related to FPL 55712 but is orally active. In normals, L-649,923 (1.0g) had no action against histamine but shifted the .LTD_4 dose-response curve to the right almost 4-fold. The side effects of colicky abdominal pain and watery diarrhoea prevented higher doses of the compound being administered[25]. The same dose of L-649,923 had a small protective effect against the early response of asthmatic patients to antigen challenge but had no effect against the late phase[26].

57

LY 171883 is also structurally related to FPL 55712[27] and has been shown in normals to shift the dose-response to inhaled LTD_4 to the right by slightly more than L-649,923[28]. In a long-term study in asthmatics, LY 171,883 was shown to produce a significant reduction in symptom score, a decrease in usage of $_2$ agonists and an increase in FEV_1[29].

Another LTD_4 antagonist based on the structure of FPL 55712, L-648,051, has been given by inhalation to normal subjects against inhaled LTD_4. In a dose of 1.6mg, L-648,051 partially inhibited the bronchoconstriction induced by LTD_4 and shortened its duration. L-648,051 did not have any unwanted side effects[30].

Three new LTD_4 antagonists have recently been described, ICI 198,615[31,] L 660,711[32] and SK+F 104,353[33]. ICI 198,615 and L 660,711 are novel compounds while SK+F 104,353 is an analogue of LTD_4. These have high pA_2 values in guinea-pig trachea and good receptor binding. In normal man, SK+F 104,353 given by inhalation antagonised inhaled LTD_4 and was active for over 4 hours[34].

ACTIONS OF LEUKOTRIENES IN THE CARDIOVASCULAR SYSTEM

Leukotrienes C_4, D_4 and E_4 are able to alter the calibre of blood vessels and their actions in the cardiovascular systems of various animal species have been well documented (see[3,4]. In most species, cysteinyl-containing LTs reduce blood flow except perhaps in the skin. It is of particular interest that, in man, intracoronary LTD_4 causes an increase in coronary vascular resistance and a reduction in mean arterial blood pressure[35].

CARDIAC ACTIONS OF LEUKOTRIENES IN VITRO

Leukotrienes C_4, D_4 and E_4 cause a decrease in coronary flow or increase in perfusion pressure accompanied by a reduction in the ventricular developed tension in guinea-pig or rat isolated hearts in vitro[36]. In hearts from sensitized guinea pigs, challenge with antigen results in cardiac anaphylaxis, the signs of which include decrease in coronary flow, reduction in developed tension, dysrhythmias, sinus tachycardia and left ventricular failure. This is accompanied by a release of histamine, LTs (mainly LTC_4) and thromboxane A_2[37,38,39]. Treatment of sensitized hearts with indomethacin prior to challenge exacerbates the signs of cardiac anaphylaxis (Fig.1) and increases release of LTC_4 (Table 2) but inhibits production of TxB_2 (Table 3) and the early phase of increased perfusion pressure[40]. On the other hand, prior administration of a 5-lipoxygenase inhibitor, CGS 8515, to the hearts, significantly protects against cardiac anaphylaxis[40]. These results suggest that LTC_4 contributes significantly to the signs of cardiac anaphylaxis, particularly in the late phase[40]. It is of interest that immunological challenge of chopped blood vessels stimulates LT release (see above) and suggest that the coronary vasculature may be a source of LTs generated in cardiac anaphylaxis.

Intracoronary injection of platelet activating factor (PAF) closely mimics cardiac anaphylaxis[41] and stimulates generation of LTC_4 and LTB_4 into the cardiac effluent of guinea-pig hearts[42]. CGS 8515 inhibits PAF-induced release of LTC_4 and the later phase of PAF-induced reduction in flow[43] which shows that LTC_4 accounts for part of the cardiac dysfunction caused by PAF.

Table 2. Time-course of the anaphylactic release of LTC_4 following ovalbumen challenge in actively sensitized guinea-pig hearts. (n=5-8)

Treatment of Sensitized Hearts	LTC_4 Released (pmol)			
	Time (minute)			
	1	2	3	4
Control	2.40 ± 0.0	6.20 ± 0.4	3.15 ± 0.2	2.10 ± 0.6
Indomethacin (2.8 uM)	6.10 ± 0.8	8.70 ± 0.9	8.80 ± 1.2	7.40 ± 0.1
CGS 8515 (1.0 uM)	1.80 ± 0.6	1.90 ± 0.3	2.20 ± 1.0	1.72 ± 0.7

Table 3. Time-course of the anaphylactic release of TxB_2 following ovalbumen challenge in actively sensitized guinea pig hearts. (n=4-5)

Treatment of Sensitized Hearts	TxB_2 Released (pmol)			
	Time (minute)			
	1	2	3	4
Control	13.21 ± 1.5	5.82 ± 3.8	4.22 ± 3.5	4.20 ± 3.2
Indomethacin (2.8 uM)	4.12 ± 2.1	2.12 ± 2.2	1.86 ± 2.0	1.28 ± 2.4
CGS 8515 (1.0 uM)	9.58 ± 2.0	7.66 ± 2.0	4.22 ± 3.1	3.56 ± 3.12

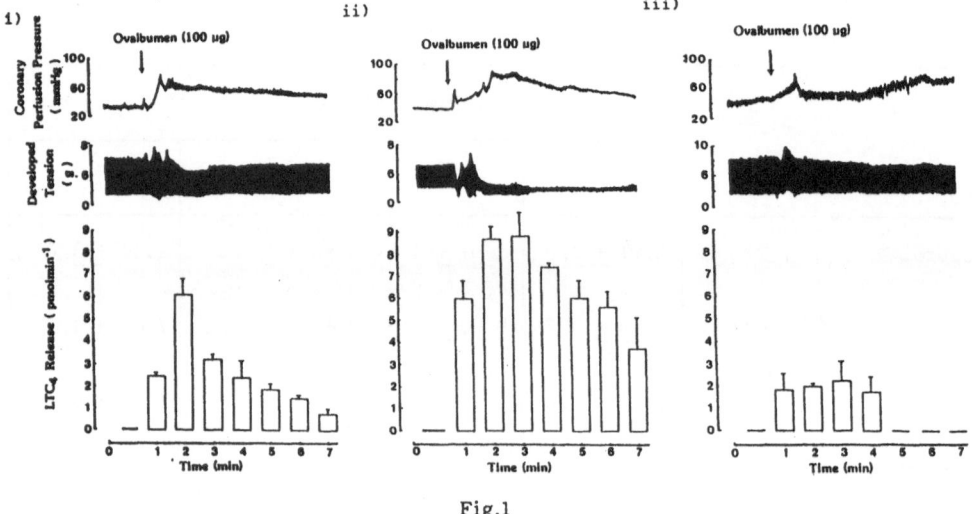

Fig.1

(i) Cardiac anaphylaxis induced by ovalbumen 100 μg in control, untreated hearts from guinea pigs sensitized to ovalbumen.
Upper panel: representative tracing of biphasic increase in coronary perfusion pressure (mmHg), dysrhythmias and reduction in cardiac developed tension (g)
Lower panel: concentration (pmol min^{-1}) of LTC_4 in cardiac effluent collected at one minute intervals (n=4)

(ii) Cardiac anaphylaxis in sensitized hearts pre-treated with indomethacin 2.8μM.
Upper panel: representative tracing showing exaggerated late phase of increased perfusion pressure, increased dysrhythmias and increased reduction in cardiac developed tension (g)
Lower panel: the peak output and duration of LTC_4 release into the cardiac effluent are increased (n=4)

(iii) Cardiac anaphylaxis in sensitized hearts pre-treated with indomethacin 2.8μM and CGS 8515 1μM.
Upper panel: representative tracing showing reduced changes in coronary perfusion pressure and cardiac developed tension
Lower panel: the peak output and duration of LTC_4 release into the cardiac effluent are reduced (n=4)

CONCLUSION

In conclusion, LTs have potent actions in the lung and cardiovascular system which suggest they may contribute to human cardiovascular and respiratory disease. For instance, in addition to constricting airway smooth muscle, they may contribute to inflammation of the airways. The availability of new, potent, selective antagonists of cysteinyl LTs which have been shown to be active in man should allow us to determine the role(s) of LTs in human disease.

REFERENCES

1. Samuelsson, B. 1983. Leukotrienes: a new class of mediators of immediate hypersensitivity reactions and inflammation. *Adv. Prostaglandin,Thromboxane, Leukotriene Res.* 11:1-13.

2. Brocklehurst, W.E. 1960. The release of histamine and formation of a slow-reacting substance (SRS-A) during anaphylactic shock. *J. Physiol.* 151:416-435.

3. Piper, P.J. 1984. Formation and actions of leukotrienes. *Phys. Rev.* 64:744-761.

4. Piper, P.J., and M.N. Samhoun. 1987. Leukotrienes. *Brit. Med. Bull.* 43(2):297-311.

5. Dahlen, S-E., G. Hansson, P. Hedqvist, T. Bjorck, E. Granstrom, and B. Dahlen. 1983. Allergen challenge of lung tissue from asthmatics elicits bronchial contraction that correlates with the release of leukotrienes C_4, D_4 and E_4. *Proc. Natl. Acad. Sci. USA* 80:1712-1716.

6. Barnett, K., and P.J. Piper. 1985. The release of leukotrienes from large and small airways of guinea-pig and man. *Br. J. Pharmacol.* 86:642P.(Abstract)

7. Piper, P.J., L.G. Letts, and S.A. Galton. 1983. Generation of a leukotriene- -like substance from porcine vascular and other tissues. *Prostaglandins* 25:591-599.

8. Piper, P.J., M.N. Samhoun, D.M. Conroy, N.C. Barnes, J.M. Evans and J.F. Costello. 1988. Leukotrienes and human airways. *Adv. Prostaglandin, Thrombox- ane, Leukotriene Res.* (In Press)

9. Piper, P.J., and S. Levene. 1987. Human umbilical arteries and veins: Generation of leukotrienes and responses to exogenous leukotrienes. *Biol. Neonate* 52:9-15.

10. Piper, P.J., J.W. Antoniw, and A.W.B. Stanton. 1988. Release of leukotri- enes from porcine and human blood vessels by immunological and non- immunological stimuli. *Ann. NY Acad. Sci.* 524:133-141.

11. Krell, R.D., B.S. Tsai, A. Berdoulay, M. Barone, and R.E. Giles. 1983. Heterogeneity of leukotriene receptors in guinea-pig trachea. *Prostaglandins* 25:171-178.

12. Buckner, C.K., R.D. Krell, R.B. Laravuso, D.B. Coursin, P.R. Bernstein, and J.A. Will. 1986. Pharmacological evidence that human intralobar airways do not contain different receptors that mediate contractions to leukotriene C_4 and leukotriene D_4. *J. Pharmacol. Exp. Ther.* 237:558-562.

13. Samhoun, M.N., and P.J. Piper. 1984. Leukotriene F_4: Comparison of its pharmacological profile with that of the other cysteinyl-containing leukotrienes in guinea-pig ileum and lung parenchyma in vitro. *Prostaglandins* 28:623-628.

14. Bernström, K., and S. Hammarström. 1986. Metabolism of leukotriene E_4 by rat tissues: formation of N-Acetyl leukotriene E_4. *Arch. Biochem. Biophys.* 244(2):486-491.

15. Conroy, D.M., P.J. Piper, and M.N. Samhoun. 1987. The effect of N-acetyl leukotriene E_4 on guinea-pig airway smooth muscle in vitro. *Br. J. Pharmacol.* 91:365P.(Abstract)

16. Samhoun, M.N., D.M. Conroy, and P.J. Piper. 1988. Studies of the bronchoconstrictor actions of leukotrienes in vitro and their relevance to investigations in man. In Drugs affecting leukotrienes and lipoxygenase products - A potential fulfilled?. IBC Technical Services Ltd., London. 65-77.

17. Barnes, N.C., P.J. Piper, and J.F. Costello. 1984. Comparative actions of inhaled leukotriene C_4, leukotriene D_4 and histamine in normal human subjects. *Thorax* 39:500-504.

18. Barnes, N.C., and P.J. Piper. 1986. The actions of leukotrienes in human lung in vitro and in vivo. In The Leukotrienes: Their biological signficance. P.J. Piper, editor. Raven Press, New York. 199-212.

19. Holroyde, M.C., R.E.C. Altounyan, A.H. Cole, M. Dixon, and E.V. Elliott. 1981. Bronchoconstriction produced in man by leukotrienes C and D. *Lancet* II:17-18.

20. Arm, J.P., B.W. Spur, and T.H. Lee. 1987. Leukotriene E_4 (LTE_4) enhances airway histamine responsiveness in asthmatic subjects. *Thorax* 42:220. (Abstract)

21. O'Driscoll, B.R.C., and A.B. Kay. 1982. Leukotrienes and lung disease. *Thorax* 37:241.

22. Zakrzewski, J.T., N.C. Barnes, J.F. Costello, and P.J. Piper. 1987. Lipid mediators in cystic fibrosis and chronic obstructive pulmonary disease. *Am. Rev. resp. Dis.* 136:779-782.

23. Black, P.N., R.W. Fuller, G.W. Taylor, P.J. Barnes, and C.T. Dollery. 1988. Bronchial reactivity is not increased after inhalation of leukotriene B_4 and Prostaglandin D_2. *Br. J. Pharmacol.* (In Press)

24. Lee, T.H., M.J. Walport, A.H. Wilkinson, M. Turner-Warwick, and A.B. Kay. 1981. Slow-reacting substance of anaphylaxis antagonist FPL-55712 in chronic asthma. *Lancet* 2:304-305.

25. Barnes, N.C., P.J. Piper, and J.F. Costello. 1987. The effect of an oral leukotriene antagonist L-649,923 on histamine and leukotriene D_4-induced bronchoconstriction in normal man. *J. Allergy Clin. Immunol.* 79:816-818.

26. Britton, J.R., S.P. Hanley, and A.E. Tattersfield. 1987. The effect of an oral leukotriene D_4 antagonist L-649,923 on the response to inhaled antigen in asthma. *J. Allergy Clin. Immunol.* 79:811.

27. Fleisch, J.H., L.E. Rinkema, C.A. Whitesitt, and W.S. Marshall. 1986.

Pharmacologic antagonism of leukotriene mediated events. In The leukotrienes - their biological significance. P.J. Piper, editor. Raven Press, New York. 109-125.

28. Phillips, G.D., P. Rafferty, and S.T. Holgate. 1987. LY-171883 as an oral leukotriene D_4 antagonist in non-asthmatic subjects. *Thorax* 42:723.

29. Fleisch, J.H., M.L. Cloud, and W.S. Marshall. 1988. A brief review of preclinical and clinical studies with LY-171,883 and some comments on newer cysteinyl leukotriene receptor antagonists. *Ann. NY Acad. Sci.* 524:356-368.

30. Evans, J.M., N.C. Barnes, P.J. Piper, and J.F. Costello. 1988. The effect of a single dose of an inhaled leukotriene antagonist L-648,051 in mild asthma. *Br. J. Clin. Pharmacol.* (In Press)

31. Krell, R.D., R.E. Giles, Y.K. Yee, and D.W. Snyder. 1987. In vivo pharmacology of ICI 198,615: a novel potent and selective peptide leukotriene antagonist. *J. Pharmacol. Exp. Ther.* 243:557-564.

32. Zamboni, R., M. Belley, E. Champion, L. Charette, R. Dehaven, R. Frenette, A.W. Ford-Hutchinson, J.Y Gauthier, and T.R. Jones. 1988. L-660,711, a potent orally active LTD_4 antagonist. *Adv. Prostaglandin,Thromboxane,Leukotriene Res.* (In Press)

33. Hay, D.W.P., R.M. Muccitelli, S.S. Tucker, L.M. Vickery-Clark, and T.J. Torphy. 1987. Pharmacological profile of SK&F 104,353: a novel, potent and selective peptidoleukotriene receptor antagonist in guinea-pig and human airways. *J. Pharmacol. Exp. Ther.* 243:474-481.

34. Evans, J.M., N.C. Barnes, J.T. Zakrzewski, H.P. Glenny, P.J. Piper, and J.F. Costello. 1988. Effects of an inhaled leukotriene (LT) antagonist, SK&F 104,353-Z_2 on LTD_4- and histamine-induced bronchoconstriction in normal man. *Br. J. Pharmacol.* (In Press)

35. Marone, G., A. Giordano, R. Cirillo, M. Triggiani, and C. Vigorito. 1988. Cardiovascular and metabolic effects of peptide leukotrienes in man. *Ann. NY Acad. Sci.* 524:321-333.

36. Letts, L.G., and P.J. Piper. 1982. The actions of leukotrienes C4 and D4 on guinea-pig isolated hearts. *Br. J. Pharmacol.* 76:169-176.

37. Levi, R. 1972. Effects of exogenous and immunologically released histamine on the isolated heart: a quantitative comparison. *J. Pharmacol. Exp. Ther.* 182:227-238.

38. Liebig, R., W. Bernauer, and B.A. Peskar. 1975. Prostaglandin, slowreacting substance and histamine release from anaphylactic guinea-pig hearts and its pharmacological modification. *Naunyn – Schmiedeberg's Arch. Pharmacol.* 289:65-76.

39. Allan, G., and R. Levi. 1981. Thromboxane and prostacyclin release during cardiac immediate hypersensitivity reactions in vitro. *J. Pharmacol. Exp. Ther.* 217:57-61.

40. Piper, P.J., and H.B. Yaacob. 1988. Release of leukotrienes in cardiac anaphylaxis and its inhibition by a lipoxygenase inhibitor, CGS 8515. *Br. J. Pharmacol.* 93:111P.

41. Levi, R., J.A. Burke, Z-G. Guo, Y. Hattori, C.M. Hoppen, L.M. McManus, D.J.

Hanahan, and R.N. Pinckard. 1984. Acetyl Glyceryl Ether Phosphorylcholine (AGEPC): A putative mediator of cardiac anaphylaxis in guinea pig. *Circ. Res.* 54:117-124.

42. Piper, P.J., and A.G. Stewart. 1986. Coronary vasoconstriction in the rat, isolated perfused heart induced by platelet-activating factor is mediated by leukotriene C4. *Br. J. Pharmacol.* 88:595-605.

43. Yaacob, H.B., and P.J. Piper. 1988. (UnPub)

BLOOD PLATELETS, ASPIRIN AND PREVENTION

OF VASCULAR DISEASE

Giovanni de Gaetano and Chiara Cerletti

Istituto di Ricerche Farmacologiche Mario Negri
Consorzio Mario Negri Sud - 66030 Santa Maria Imbaro, Italy

BACKGROUND

Early studies of aspirin in the prophylaxis of arterial thrombosis

"In 40 years as a general practitioner, I have been especially interested in the possibility that some simple and harmless agent may be effective against the two major causes of death and disability among the persons who have most to contribute to our civilization. When aspirin appeared to offer such protection, I urged my friends and patients to adopt the practice of taking aspirin, one or two 5 gr. tablets daily. Surely the practice could do no harm. It might prove life-saving. To date, approximately 8,000 men have adopted this regime, with a surprising result. Not a single case of detectable coronary or cerebral thrombosis has occurred among patients who faithfully have adhered to this regime. Sufficient time has elapsed since the start of this program for me to report that aspirin administration offers a safe and sure method of prophylaxis against thrombosis" (Craven, 1956).

"Overall, there was a 47% reduction in the risk of total myocardial infarction, which is statistically significant. This includes significant benefits of aspirin on both non fatal and fatal events" (Steering Committee of the Physicians' Health Study Research Group, 1988).

Thirty - two years elapsed between the reports of these two clinical trials on the prevention of cardiovascular events by aspirin. For different reasons neither study can be taken as a case for the generalised use of aspirin for the primary prevention of vascular mortality in apparently healthy people (de Gaetano, 1988). However, both studies indicate the long-lasting interest of physicians and pharmacologists in this almost 90 years old remedy as an antithrombotic drug. The hemorrhagic potential of aspirin (acetylsalicylic acid) as a consequence of its influence on hemostasis was described many years ago (Beaumont et al, 1955) and was in fact the empyrical observation on which Dr. Craven (1956) based his decision to give aspirin to his patients. Dr. Craven thought that aspirin would act as an anticoagulant in view of the structural similarity between salicylic acid and dicumarol. He realized however that the amounts of aspirin taken under the prescribed regimen were insufficient to cause lowering of prothrombin time, but argued that electroshock or quinine were effective means of treating the confused or the malarian patients despite the fact that the mechanism of action for both therapeutic procedure was as yet unknown.

Studies on the inhibitory effects of aspirin on platelet function and prostaglandin synthesis

We don't know whether Dr. Craven became acquainted by the end of the Sixties of a number of studies showing the inhibitory effect of aspirin on platelet aggregation and the concomitant release reaction (Weiss and Aledort, 1967; O' Brien, 1968; Zucker and Peterson, 1968; Evans et al, 1968). Aspirin was active not only *in vitro* but also exerted a long-lasting (at least 24-48 hours) antiplatelet effect in man after administration of doses as low as 150 mg. Salicylate was virtually inactive. This original observation suggested that the effect of aspirin on platelets was linked to an irreversible acetylating process, which was demonstrated few years later (Roth et al, 1975).

In 1971 aspirin, but not salicylate, was shown to exert a long-lasting inhibition of prostaglandin formation in platelets (Smith and Willis, 1971; Kocsis et al, 1973). The biochemistry of arachidonic acid metabolism in platelets and in vascular cells was established in the following years (Silver, 1981; Moncada and Vane, 1979).

The "aspirin dilemma"

When it was shown that aspirin prevented the formation of two compounds with opposite biological effects -namely the platelet aggregatory thromboxane A_2 in platelets (Hamberg et al, 1975; Patrignani et al, 1982) and the antiaggregatory prostaglandin I_2, prostacyclin, in vascular cells (Villa and de Gaetano, 1977; Weksler at al, 1983; FitzGerald et al, 1983)- an "aspirin dilemma" emerged (Marcus, 1977; de Gaetano et al, 1982). Possibly, the clinical relevance of this "dilemma" although conceptually stimulating, has been overemphasised. In fact there was no significant difference between the effects on vascular events of different doses of aspirin, when randomised trials in patients with vascular disease were reviewed (Antiplatelet Trialists' Collaboration, 1988), despite the assumption that low dose aspirin would suppress thromboxane generation while sparing prostacyclin synthesis.

A possible explanation of the Antiplatelet Trialists' Collaboration (1988) results can be found in more recent data indicative of presystemic inhibition of platelets after oral aspirin (Siebert et al, 1983; Pedersen and FitzGerald, 1984; de Gaetano et al, 1984). Oral aspirin can be extensively hydrolysed to salicylate in the stomach and liver (first pass) before it enters the systemic circulation. Presystemic acetylation of platelets thus occurs during aspirin absorption, with a concomitant sparing of peripheral vascular cyclo-oxygenase mainly exposed to salicylate (Cerletti et al, 1986). This "biochemical selectivity" of oral aspirin (Pedersen and FitzGerald, 1984) as an inhibitor of platelet versus vascular cyclo-oxygenase activity is reduced by elimination of the first pass hepatic metabolism by portacaval shunt (Gambino et al, 1988). The possibility that aspirin exerts an antithrombotic effect by mechanism(s) different from platelet inhibition has been suggested on the basis of experimental findings, but its clinical relevance remains to be established (de Gaetano et al, 1985).

CURRENT STATUS

On the basis of its antiplatelet effect, aspirin has been assessed over the past decade in more than 25,000 patients with a history of myocardial infarction, stroke, unstable angina or transient ischemic attacks.

Secondary prevention of vascular disease by aspirin: a metanalysis

A metanalysis of 25 randomised trials of long-term antiplatelet treatment for secondary prevention of vascular disease included 19 trials in which aspirin was used (at doses ranging between 300 and 1500 g daily) (Antiplatelet Trialists' Collaboration, 1988). As there was no significant difference between the effects of the different drugs used, the results of this metanalysis can be essentially attributed to aspirin. This drug reduced mortality due to vascular disease by 15% and non-fatal vascular events (myocardial infarction and stroke) by 30%. The antithrombotic mechanism of aspirin is indirectly supported by the lack of any apparent effect on mortality rate for non vascular disease.

The observed benefit associated with aspirin in patients with unstable angina was greater than that in patients with myocardial infarction (36% vs 25% reduction in fatal and non fatal vascular events). This difference however was not significant, possibly because only two trials on unstable angina could be analysed. Interestingly enough, patients with a history of cerebrovascular disease had a reduction of non fatal strokes of 22%, and those with a history of myocardial infarction of 42%. Non fatal myocardial infarction was reduced by 31% in patients with previous infarction and by 35% in those with angina and cerebrovascular disease. It seems therefore that aspirin treatment is able to protect patients who suffered vascular disease in one district not only from a second event in the same district, but also from a primary event in other districts.

Altogheter the metanalysis indicates that aspirin reduces the incidence of vascular disease in patients at particular risk of a new occlusive vascular event. If 1,000 patients with established vascular disease are treated with aspirin for two years, 10 of 60 fatal and 20 of 60 non-fatal vascular events would be averted; 20 of 120 fatal and 30 of 90 non-fatal events would be avoided in patients discharged from hospital after myocardial infarction.

The ISIS-2 trial of aspirin and streptokinase

Very recently, the results of the Second International Study of Infarct Survival (ISIS-2) were presented (ISIS-2 Collaborative Group, 1988).   ISIS-2 has assessed for the first time the separate and combined effects of oral aspirin (160 mg/day for a month) and of i.v. streptokinase (a single infusion of 1.5 MU over 60 min) in 17,000 patients with acute myocardial infarction. Each agent produced a significant reduction in 5-week vascular mortality and their combination was significantly better than either drug alone. Aspirin also significantly reduced non-fatal reinfarction and non-fatal stroke and was not associated with any increase in cerebral hemorrhage.

The excess of non-fatal reinfarction, reported when streptokinase was used alone, was entirely avoided by the addition of aspirin. The differences in early mortality produced by aspirin and streptokinase persisted at least 15 months (average).

This is the largest clinical trial on an antiplatelet drug completed up to date; it is also the first single trial in which a significant clinical benefit of aspirin could be shown in patients with myocardial infarction. The dose used was half the lowest dose of the drug which appeared to be effective according to the metanalysis discussed above. At variance with all other "old" trials, patients were treated with aspirin as soon as myocardial infarction was suspected (not necessarily established). The enormous clinical relevance of this finding needs not to be underlined. From a physiopathological point of view, it would be of interest to know whether aspirin and streptokinase were effective in comparable sub-groups of patients or whether a peculiar clinical and/or pathological subset was "selected" by either drug. It seems reasonable to envisage coronary occlusion underlying myocardial infarction as a dynamic process where activation of platelets and of the fibrinolytic system contributes to alternate cycles of thrombus formation and dissolution. These cycles can be interrupted with an antiplatelet or a fibrinolytic agent. Association of both treatments would then result in mutual potentiation. Alternatively, both aspirin and streptokinase might exert other relevant pharmacological effects: one should mention, as an example, the antiplatelet effects of fibrin(ogen) degradation products formed by fibrinolysis activation (Buczko et al, 1976) or the leukocyte-mediated activation of fibrinolysis by aspirin (Moroz, 1977).

Primary prevention of vascular disease by aspirin

The possibility that prophylactic aspirin would prevent some thrombotic events in apparently healthy people has been recently assessed in America and Britain (Steering Committee of the Physicians' Health Study Research Group, 1988; Peto et al, 1988).

From about 60,000 male US doctors (aged 40-84 years) 22,000 volunteers were randomly assigned to receive every other day either buffered aspirin (325 mg) or placebo. After an average follow-up of about 5 years, there were 104 myocardial infarctions (5 fatal) in the aspirin group and 189 (18 fatal) in the control group, a statistically significant difference. In the aspirin group, despite the reduction in fatal myocardial infarction, which was possibly the result of the low non-fatal myocardial infarction rate, the overall mortality due to vascular disease was not reduced. Total mortality was also unaffected by drug treatment. The selection procedure used in this trial was the most likely reason for the exceptionally low cardiovascular mortality rate among participants (a ratio of about 1 to 8) in respect to a comparable unselected population. Indeed a highly motivated, rather homogeneous population with apparently no risk factor for vascular disease (except being male aged over 40) was selected for this trial. This data indicates that reduction of known risk factors for atherosclerosis complications results in a dramatic prevention of primary cardiovascular fatal events. It is noteworthy that aspirin -with the limitations mentioned above- is still able to exert some beneficial effects on myocardial infarction in very healthy people.

The reduction in fatal myocardial infarction (5 in the aspirin group versus 18 controls) was not accompanied by a decrease in sudden deaths, which were indeed slightly more frequent in the aspirin group (13 versus 9).This finding is difficult to reconcile with the viewpoint that platelet thrombi may be implicated in sudden death (Silver, 1981).

The ischemic stroke rate was not affected by aspirin, which does not accord with the finding that non-fatal strokes were significantly reduced by antiplatelet treatment in myocardial infarction (Antiplatelet Trialists' Colaboration, 1988; ISIS-2 Collaborative Group, 1988). The total number of strokes was slightly increased in aspirin-takers (80 versus 70 in controls). Hemorrhagic strokes were double those in controls (13 versus 6) and there was an unfortunate though small increase in fatal cerebral hemorrhage (6 versus 2): therefore the risk-benefit balance of aspirin treatment in healthy people needs to be evaluated accurately.

Doubts about the value of aspirin in the primary prevention of cardiovascular mortality and its hemorrhagic potential at cerebrovascular level were lately substantiated by the findings of a similar British trial in male doctors (Peto et al, 1988).

When the data from the American and the British trials are combined (by simple addition of data), 646 subjects out of about 27,000 died (225 from vascular disease and 421 from non-vascular disease), in contrast to about 3,000 patients of the 29,000 in the metanalysis of the Antiplatelet Trialists' Collaboration (1988). In this report there were 497 deaths from non-vascular disease and 2,431 from vascular disease: treatment with aspirin (or other antiplatelet drugs) reduced the vascular mortality rate by 15% (a small but statistically significant difference). It is therefore not surprising that because of the very low event rate in both doctors' trials, no significant effect of aspirin was seen, such as that shown by metanalysis in patients with vascular disease.

If the data of the two primary prevention trials are applied to the general population, 1,000 healthy men (aged over 40) would have to take aspirin for five years to avert 8 of the 17 myocardial infarcts expected during that time (a reduction of about 50%). Since these 17 subjects could not be identified before treatment, 983 people would have to take aspirin, in whom myocardial infarction would not develop, even without the drug. One death from myocardial infarction would be avoided for about 850 healthy people given aspirin for five years.

At present there is no case for the generalised use of aspirin at any dose for the primary prevention of vascular disease in apparently healthy people. The value and safety of aspirin should be assessed in a representative sample of a healthy population or in healthy subjects at increased risk for cardiovascular disease.

FUTURE DIRECTIONS

The clinical efficacy of aspirin as an antithrombotic drug becomes to be established. Several questions however remain to be answered.

1. Would a more accurate selection of patients with vascular disease (particularly those with cerebrovascular disease) result in improved therapeutic benefit of aspirin?

2. Would administration of aspirin after a vascular event, earlier (hours, days) than that used in previous trials (weeks, months) result in the selection of patients more susceptible to the antithrombotic effect of aspirin (as it occurred in the ISIS-2 trial)?

3. Would doses of aspirin substantially lower than 160-320 mg per day exert comparable or even greater therapeutic benefits than that shown by the ISIS-2 trial or the metanalysis? Should aspirin be administered in single daily doses? Would different pharmaceutical preparations of aspirin be equally effective in thrombosis prevention? In particular, would the "biochemical selectivity" (Pedersen and FitzGerald, 1984; Cerletti et al, 1986) be enhanced by slow release or enteric-coated preparations, thus increasing benefits and reducing risks of aspirin?

4. Is aspirin of real benefit in the primary prevention of vascular disease?

5. Do antiplatelet drugs other than aspirin with mechanism of action similar or different from aspirin share its antithrombotic effect? Does aspirin exert its antithrombotic effect (solely) through an antiplatelet mechanism?

ACKNOWLEDGMENTS

The Authors thank all their coworkers who contributed to the research on aspirin performed at Mario Negri Institute during the past 15 years.

Ms. Silvia Falcone helped prepare the manuscript.

This work was partially supported by the Italian National Research Council (CNR, Convenzione CNR - Consorzio Mario Negri Sud).

REFERENCES

Antiplatelet Trialists' Collaboration. Secondary prevention of vascular disease by prolonged antiplatelet treatment. Br Med J 1988; 296: 320-331.

Beaumont JL, Caen J, Bernard J. Action hémorrhagipare de l'acide acétylsalicylique au cours des maladies du sang. Bull Soc Med Hôp Paris 1955;71:1087.

Buczko W, de Gaetano G, Franco R, Donati MB. Biological properties of dialysable peptides derived from plasmin digestion of bovine fibrinogen preparations. Thromb Diath Haemorrh 1976; 35:651-657.

Cerletti C, Gambino MC, Garattini S, de Gaetano G. Biochemical selectivity of oral versus intravenous aspirin in rats. Inhibition by oral aspirin of cyclo-oxygenase activity in platelets and presystemic but not systemic vessels. J Clin Invest 1986; 78: 323-326.

Craven LL. Experiences with aspirin (acetylsalicylic acid) in the non-specific prophylaxis of coronary thrombosis. Mississippi Valley Med J 1956; 75: 38-44.

de Gaetano G. Primary prevention of vascular disease by aspirin. Lancet 1988; 1: 1093-1094.

de Gaetano G, Cerletti C, Bertelè V. Pharmacology of antiplatelet drugs and clinical trials on thrombosis prevention: a difficult link. Lancet 1982;II: 974-977.

de Gaetano G, Cerletti C, Dejana E, Latini R, Villa S. The "aspirin dilemma": new points for discussion. Thromb Haemost 1984; 52:215.

de Gaetano G, Cerletti C, Dejana E, Latini R. Platelets and vascular occlusion. Pharmacology of platelet inhibition in humans: Implication sof the salicylate-aspirin interaction. Circulation 1985; 72:1185-1193.

Evans G, Packham MA, Nishizawa EE, Mustard JF, Murphy EA. The effect of acetylsalicylic acid on platelet function. J Exp Med 1968; 128:887-94.

FitzGerald GA, Oates JA, Hawiger J, Maas RL, Roberts II LJ, Lawson JA, Brash AR. Endogenous biosynthesis of prostacyclin and thromboxane and platelet function during administration of aspirin in man. J Clin Invest 1983; 71:676-88.

Gambino MC, Passaghe S, Chen ZM, Bucchi F, Gori G, Latini R, de Gaetano G, Cerletti C. Selectivity of oral aspirin as an inhibitor of platelet vs. vascular cyclo-oxygenase activity is reduced by portacaval shunt in rats. J Pharmacol Exp Ther 1988; 245:287-290.

Hamberg M, Svensson J, Samuelsson B. Thromboxanes: a new group of biologically active compounds derived from prostaglandin endoperoxides. Proc Natl Acad Sci USA 1975; 72:2994-24.

ISIS-2 Collaborative Group. Randomised trial of intravenous streptokinase, oral aspirin, both or neither among 17,189 cases of suspected acute myocardial infarction. Lancet 1988; 2: 349-360.

Kocsis JJ, Hernandovich J, Silver MJ, Smith JB, Ingerman C. Duration of inhibition of platelet prostaglandin formation and aggregation by ingested aspirin or indomethacin. Prostaglandins 1973; 3:141-44.

Marcus AJ. Aspirin and thromboembolism: A possible dilemma. N Engl J Med 1977; 297:1284-85.

Moncada S, Vane JR, Arachidonic acid metabolites and interactions between platelets and blood-vessel wall. N Engl J Med 1979; 300: 1142-1147.

Moroz LA. Increased blood fibrinolytic activity after aspirin ingestion. N Engl J Med 1977; 296:525.

O' Brien JR. Effects of salicylates on human platelets. Lancet 1968; i:779-83.

Patrignani P, Filabozzi P, Patrono C. Selective cumulative inhibition of platelet thromboxane production by low-dose aspirin in healthy subjects. J Clin Invest 1982;69:1366-1372.

Pedersen AK, FitzGerald GA. A dose-related kinetics of aspirin. Presystemic acetylation of platelet cyclo-oxygenase. N Engl J Med 1984; 311: 1206-1211.

Peto R, Gray R, Collins R, Wheatley K, Hennekens C, Jamrozik K, Warlow C, Hafner B, Thompson E, Norton S, Gilliland J, Doll R. Randomised trial of prophylactic daily aspirin in British male doctors. Br Med J 1988; 296: 313-316.

Roth GJ, Stanford N, Majerus PW. Acetylation of prostaglandin synthase by aspirin. Proc Natl Acad Sci USA1975; 72:3073-76.

Siebert DJ, Bochner F, Imhoff DM, Watts S, Lloyd JV, Field J , Gabb BW. Aspirin kinetics and platelet aggregation in man. Clin Pharmacol Ther 1983; 33:367-374.

Silver MJ. Mechanisms of hemostasis and therapy of thrombosis:New concepts based on the metabolism of arachidonic acid by platelets and endothelial cells. Adv Pharmacol Chemother 1981; 18:1-47.

Smith JB, Willis AL. Aspirin selectivity inhibits prostaglandin production in human platelets. Nature New Biol 1971;231:235-37.

Steering Committee of the Physicians' Health Study Research Group. Preliminary report: findings from the aspirin component of the ongoing physician's health study. N Engl J Med 1988; 318: 262-264.

Villa S, de Gaetano G. Prostacyclin-like activity in rat vascular tissues. Fast, long-lasting inhibition by treatment with lysine acetylsalicylate. Prostaglandins 1977; 14:1117-24.

Weiss HJ, Aledort LM. Impaired platelet connective-tissue interaction in man after aspirin ingestion. Lancet 1967; 2: 495-497.

Weksler BB, Pett SB, Alonso D, Richter RC, Stelzer P, Subramanian V, Tack-Goldman K, Gay WA Jr. Differential inhibition by aspirin of vascular and platelet prostaglandin synthesis in atherosclerotic patients. N Engl J Med 1983; 308:800-805.

Zucker MB, Peterson J. Inhibition of adenosine diphosphate-induced secondary aggregation and other functions by acetylsalicylic acid ingestion. Proc Soc Exp Biol Med 1968; 127:547-51.

CARDIOPROTECTIVE EFFECTS OF PROSTACYCLIN ANALOGUES

Fiona M. McDonald

Research Laboratories of Schering AG, Berlin (West) and Bergkamen, Müllerstraße 170-178, D-1000 Berlin 65 (West), FRG

In recent years, a considerable amount of evidence has accumulated suggesting that prostacyclin and prostacyclin analogues show cardioprotective activity in a number of different models of myocardial injury. Cardioprotective effects may be manifest in a variety of ways, including biochemical (e.g. conservation/improved recovery of mitochondrial oxidative function), morphological (preservation of myocyte ultrastructure), functional (enhancement of local or global mechanical performance) and electrical (anti-arrhythmic) protection. This has resulted in a multitude of parameters being used to assess both the extent of myocardial injury and the degree of myocardial protection. Tables 1 and 2 summarise some of the situations in which effects of prostacyclin or prostacyclin analogues have been seen, and interpreted as cardioprotection.

Table 1. Cardioprotective effects of prostacyclin analogues in vitro

	References
Improved functional recovery during reperfusion after prolonged cold or short-term warm cardioplegia, or global ischaemia	1,2,3,4,5
Preservation of nerve stimulation-induced noradrenaline release following ischaemia and reperfusion	1
Reduced oxidative stress during ischaemia and reperfusion	2
Increased CP:P_i radio during reperfusion after global ischaemia	6
Reduced creatine kinase release during reoxygenation after hypoxic perfusion	7
Protection against arrhythmias induced by hypoxia and reoxygenation, aconitine or cardiac glycosides	7,8,9

Table 2. Cardioprotective effects of prostacyclin analogues in vivo

	References
Infarct size reduction following ischaemia, ischaemia and reperfusion or coronary embolisation	10,11,12,13,14
Protection against isoprenaline-induced necrosis	15
Enhanced recovery of regional myocardial function during reperfusion following ischaemia	16,17
Preservation of myocardial CK and SOD activity following ischaemia and reperfusion	18,19,20,21,22
Amelioration of ischaemia-induced reductions in membrane phospholipids and intraneuronal catecholamines	19,23,24
Reduction of ischaemia-induced increases in cAMP and free lysosomal enzymes	21,22,23,25
Reduction in ischaemia-induced cardiac mitochondrial dysfunction	25
Improved survival of cardiac allografts	26,27
Reduction in coronary thrombus formation, enhancement of streptokinase-induced thrombolysis	28,29
Prevention of cyclic reductions in coronary flow in the presence of coronary stenosis	30,31
Antiarrhythmic effects against ischaemia/ reperfusion-induced and digoxin-induced arrhythmias	6,8,14,32,33
Reduction of ischaemia-induced ST-elevation	14,20,22,24

Whereas many of these effects appear to be well-established and reproducible, some others are more controversial. For example, in contrast to the improved functional recovery seen with prostacyclin analogues in a variety of in vitro ischaemia and reperfusion models[1-5], Moffat[34] and Karmazyn[35] found prostacyclin to have deleterious effects on recovery of function in isolated hearts.

Cardioprotection in ischaemia-reperfusion situations

A large part of the experimental evidence for cardioprotective effects of prostacyclin analogues has been obtained in models of myocardial ischaemia and reperfusion (see Tables 1 and 2). This reflects the general clinical situations in which there is probably the greatest scope for the application of cardioprotective agents, e.g. acute myocardial infarction, angina pectoris, cardiac transplantation.

During myocardial ischaemia, cardiomyocytes in the underperfused region show progressive changes from the normal state to a state of irreversible injury. The rate at which this progression occurs is primarily dependent on the extent of coronary collateral blood flow during

ischaemia[36]. Therefore species with virtually no coronary collateral
vessels, such as the rabbit and pig, develop severe ischaemia on coronary occlusion, with rapid progression to irreversible injury. In the
guinea pig, on the other hand, collateral blood flow is so great that
coronary artery occlusion does not normally lead to irreversible injury
and necrosis. The animal most widely used in such studies, the dog,
takes an intermediate position, with relatively large interindividual
variations in collateral development. The normal human heart has only
poorly developed coronary collaterals, but repetitive ischaemic episodes (as in angina pectoris) may lead to extensive collateralisation.

The temporal progression of injury during ischaemia means that
there is a "time window" during which cells which are not yet irreversibly injured may be salvaged by therapeutic intervention. The primary
treatment of myocardial ischaemia must remain the re-establishment of
adequate blood flow. Reperfusion may, however, in some situations
represent a "double-edged sword", in that long-term tissue viability is
not possible in the absence of reperfusion, but reperfusion itself may
lead to the death of some cardiomyocytes which, at the time of reperfusion, were not yet irreversibly injured. Cardioprotective effects
might therefore be expected with substances which extend the "time
window" for reperfusion (by reducing the severity of ischaemia or
increasing the ischaemia tolerance of the cardiomyocytes) and/or reduce
the extent of reperfusion injury.

How important are the "classical" effects of prostacyclin analogues
(vasodilatation, inhibition of platelet activation) for cardioprotection in ischaemia-reperfusion situations?

Clinical myocardial infarction usually results from intracoronary
thrombus formation, often at a site of plaque rupture, possibly accompanied by vasoconstriction. Figure 1 shows a simplified schematic
representation of this situation, and demonstrates the self-amplifying
nature of these events.

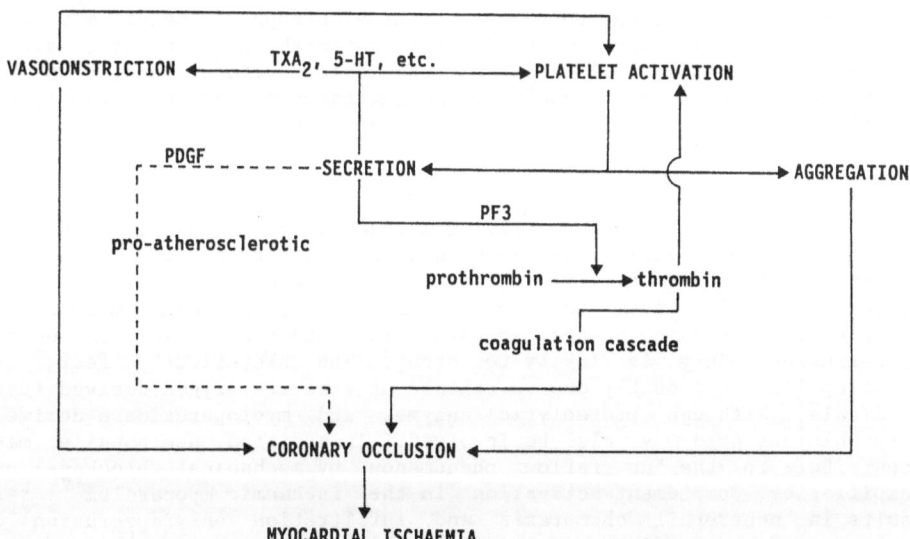

Figure 1. Schematic representation of events involved in the initiation
of acute myocardial infarction.

Use of a prostacyclin analogue to interrupt this vicious cycle of vasoconstriction and platelet activation might therefore be expected to
result in beneficial effects in this situation. However, these effects
alone do not seem to be sufficient explanation for the cardioprotective
effects of prostacyclin analogues in ischaemia-reperfusion. Improved
functional recovery is seen using doses of the prostacyclin analogue
iloprost which cause relatively little systemic vasodilatation (and
consequent reduction in afterload) and no increase in collateral blood
flow to the ischaemic myocardium[16]. This protective effect was not seen
using equihypotensive doses of sodium nitroprusside. Beneficial effects
of iloprost on functional recovery and infarct size have also been
shown for species with minimal coronary collateral development (pig[17],
rabbit[10]), thus excluding increases in collateral blood flow during
ischaemia as the primary underlying protective mechanism in this situation.

A primary role for platelets in the development of myocardial
infarction in models of non-thrombotic coronary occlusion seems doubt-
ful, as infarct size is not reduced in dogs made acutely thrombocyto-
penic before the ischaemic insult[37,38].

These findings would appear to rule out vasodilatation and inhibition of platelet activation as being the sole mechanisms underlying the
cardioprotective effects of prostacyclin analogues in ischaemia-reperfusion situations.

Other possible mechanisms involved in the cardioprotective effects of
prostacyclin analogues

Figure 2 summarises some of the possible mechanisms involved in prosta-
cyclin-induced cardioprotection.

In addition to vasodilatation and inhibition of platelet activation, a number of other actions have been described for prostacyclin
and prostacyclin-analogues. "Membrane stabilisation", assessed on the
basis of washout of labelled lipids, has been described for iloprost[5].
This effect is different to the classical electrophysiological membrane
stabilisation, as seen with Class I antiarrhythmic agents, since
prostacyclin analogues do not reduce the maximum rate of depolarisation
in atrial or ventricular muscle[39]. The increase in lysosomal stabilisation[21-23,25], and preservation of intraneuronal catecholamines[23,24]
seen with prostacyclin analogues may also reflect a generalised membrane stabilisation.

However, a principal underlying mechanism for the cardioprotective
actions of prostacyclin analogues in ischaemia-reperfusion situations
appears to be their ability to attenuate neutrophil activation. Activated neutrophils seem to play a central role in many models of
ischaemia-reperfusion damage, in particular under conditions in which
reperfusion injury is likely to occur. The deleterious effects of
neutrophils are probably due to release of reactive oxygen-derived free
radicals, although proteolytic enzymes and myeloperoxidase-derived
hypochlorous acid may also be involved. In addition, neutrophils may
contribute to the "no reflow" phenomenon by mechanical blockage of
capillaries. Complement activation in the ischaemic myocardium[40] results in neutrophil chemotaxis and infiltration on reperfusion[41].
Release of leukotrienes from neutrophils will amplify leucocyte
chemotaxis and may cause vasoconstriction and leakage of plasma proteins[42]. A number of studies have shown a reduction in infarct size or
improved myocardial functional recovery in animals made acutely

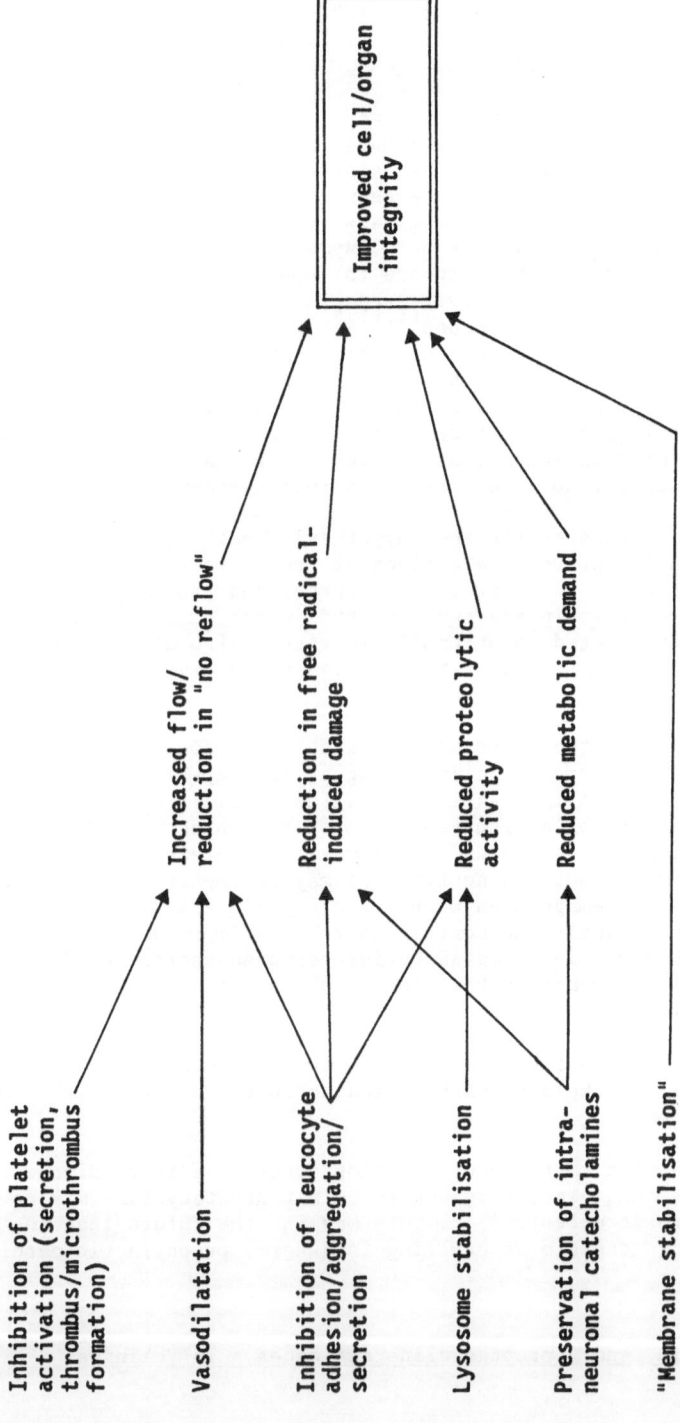

Figure 2. Possible mechanisms involved in cardioprotective effects of prostacyclins

neutropenic prior to ischaemia[43-45], or treated with antibody to the glycoprotein Mo1 (which is expressed on the surface of activated neutrophils and promotes $C3_{bi}$ binding and neutrophil adhesion)[46], or with scavengers of reactive oxygen species[47-50]. In investigations carried out under conditions in which reperfusion injury is less likely to occur (e.g. reperfusion after prolonged ischaemia) such treatment appears less successful[45,51].

Prostacyclin and the prostacyclin analogue iloprost have been shown to reduce neutrophil accumulation in ischaemic-reperfused myocardium, and this effect was associated with reduction in infarct size of similar magnitude to those seen in neutropenic animals[11,12]. In these studies, reductions were also seen in neutrophil accumulation following intradermal injection of zymosan-activated plasma (C5a), and in superoxide burst in response to opsonised zymosan in neutrophil suspensions in vitro. However, reductions in O_2^- production seen with prostacyclin and its analogues[11,12,52] require very high concentrations (μM and more) compared to the concentrations at which vasodilatation and inhibition of platelet aggregation occur (nM). Inhibition of neutrophil aggregation[53] and reductions in neutrophil adhesion to the endothelial surface in vitro[54] and in vivo[55] are seen at pharmacologically relevant concentrations. Belch et al. also found prostacyclin, but not iloprost, to have direct superoxide scavenging effects[53].

Further support for the hypothesis that neutrophil effects are involved in the protective actions of prostacyclin analogues comes from the finding that, in contrast to iloprost and prostacyclin itself, the 5-fluoro prostacyclin analogue SC 39902 which did not reduce O_2^- production from stimulated neutrophils in vitro also did not significantly reduce infarct size in dogs after coronary artery occlusion and reperfusion[11].

Summarising the experimental data, therefore, it seems clear that prostacyclin and prostacyclin analogues are capable of exerting cardio-protective effects in a variety of situations. It also appears that no single mechanism of action can be proposed which will account for all the protective effects seen in the various systems studied - for example, although effects on neutrophils may be important for the reduction in reperfusion damage seen with prostacyclin analogues in vivo, these effects are unlikely to contribute to the improvements in functional recovery observed in isolated buffer-perfused hearts in vitro. It seems more plausible to assume that these substances exert a relatively wide spectrum of effects, each of which may to a greater or lesser extent contribute to the overall cardioprotective activity. It follows from this that the principal mechanism unterlying an observed cardioprotective effect is likely to vary depending on the experimental model under consideration.

In addition to the acute cardioprotective effects discussed above, evidence is accumulating to suggest that prostacyclins may have anti-atherosclerotic effects[56-58]. This may in the future lead to development of drugs capable of exerting long-term, prophylactic cardioprotection.

Prostacyclin and prostacyclin analogues in clinical myocardial ischaemia

The effects of prostacyclin analogues in clinical myocardial ischaemia have not, as yet, been extensively investigated. Bugiardini et al. have shown that iloprost increases exercise capacity in patients

with stable angina pectoris[59]. However, as with other coronary vaso-
dilators, prostacyclins may induce myocardial ischaemia in susceptible
patients[60]. Prostacyclin and iloprost have been shown to be well toler-
ated in patients with acute myocardial infarction[61-63]. Henriksson et
al. have shown reductions in peak activity of creatine kinase and
lactate dehydrogenase in plasma from patients receiving prostacyclin
within 6 h of the onset of symptoms, implying a reduction in the extent
of myocardial injury[62]. These studies, however, have all been carried
out on relatively small numbers of patients, and an adequate evaluation
of the therapeutic efficacy of these substances will only be possible
when data from large-scale controlled studies become available.

References

1. K. Schrör and K. Funke, Prostaglandins and myocardial
    noradrenaline overflow after sympathetic nerve stimulation
    during ischemia and reperfusion, J. Cardiovasc. Pharmacol. 7
    (Suppl. 5): S50 (1985).

2. R. Ferrati, A. Cargnoni, S. Curello, C. Ceconi and E. Pasini,
    Protective effects of iloprost during myocardial ischaemia and
    reperfusion, J. Mol. Cell. Cardiol. 20 (Suppl. V):S41 (1988).

3. W.H. van Gilst, P.W. Boonstra, J.A. Terpstra, C.R.H. Wildevuur and
    C.D.J. de Langen, Improved recovery of cardiac function after
    24 h of hypothermic arrest in the isolated rat heart: compari-
    son of a prostacyclin analogue (ZK 36 374) and a calcium entry
    blocker (diltiazem), J. Cardiovasc. Pharmacol. 7:520 (1985).

4. F. Nomura, H. Matsuda, H. Hirose, S. Nakano, S. Maeda, M. Ohtani,
    M. Kaneko, K. Kadoba and Y. Kawashima, Assessment of myocardial
    protective effects of a new prostacyclin analogue, OP-41483,
    Surg. Forum 37:265 (1986).

5. E.F. Smith III, G. Kloster, G. Stöcklin and K. Schrör, Effect of
    iloprost (ZK 36 374) on membrane integrity in ischemic rabbit
    hearts, Biomed. Biochim. Acta 43:S155 (1984).

6. M. Pissarek, W. Gründer and T. Keller, 31-P-NMR-spectroscopy on
    ischemic and reperfused rat hearts: effects of iloprost,
    Biomed. Biochim. Acta 46:S564 (1987).

7. B. Müller, J. Schneider, H.H. Hennies and L. Flohé,
    Cardioprotective actions of the new stable epoprostenol ana-
    logue CG 4203 in rat models of cardiac hypoxia and ischemia,
    Arzneim.-Forsch./Drug Res. 34:1506 (1984).

8. H.E. Aksulu, Z.S. Ercan and R.K. Türker, Further studies on the
    antiarrhythmic effect of iloprost, Arch. Int. Pharmacodyn.
    Ther. 277:223 (1985).

9. M. Metin, Ö. Dörtlemez, H. Dörtlemez, F. Akar, Z.S. Erca and R.K.
    Türker, Prevention by a carbacyclin analogue (ZK 36 374) of
    digoxin-induced ventricular extrasystoles in guinea-pig myo-
    cardium, Eur. J. Pharmcol. 98:125 (1984).

10. M. Chiariello, P. Golino, M. Cappelli-Bigazzi, G. Ambrosio,
    I. Tritto and M. Salvatore, Reduction in infarct size by the
    prostacyclin analogue iloprost (ZK 36374) after experimental
    coronary artery occlusion-reperfusion, Am. Heart J. 115:499
    (1988).

11. P.J. Simpson, S.E. Mitsos, A. Ventura, K.P. Gallagher,
    J.C. Fantone, G.D. Abrams, M.A. Schork and B.R. Lucchesi,
    Prostacyclin protects ischemic reperfused myocardium in the dog
    by inhibition of neutrophile activation, Am. Heart J. 113:129
    (1987).

12. P.J. Simpson, J. Mickelson, J.C. Fantone, K.P. Gallagher and
    B.R. Lucchesi, Iloprost inhibits neutrophil function in vitro

and in vivo and limits experimental infarct size in canine heart, Circ. Res. 60:666 (1987).

13. F.M. Lupinetti, V.A. Starnes, K.A. Laws, J.C. Collins and J.W. Hammon, Prostacyclin reduction of regional ischemic injury in the canine myocardium, J. Surg. Res. 41:146 (1986).

14. C.D.J. de Langen, W.H. van Gilst and H. Wessling, Sustained protection by iloprost of the porcine heart in the acute and chronic phases of myocardial infarction, J. Cardiovasc. Pharmacol. 7:924 (1985).

15. P.S. Körmöczy, C. Vértesi, E. Mikus, L. Tardos and G. Kovács, Cardioprotective effect of prostacyclin and 7-oxo-PGI$_2$ in rats against chronic isoproterenol damage, Prostaglandins 33:505 (1987).

16. N.E. Farber, G.M. Pieper, J.P. Thomas and G.J. Gross, Beneficial effects of iloprost in the stunned canine myocardium, Circ. Res. 62:204 (1988).

17. W.J. van der Giessen, B. Schoutsen, J.G.P. Tijssen and P.D. Verdouw, Iloprost (ZK 36374) enhances recovery of regional myocardial function during reperfusion after coronary artery occlusion in the pig, Br. J. Pharmac. 87:23 (1986).

18. C. Thiemermann, E. Steinhagen-Thiessen and K. Schrör, Inhibition of oxygen-centered free radical formation by the stable prostacyclin-mimetic iloprost (ZK 36 374) in acute myocardial ischemia, J. Cardiovasc. Pharmacol. 6:365 (1984).

19. H. Darius, J.A. Osborne, D.K. Reibel and A.M. Lefer, Protective actions of a stable prostacyclin analog in ischemia induced membrane damage in rat myocardium, J. Mol. Cell. Cardiol. 19:243 (1987).

20. H. Darius, T. Thomsen and K. Schrör, Cardiovascular actions in vitro and cardioprotective effects in vivo of nileprost, a mixed type PGI$_2$/PGE$_2$ agonist, J. Cardiovasc. Pharmacol. 10:144 (1987).

21. E.F. Smith III, W. Gallenkämper, R. Beckmann, T. Thomsen, G. Mannesmann and K. Schrör, Early and late administration of a PGI$_2$-analogue, ZK 36 374 (iloprost): effects on myocardial preservation, collateral blood flow and infarct size, Cardiovasc. Res. 18:163 (1984).

22. K. Schrör, H. Darius, R. Ohlendorf, R. Matzky and W. Klaus, Dissociation of antiplatelet effects from myocardial cytoprotective activity during acute myocardial ischemia in cats by a new carbacyclin derivtive (ZK 36 375), J. Cardiovasc. Pharmacol. 4:554 (1982).

23. K. Schrör, K. Addicks, H. Darius, R. Ohlendorf and P. Rösen, PGI$_2$ inhibits ischemia-induced platelet activation and prevents myocardial damage by inhibition of catecholamine release from adrenergic nerve terminals. Evidence for cAMP as common denominator, Thromb. Res. 21:175 (1981).

24. K. Schrör, R. Ohlendorf and H. Darius, Beneficial effects of a new carbacyclin derivative, ZK 36 374, in acute myocardial ischemia, J. Pharmacol. Exp. Ther. 219:243 (1981).

25. N. Hieda, Y. Toki, S. Sugiyama, T. Ito, T. Satake and T. Ozawa, Prostaglandin I$_2$ analogue and propranolol prevent ischaemia induced mitochondrial dysfunction through the stabilisation of lysosomal membranes, Cardiovasc. Res. 22:219 (1988).

26. J.R. Rowles and M.L. Foegh, The synergistic effect of cyclosporine and iloprost on survival of rat cardiac allografts, Transplantation 42:94 (1986).

27. J.F. Shaw, Prolongation of rat allograft survival by treatment

with prostacyclin or aspirin during acute rejection. Transplantation 35:526 (1983).

28. W.J. van der Giessen, W.J. Mooi, A.M. Rutteman, L. Berk and P.D. Verdouw, The effects of the stable prostacyclin analogue ZK 36 374 on experimental coronary thrombosis in the pig, Thromb. Res. 36:45 (1984).

29. W.A. Schumacher, E.C. Lee and B.R. Lucchesi, Augmentation of streptokinase-induced thrombolysis by heparin and prostacyclin, J. Cardiovasc. Pharmacol. 7:739 (1985).

30. Y. Uchida and S. Murao, Effects of a prostaglandin I_2 analogue, ZK 36374, on recurring reduction of coronary blood flow, Jap. Heart J. 24:641 (1983).

31. Y. Uchida and S. Murao, Effect of prostaglandin I_2 on cyclical reduction of coronary blood flow. Jap. Circ. J. 43:645 (1979).

32. B. Müller, B. Maass, S. Stürzebecher and W. Skuballa, Antifibrillatory action of the stable orally active prostacyclin analogues iloprost and ZK 96 480 in rats after coronary artery ligation, Biomed. Biochim. Acta 43:S175 (1984).

33. S.J. Coker and J.R. Parratt, Prostacyclin - antiarrhythmic or arrhythmogenic? Comparison of the effects of intravenous and intracoronary prostacyclin and ZK 36374 during coronary artery occlusion and reperfusion in anaesthetised greyhounds, J. Cardiovasc. Pharmacol. 5:557 (1983).

34. M.P. Moffat, Concentration-dependent effects of prostacyclin on the response of the isolated guinea pig heart to ischemia and reperfusion: possible involvement of the slow inward current, J. Pharmacol. Exp. Ther. 242:292 (1987).

35. M. Karmazyn, Contribution of prostaglandins to reperfusion-induced ventricular failure in isolated rat hearts, Am. J. Physiol. 251:H133 (1986).

36. M.P. Maxwell, D.J. Hearse and D.M. Yellon, Species variation in the coronary collateral circulation during regional myocardial ischaemia: a critical determinant of the rate of evolution and extent of myocardial infarction, Cardiovasc. Res. 21:737 (1987).

37. K.M. Mullane and J.C. McGiff, Platelet depletion and infarct size in an occlusion-reperfusion model of myocardial ischemia in anesthetized dogs, J. Cardiovasc. Pharmacol. 7:733 (1985).

38. S.R. Jolly, W.A. Schumacher, S.L. Kungel, G.D. Abrams, J. Liddicoat and B.R. Lucchesi, Platelet depletion in experimental myocardial infarction, Basic Res. Cardiol. 80:269 (1985).

39. V. Kecskemeti, Cardiac electrophysiological effects of prostacyclin analogues, 7-oxo-PGI_2 and iloprost. Biomed. Biochim. Acta 46:S460 (1987).

40. R.D. Rossen, J.L. Swain, L.H. Michael, S. Weakley, E. Giannini and M.L. Entman, Selective accumulation of the first component of complement and leucocytes in ischemic canine heart muscle. A possible initiator of an extra myocardial mechanism of ischemic injury, Circ. Res. 57:119 (1985).

41. K.M. Mullane, R. Kraemer and B. Smith, Myeloperoxidase activity as a quantitative assessment of neutrophil infiltration into ischemic myocardium, J. Pharmacol. Methods 14:157 (1985).

42. G. Feuerstein and J.M. Hallenbeck, Leukotrienes in health and disease, FASEB J. 1:186 (1987).

43. R. Engler and J.W. Covell, Granulocytes cause reperfusion ventricular dysfunction after 15-minute ischemia in the dog, Circ. Res. 61:20 (1987).

44. J.L. Romson, B.G. Hook, S.L. Kunkel, G.D. Abrams, A. Schork and B.R. Lucchesi, Reduction of the extent of ischemic myocardial injury by neutrophil depletion in the dog, Circulation 67:1016 (1983).

45. S.R. Jolly, W.J. Kane, B.G. Hook, G.D. Abrams, S.L. Kunkel and B.R. Lucchesi, Reduction of myocardial infarct size by neutrophil depletion: effect of duration of occlusion, Am. Heart J. 112:682 (1986).

46. P.J. Simpson, R.F. Todd III, J.C. Fantone, J.K. Michelson, J.D. Griffin and B.R. Lucchesi, Reduction of experimental canine myocardial reperfusion injury by a monoclonal antibody (Anti-Mol, Anti-CD11b) that inhibits leukocyte adhesion, J. Clin. Invest. 81:624 (1988).

47. G. Ambrosio, L.C. Becker, G.M. Hutchins, H.F. Weisman and M.L. Weisfeldt, Reduction in experimental infarct size by recombinant human superoxide dismutase: insights into the pathophysiology of reperfusion injury, Circulation 74:1424 (1986).

48. K. Przyklenk and R.A. Kloner, Superoxide dismutase plus catalase improve contractile function in the canine model of the "stunned myocardium", Circ. Res. 58:148 (1986).

49. S.E. Mitsos, J.C. Fantone, K.P. Gallagher, K.M. Walden, P.J. Simpson, G.D. Abrams, M.A. Schork and B.R. Lucchesi, Canine myocardial reperfusion injury: protection by a free radical scavenger, N-2-mercaptopropionyl glycine, J. Cardiovasc. Pharmacol. 8:978 (1986).

50. M.L. Myers, R. Bolli, R.F. Lekich, C.J. Harley and R. Roberts, N-2-mercaptopropionylglycine improves recovery of myocardial function after reversible regional ischemia, J. Am. Coll. Cardiol. 8:1161 (1986).

51. K.P. Gallagher, A.J. Buda, D. Pace, R.A. Gerren and M Shlafer, Failure of superoxide dismutase and catalase to alter size of infarction in conscious dogs after 3 hours of occlusion followed by reperfusion, Circulation 73:1065 (1986).

52. H.J. Stahlberg, G. Loschen and L. Flohé, Effects of prostacyclin analogs on cyclic adenosine monophosphate and superoxide formation in human polymorphonuclear leukocytes stimulated by formyl-methionyl-leucyl-phenylalanine, Biol. Chem. Hoppe-Seyler 369:329 (1988).

53. J.J.F. Belch, A. Saniabadi, R. Dickson, R.D. Sturrock and C.D. Forbes, Effect of iloprost (ZK 36374) on white cell behavior, in: "Prostacyclin and Its Stable Analogue Iloprost", R.J. Gryglewski and G. Stock, eds., Springer Verlag, Berlin, Heidelberg (1987).

54. D. Fricke, D. Damerau and W. Vogt, Adhesion of guinea pig polymorphonuclear leucocytes to autologous aortic strips: influence of chemotactic factors and of pharmacological agents which affect arachidonic acid metabolism, Int. Archs. Allergy appl. Immun. 78:429 (1985).

55. B. Müller, M. Schmidtke and W. Witt, Adherence of leucocytes to electrically damaged venules in vivo. Effects of iloprost, PGE_1, indomethacin, forskolin, BW 755 C, sulotroban, hirudin, and thrombocytopenia, Eicosanoids 1:13 (1988).

56. A.L. Willis, D.L. Smith and C. Vigo, Suppression of principal atherosclerotic mechanisms by prostacyclins and other eicosanoids, Prog. Lipid Res. 25:645 (1986).

57. A.N. Orekhov, V.V. Tertov, A.V. Mazurov, E.R. Andreeva, V.S. Repin and V.N. Smirnov, "Regression" of atherosclerosis in cell culture: effects of stable prostacyclin analogues, Drug Dev. Res. 9:189 (1986).

58. H. Jellinek, G. Stock and E. Takács, Lipofundin arteriosclerosis and iloprost treatment, in: "Prostacyclin and Its Stable Analogue Iloprost", R.J. Gryglewski and G. Stock, eds., Springer Verlag, Berlin, Heidelberg (1987).

59. R. Bugiardini, M. Galvani, D. Ferrini, C. Gridelli, L. Mari, P. Puddu and S. Lenzi, Effects of iloprost, a stable prostacyclin analog, on exercise capacity and platelet aggregation in stable angina pectoris, Am. J. Cardiol. 58:453 (1986).

60. R. Bugiardini, M. Galvani, D. Ferrini, C. Gridelli, D. Tollemeto, N. Macri, P. Puddi and S. Lenzi, Myocardial ischemia during intravenous prostacyclin administration: hemodynamic findings and precautionary measures, Am. Heart J. 113:234 (1987).

61. F.J. Kiernan, J. Kluger, J.C. Regnier, M. Rutkowski and A. Fieldman, Epoprostenol sodium (prostacyclin) infusion in acute myocardial infarction, Br. Heart J. 56:428 (1986).

62. P. Henriksson, O. Edhag and A. Wennmalm, Prostacyclin infusion in patients with acute myocardial infarction, Br. Heart J. 53:173 (1985).

63. K. Swedberg, P. Held, H. Wadenvik and J. Kutti, Central haemodynamic and antiplatelet effects of iloprost - a new prostacyclin analogue - in acute myocardial infarction in man, Eur. Heart J. 8:362 (1987).

NEW PHARMACOLOGICAL AGENTS WHICH ANTAGONIZE LEUKOTRIENE D_4 AND PLATELET ACTIVATING FACTOR

Ann F. Welton and Margaret O'Donnell

Hoffmann-La Roche Inc.
340 Kingsland Avenue
Nutley, N.J. 07110

INTRODUCTION

Leukotriene D_4 (LTD_4) and Platelet Activating Factor (PAF) are two important lipid mediators of allergy and inflammation which were defined structurally in the late 1970's and early 1980's, although these substances had been identified many years earlier based on their biological activities. The structure of LTD_4 was elucidated from initial observations made during investigations ongoing in Samuelsson's laboratory in 1979 (1). Subsequently it was demonstrated that LTD_4 is one of a family of peptidoleukotriene metabolites of arachidonic acid formed by the sequential bioconversion of arachidonic acid via Δ^5-lipoxygenase and LTC_4 synthetase (a glutathione-S-transferase enzyme). Metabolism of arachidonic acid via this pathway leads to the formation of LTC_4, LTD_4, and LTE_4 (the peptidoleukotrienes) (2). LTD_4 was ultimately shown to be the major biologically active component of slow reacting substance of anaphylaxis (3), a substance originally described by Kellway and Trethewie in 1940 (4).

The biological activity of PAF was first described in the early 1970's by Benveniste et al. (5). It took 10 years for the structure to be reported almost coincidentally by Hanahan et al. (6) and Benveniste et al. (7). In these reports, PAF was described to be a phosphorylcholine derivative with either a 16 or 18 carbon fatty acid hydrocarbon alkyl group linked via an ether bond to the 1-carbon position of the phosphorylcholine and containing an acyl group at the 2-carbon position.

Recent studies of the interrelationships of PAF and the peptido-leukotrienes have demonstrated that in some cells these mediators can be formed from a common precursor, 1-O-alkyl-2-arachidonyl phosphorylcholine (8). Upon cellular stimulation, a phospholipase A_2 is activated which releases arachidonic acid and a lysophospholipid. Arachidonic acid is then metabolized to the leukotrienes while the lysophospholipid interme- diate is enzymatically acetylated at the 2-carbon position to form PAF.

Since the early 1980's, there has been a large increase in our knowledge of the cells which synthesize the peptidoleukotrienes and/or PAF (Table 1) and of the pharmacological activities associated with these mediators (Table 2).

Table 1. Cellular Sources of Peptidoleukotrienes and PAF

Peptidoleukotrienes	PAF
Mast Cell	Mast Cell
Basophil	Eosinophil
Eosinophil	Macrophage
Macrophage	Platelet
Endothelial Cell	Neutrophil
Keratinocyte	Endothelial Cell
Arterial Smooth Muscle Cell	Keratinocyte

Table 2. Biological Activities of Peptidoleukotrienes and PAF

Peptidoleukotrienes	PAF
Bronchoconstriction	Platelet Activation
Mucus Secretion	Platelet Aggregation
Decreased Mucus Velocity	Bronchoconstriction
Increased Capillary Permeability	Mucus Secretion
Increased Electrolyte Secretion in the Colon	Increased Capillary Permeability
Stimulation of Epidermal Cell Proliferation	Inflammatory Cell Chemotaxis
	Inflammatory Cell Activation
	Induction of Bronchial hyper-reactivity
	Modulation of Cellular Immune responses
	Systemic Hypotension and Shock
	Vasoconstriction
	Decreased Myocardial Contractility
	Conduction Arrythmias
	Negative Ionotropic Effects

Based upon the known biological activities of these mediators, the identity of the cells which synthesize these substances, and the presence of increased levels of these mediators in fluids or tissues associated with certain disease processes, it has been hypothesized that the peptidoleukotrienes and PAF may be important mediators of diseases such as asthma, inflammatory bowel disease, cutaneous inflammatory disorders, septic shock, and myocardial ischemia. For this reason, there has been a great deal of effort ongoing in the pharmaceutical industry to identify antagonists of these mediators as potential therapeutic agents.

The purpose of this chapter is to review the current status of the development of these types of drugs. For further information, the reader is also referred to several other reviews which have appeared on this topic in recent years (9-14).

Development of LTD$_4$ Antagonists

Based upon the known biological activities of LTD$_4$, it could be hypothesized that peptidoleukotriene antagonists may be useful in the treatment of several diseases. Most of the activity in the pharmaceutical industry, however, has focused on the potential use of LTD$_4$ antagonists in asthma. This is probably based on the fact that much of the early pharmacological characterization of LTD$_4$ concentrated on its activity in airway tissue and its identity to SRS-A. Therefore, the pharmacological model systems which have been primarily used to characterize LTD$_4$ antagonists are those which would be most applicable to antagonizing the actions of LTD$_4$ in the lung (i.e., LTD$_4$-induced contraction of guinea pig trachea, ^{3}H-LTD$_4$ binding to lung homogenate membranes, and LTD$_4$-induced bronchoconstriction in guinea pigs in vivo).

Over the past 10 years, several categories of LTD$_4$ antagonists have been identified. These include:

1) acetophenone-like compounds

2) quinoline-based compounds

3) leukotriene analogs

4) indazole-indole-based analogs

5) other structural types.

The structures of the most potent compounds in each of these categories are shown in Figure 1. The profiles of these compounds in in vitro and in vivo test systems are presented in Table 3. Many of these compounds were comparatively evaluated in our laboratories; however, the results denoted with an asterisk in Table 3 were obtained from published values which, in some cases, were determined under different experimental conditions than were used in our laboratories.

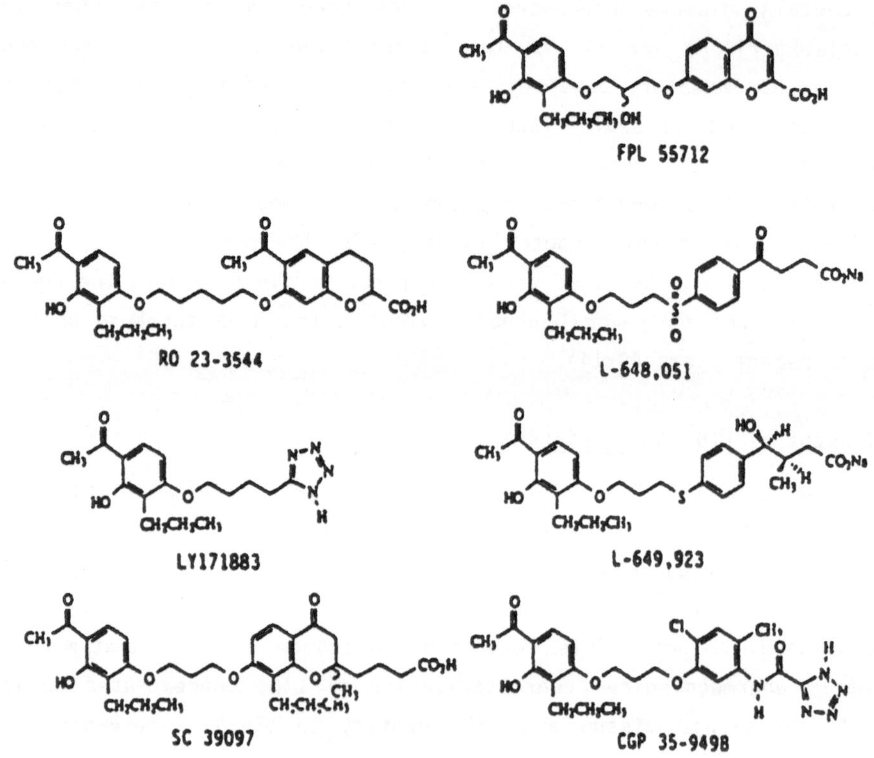

FPL 55712

RO 23-3544

L-648,051

LY171883

L-649,923

SC 39097

CGP 35-949B

Acetophenone-Like Compounds

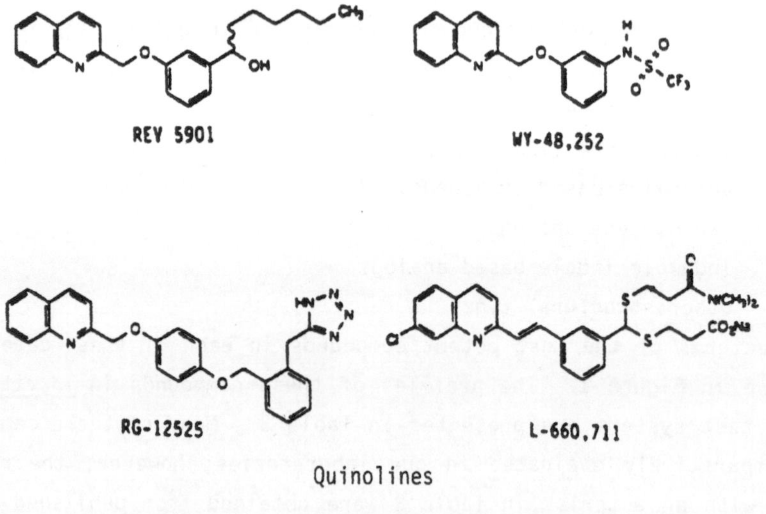

REV 5901

WY-48,252

RG-12525

L-660,711

Quinolines

Figure 1. Leukotriene D$_4$ Antagonists

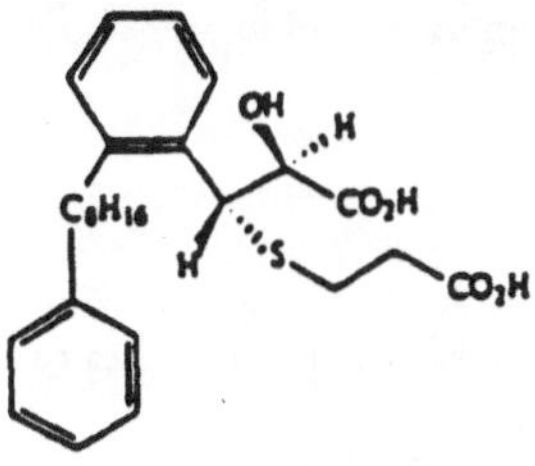

SKF 104,353

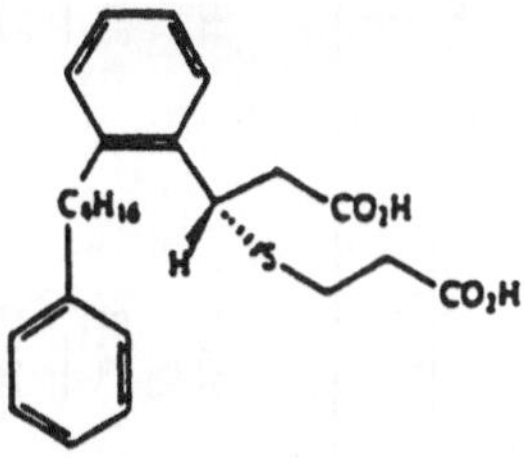

SKF 106,203

Leukotriene Analogs

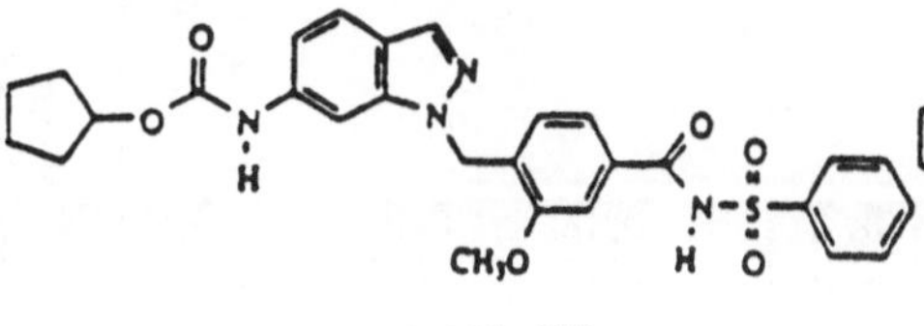

ICI 198,615

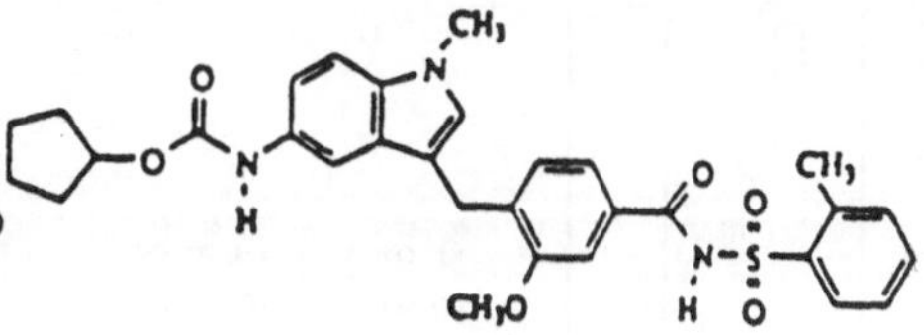

ICI 204,219

Indazole-Indoles

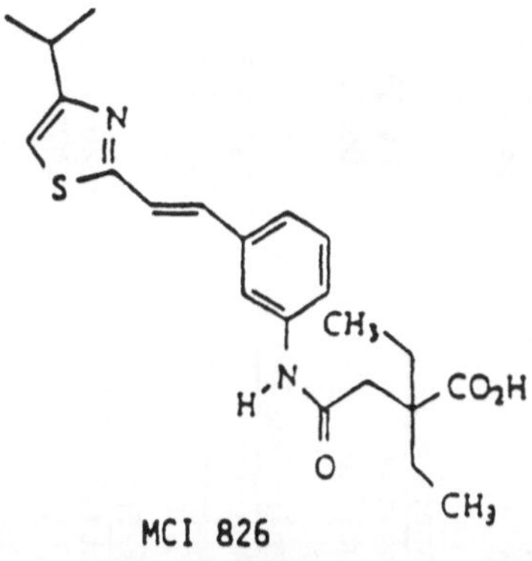

MCI 826

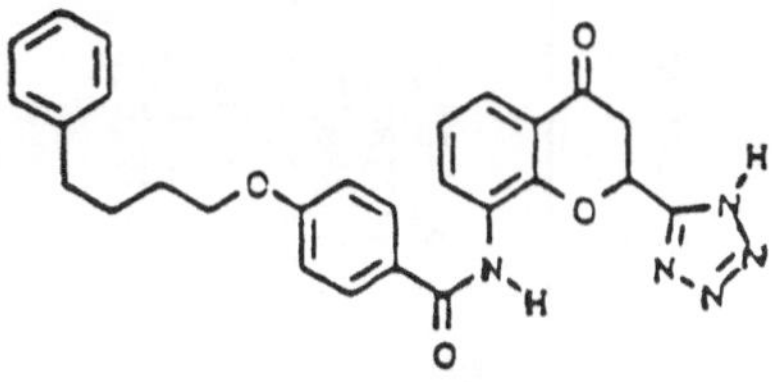

ONO 1078

Other Compounds

Figure 1. (Continued)

Table 3. Comparison of LTD$_4$ Antagonists

Pharmaceutical Company	Compound	LTD$_4$ Binding[a] IC$_{50}$ (μM)	Guinea Pig Trachea pA$_2$	LTD$_4$-induced bronchoconstriction in guinea pigs ID$_{50}$ (mg/kg)[b]		Reference
				Intravenous	Oral	
Acetophenone-like						
Fison	FPL 55712	3	6.4*	2	Inact[c]	18
Lilly	LY171883	10	6.9*	5	27	19
Searle	SC 39097	2	---	0.4*	3.8*	20
Ciba Geigy	CGP 35-949B	1	---	10	---	---
Roche	Ro 23-3544	5	6.1	5	Inact[c]	21
Merck	L-648,051	>10	7.3*	6	---	22
Merck	L-649,923	>10	7.2*	6	5*	23
Quinoline-Based						
Rorer	REV 5901	4	---	---	30*	24
Wyeth	Wy-48,252	6	7.6*	0.1*	0.1*	25
Merck	L-660,711	0.001*	9.4*	2*	0.2*	26-28
Rorer	RG-12525	0.003*	---	---	2*	29
Leukotriene Analogs						
Smithkline	SKF 104,353	0.005*	8.6*	---	---	30,31
Smithkline	SKF 106,203	---	7.6*	1.1*	2.2*	69
Indazole-Indole-Based						
ICI America	ICI 198,615	0.001	10.1*	0.03	27	32
ICI America	ICI 204,219	0.0001	9.5*	0.03	1.4	33
Novel Chemicals						
Mitsubishi	MCI-826	0.007	---	0.04	0.16	---
ONO	ONO 1078	0.01	7.5*	0.25	2.6	34

[a] LTD$_4$ binding assay methodology; Hogaboom et al., Biochem. Biophys. Res. Commun. 116, 1136, 1983.
[b] LTD$_4$ bronchoconstriction assay methodology; O'Donnell and Welton; Agents Actions 14, 43, 1984.
[c] Inact = no significant inhibition at 30 mg/kg. *Results estimated from published values.

Most of the acetophenone compounds were synthesized and reported in the years between 1980 and 1987. These compounds were follow-ups to FPL 55712, an acetophenone which was identified in the 1970's as being an SRS-A antagonist with a short duration of action and poor bioavailability (15-17). Some of the back-up acetophenones were viewed as improvements upon FPL 55712 because they were orally active (LY171883, SC 39097, and L-649,923) or more active than FPL 55712 by the inhalation route (Ro 23-3544 and L-648,051). It should be noted from the data presented in Table 3, however, that the follow-up compounds, in general, were not significantly more potent that FPL 55712 in in vitro binding or bioassay systems or in vivo by the intravenous route of administration.

Three of these acetophenones (LY171883, L-649,923 and L-648,051) have recently undergone clinical trials (see Table 4) in normal subjects (challenged with LTD_4) and asthmatic subjects (challenged with antigen). The general design of human studies with LTD_4 antagonists has been to first evaluate the pharmacological activity of the compound in man in an LTD_4-induced bronchoconstriction study prior to evaluating the activity of the compound against antigen-induced bronchoconstriction in man. A 50 to 100-fold shift in the LTD_4 bronchoconstriction dose-response curve is believed to be needed to expect optimum activity vs. antigen challenge. Although L-649,923 (1 gram, oral), L-648,051 (1.6 mg, aerosol), and LY171883 (400 mg, oral) only produced a 3-to 6-fold shift in the LTD_4-induced bronchoconstriction studies, these compounds were still evaluated in an antigen-challenge study and exhibited modest inhibition. In light of the apparent weak antagonistic activity of these compounds at the doses tested in LTD_4-challenged normal subjects, these modest effects vs. an antigen-challenge should be viewed as a promising indication of the eventual utility of LTD_4 antagonists in asthma. In any case, from these studies with the "first generation" acetophenone LTD_4 antagonists, it became evident that more potent compounds were necessary to conceptually evaluate the role of LTD_4 in mediating asthma.

In this regard, two quinolines (Table 3) seem to have promising potency based on very recent reports. These are L-660,711 and RG-12525 from Merck and Rorer, respectively. These compounds are currently in clinical study.

Two LTD_4 antagonists, SKF 104,353 and SKF 106,203, disclosed by scientists at Smith-Kline were derived from studies designed to synthesize LTD_4 analogs with antagonistic activity. These compounds have also demonstrated improved potency over the "first generation" acetophenones in in vitro model systems. Moreover SKF 104,353 (0.8 mg, aerosol) has shown promising clinical activity vs. LTD_4 challenge in normal subjects

Table 4. Clinical trials with leukotriene antagonists in normal and asthmatic subjects

Study	Compound	Dose	Challenge	Effect	Adverse Reactions
Normal Subjects					
Barnes, 1987 (35)	Merck L-649,923	1 gm oral	LTD	3.8-fold rightward shift of a LTD dose-response curve; n=12.	colicky, abdominal pain and diarrhea (45%)
Biollaz, 1988 (36)	Merck L-648,051	1.6 mg aerosol	LTD	4-fold rightward shift of a LTD dose-response curve; n=16.	mild irritation (13%) cough, dyspnea
Phillips, 1988 (37)	Lilly LY171883	400 mg oral	LTD	6-fold rightward shift of a LTD dose-response curve; n=12.	none
Barnes, 1988 (38)	Rorer REV-5901	1 gm oral	LTD	no effect; n=8.	nausea (25%)
Evans, 1988 (39)	Smithkline SKF 104,353	0.8 mg aerosol	LTD	48% protection of LTD-Induced fall in sGaw; 41% inhibition of LTD_4-induced decrease in $Vmax_{30}$; n=8.	none
Asthmatic Subjects					
Britton, 1987 (40)	Merck L-649,923	1 gm oral	allergen	early phase - very slight protection late phase - no protection; n=8.	---
Barnes, 1988 (38)	Merck L-648,051	1.6 mg aerosol	allergen	33% protection of antigen-induced decrease in Vmax 30; n=8.	---
Israel, 1988 (41)	Lilly LY171883	600 mg oral bid for 2 weeks	cold air	2-fold rightward shift; improvement in chest tightness; n=19.	
Fleisch, 1988 (42)	Lilly LY171883	600 mg oral bid for 6 weeks	none	small, but gradual improvement in lung function (FEV), and wheezing; decrease in concomitant broncho-dilator dosage; improvements in symptoms; n=138.	---
Mathur, 1986 (43)	Lilly LY171883	600 mg oral bid for 5d	allergen	inhibition of late phase broncho-constrictor response; n=8.	---

(Table 4) and this compound may also be evaluated in the future vs. antigen challenge. SKF 106,203 appears, however, to be a follow-up compound with a longer biological half-life in vivo and improved bio-availability and it is anticipated that this compound will be developed by the oral route of administration.

Among the newer "second generation" LTD_4 antagonists, ICI 204,219 and MCI-826 are also quite promising compounds based on their potent oral activity and duration of action in preclinical animal models. These compounds, too, appear to be undergoing clinical evaluation for use in asthma. Thus, it appears that many of the "second generation" compounds are markedly more potent than the early acetophenone-based compounds which were evaluated in man. It is hoped that in the next few years the compounds now undergoing clinical evaluation will conclusively answer the question of the role of LTD_4 in asthma and the therapeutic utility of an LTD_4 antagonist in treating this disease.

Development of PAF Antagonists

The chemical approaches used by most pharmaceutical companies to develop antagonists of PAF can be loosely categorized into 4 types (structures of representative compounds for each of these categories are shown in Figure 2)

1) analogs of PAF
2) natural products (ginkgolides and kadsurenone-analogs)
3) triazolodiazepines
4) pyridines

Since 1985, numerous PAF antagonists have been described in the litera-ture (44-61). In Table 5, the in vitro and in vivo profiles of 18 of these antagonists in a number of model systems are compared. Many of these compounds have been comparatively evaluated in our laboratories; however, the results indicated with an asterisk in Table 5 were taken from published values which in some cases were determined under different experimental conditions than are used in our laboratories.

A key structural modification which resulted in PAF analogs with antagonistic activity was the replacement of the choline at the 3-carbon position of PAF with a thiazolium moiety. This was first described in the Takeda antagonist, CV 3988. Other changes in the chemical structures indicated in Figure 2 were made to stabilize the compounds to metabolism. In general, two problems have hindered the development of PAF analogs as PAF antagonists, however. These include the observation that at high concentrations many of these compounds exhibit agonistic activity and the fact that these compounds seem, in general, to have poor bioavailability.

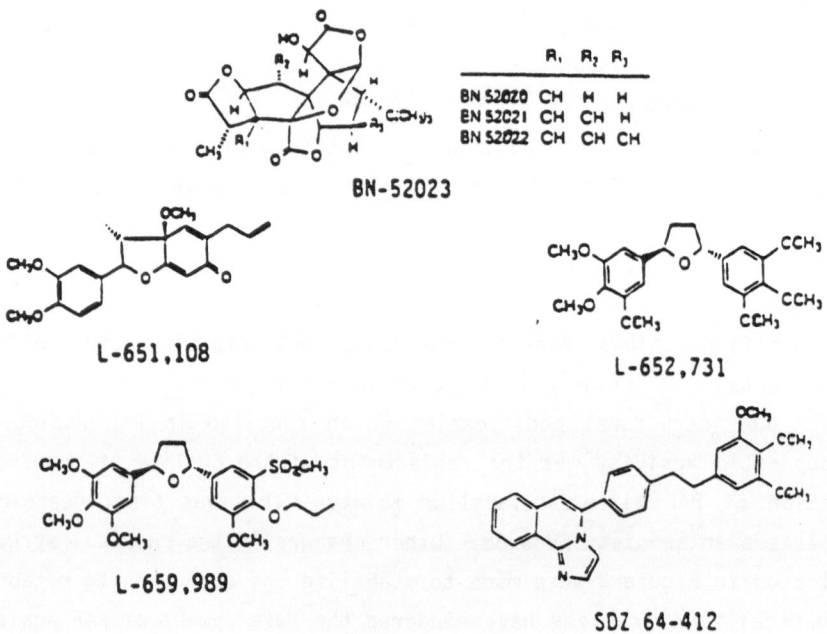

CV-3988

CV-6209

SDZ 63-072

SDZ 63-119

RO 19-3704

PAF Analogs

BN-52023

	R₁	R₂	R₃
BN 52020	CH	H	H
BN 52021	CH	CH	H
BN 52022	CH	CH	CH

L-651,108

L-652,731

L-659,989

SDZ 64-412

Natural Products

Figure 2. PAF Antagonists

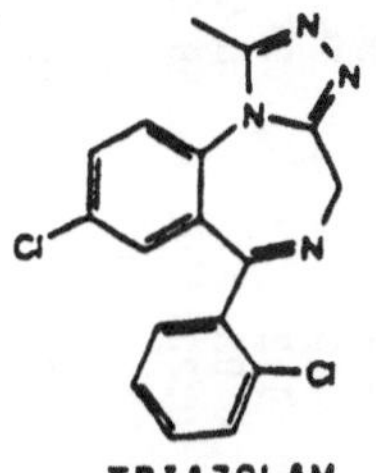

TRIAZOLAM

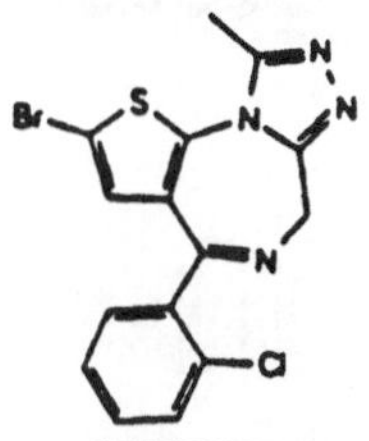

BROTIZOLAM

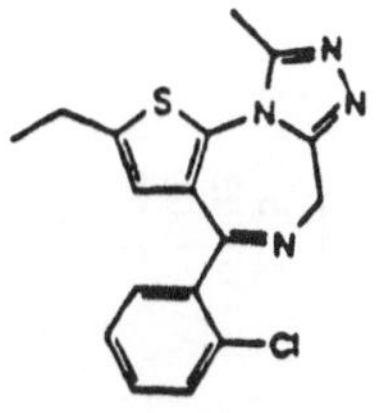

ETIZOLAM

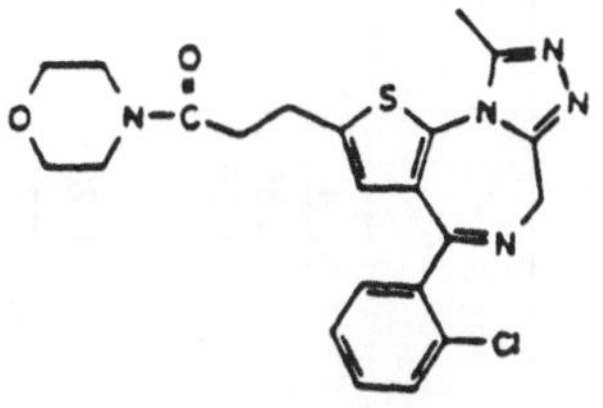

WEB 2086

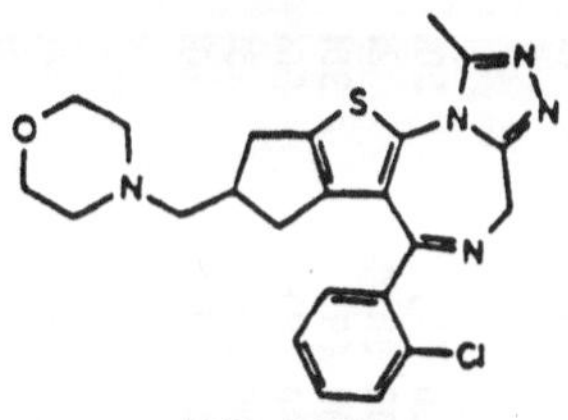

STY 2108

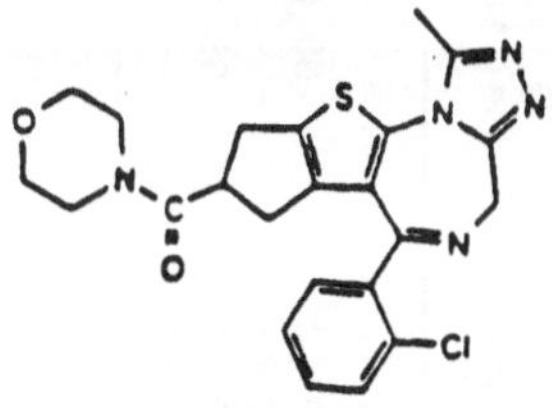

WEB 2170

Triazolodiazepines

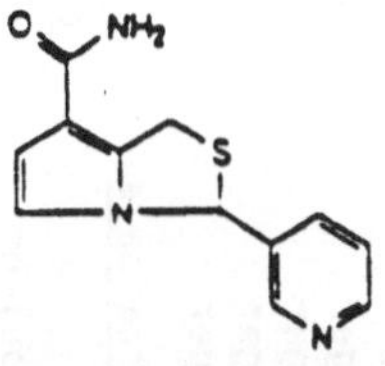

48740 RP

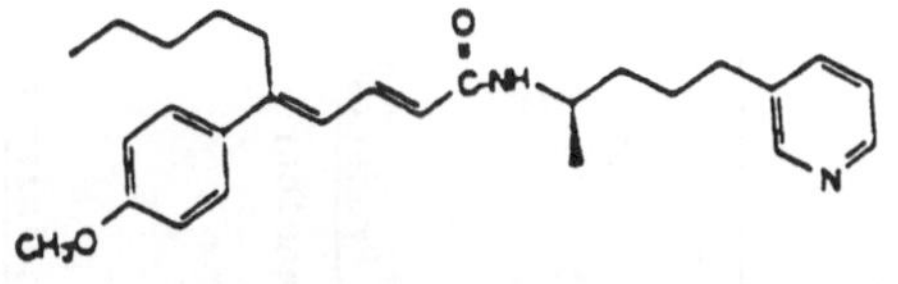

RO 24-0238

Pyridines

Figure 2. (Continued)

Table 5. Comparison of PAF Antagonists

Pharmaceutical Company	Compound	PAF Aggregation[a] IC_{50} (nM) Rabbit (R) or Human (H) Platelets	PAF Binding[b] IC_{50} (nM) Dog (D)	PAF-Induced Bronchoconstriction in Guinea Pigs ID_{50} (mg/kg)[c] Intravenous	Oral	Reference
PAF Analogs						
Takeda	CV-3988	3200 (R)	700 (D)	1	Inact[d]	44,45
Takeda	CV-6209	170 (H)*	--	--	---	46
Roche	Ro 19-3704	70 (R)	95 (D)	0.2	Inact[d]	47
Sandoz	SDZ 63-072	4700 (R)	---	0.3*	50*	48
Sandoz	SDZ 63-119	400 (R)	---	0.1*	20*	48
Natural Products						
Ipsen Beaufour	BN 52021	500 (R)	800 (D)	0.28	---	49,50
Merck	L-651,108	500 (R)	>1000 (D)	---	---	51
Merck	L-652,731	400 (R)	180 (D)	---	---	52
Merck	L-659,989	1.7 (R)*	95 (D)	0.16	1.6	53
Sandoz	SDZ 64-412	60 (H)*	60 (H)*	0.06*	16*	54
Triazolodiazepines						
Upjohn	Triazolam	2000 (R)	500 (D)	--	200	55
Yoshitomi	Etizolam	3800 (R)*	22 (R)*	--	---	56
Boehringer	Brotizolam	200 (R)	300 (D)	0.5	10	55
Boehringer	WEB 2086	180 (H)	200 (D)	0.03	1.2	57
Boehringer	WEB 2170	300 (H)*	130 (D)	0.02	0.03	58,59
Boehringer	STY 2108	40 (H)*	180 (D)	0.02	0.22	58,59
Novel Chemicals						
Roche	Ro 24-0238	3800 (H)	40 (D)	0.06	16	60
Rhone Poulenc	48740 RP	3000 (R)	38 (H)*	3*	---	61

[a] PAF aggregation assay methodology; Lagente et al., Br. J. Pharmacol. 94, 27, 1988.
[b] PAF binding assay methodology; Janero et al., Thrombosis Res. 50, 789, 1988.
[c] PAF bronchoconstriction assay methodology; Tilley et al., J. Med. Chem. Submitted.
[d] Inact = no significant inhibition at 50 mg/kg. *Results estimated from published values.

Leads from natural products for two types of PAF antagonist have been found in the extracts from plants used to treat inflammatory disorders, asthma, and other lung diseases. These include Kadsurenone (L-651, 108) which was isolated from the Chinese medicinal herb, haifenteng, by scientists at Merck and is a natural tetrahydrofuran. Three other synthetic compounds, L-652,731, L-659,989, and SDZ 64-412, evolved from the structure of Kadsurenone. It is believed the latter two compounds are in clinical development. Also, several ginkgolides (e.g. BN 52021), which are natural products extracted from the leaves of the Ginkgo biloba tree and which were isolated by investigators at Ipsen-Beaufour, exhibit PAF antagonistic activity. A mixture of these ginkgolides, BN 52063, is undergoing clinical evaluation (see below).

Screening studies led to the discovery that several triazolobenzodiazepines such as triazolam, etizolam and brotizolam are PAF antagonists. Based on these leads, scientists at Boehringer-Ingelheim synthesized a number of analogs and, from these efforts, WEB 2086 evolved. WEB 2086 is a very potent PAF antagonist which is free of the sedative and anxiolytic activities of its predecessors. Two follow-up compounds, STY 2108 and WEB 2170, also identified by scientists at Boehringer-Ingelheim, are even more potent than WEB 2086.

Under the fourth classification of PAF antagonists are listed the Roche compound, Ro 24-0238, which is a dual acting agent combining potent PAF antagonism with thromboxane synthase inhibitory activity, and a Rhone Poulenc compound, 48740 RP.

Phase 1 clinical trials have been conducted with 4 chemically dissimilar PAF antagonists in normal subjects (Table 6). These include BN 52063 (a mixture of 3 ginkgolides of which BN 52021 is the active component), CV-3988, WEB 2086, and 48740 RP. The general design of these studies consists of an evaluation of both safety and pharmacological activity (ex vivo measurement of antagonism of PAF-induced platelet aggregation) in Phase I studies. Indeed, all 4 compounds tested in normal volunteers inhibited ex vivo PAF-induced platelet aggregation with WEB 2086 being the most potent by the intravenous, oral, and aerosol route of administration. BN 52063 is the only PAF antagonist for which results are available from additional clinical studies. It has been shown to inhibit PAF-induced skin responses and to inhibit allergen-induced bronchoconstriction (causing a 7-fold shift of an allergen dose-response curve). These results with BN 52063 are very promising and support the utility of PAF antagonists in treating asthma. Presently WEB 2086, a more potent PAF antagonist than BN 52063, is believed to be in

Table 6. Clinical trials with PAF antagonists in normal and asthmatic subjects

Study	Compound	Dose	Challenge	Effect	Adverse Reactions
Normal Subjects					
Arnout, 1988 (62)	Takeda CV-3988	0.75-2 mg/kg intravenous	PAF-induced ex vivo platelet aggregation	The highest dose produced a 360% increase in the threshold aggregating concentration of PAF and a plasma concentration of 6,400 ng/ml (10 μM); n=12.	No changes in blood pressure, pulse or respiratory rate; insignificant changes in plasma hemaglobin and serum heptoglobin indicating slight hemolysis
Adamus, 1988 (63)	Boehringer-Ingelheim WEB 2086	0.5, 2, 10, 20 or 50 mg iv infusion	PAF-induced ex vivo platelet aggregation	Dose-related inhibition of ex vivo platelet aggregation (0.5 mg dose produced 68% inhibition); n=8.	No clinically significant drug-related effects on vital parameters or adverse reactions
Adamus, 1988 (64)	Boehringer-Ingelheim WEB 2086	0.05, 0.25, 0.5 or 1.0 mg inhaled	PAF-induced ex vivo platelet aggregation	Dose-related inhibition of ex vivo platelet aggregation (0.5 mg and 1.0 mg produced 46% and 64% inhibition respectively); n=8.	None
Adamus, 1988 (64)	Boehringer-Ingelheim WEB 2086	1.25, 5, 20, 100, 200 or 400 mg oral	PAF-induced ex vivo platelet aggregation	Dose-related inhibition of ex vivo platelet aggregation (1.25 mg and 20 mg produced 62% and 100%, respectively); n=6.	None
Pinquier, 1988 (65)	Rhone Poulenc 48740 RP	250, 500 or 1000 mg oral	PAF-induced ex vivo platelet aggregation	Dose-related inhibition of ex vivo platelet aggregation (250, 500 and 1000 mg produced 41, 41 and 79% inhibition, respectively); n=29.	None
Guinot, 1986 (66)	Ipsen-Beaufour BN 52063	80 mg oral	PAF-induced wheal and flare reaction	80 mg dose produced 74% inhibition of acute wheal response and 66% inhibition of flare response; n=5.	Headache (80%)
Chung, 1987 (67)	Ipsen-Beaufour BN 52063	80 or 120 mg oral	PAF-induced skin response and ex vivo platelet aggregation	Dose-related inhibition of acute wheal and flare response (maximum inhibition 60%); dose-related inhibition of ex vivo platelet aggregation; n=6.	Drowsiness (17%)
Asthmatic Subjects					
Guinot, 1987 (68)	Ipsen-Beaufour BN 52063	40 mg tid for 3 d oral	Bronchial provocation with allergen	Inhibition of immediate broncho-constrictor response (7-fold shift of allergen dose-response curve); n=8.	None

Phase 2 study in asthmatics. The results of studies with this compound should also help define the role of PAF in the pathogenesis of bronchial asthma.

Conclusion

Over the last 10 years the pharmaceutical industry has identified potent LTD_4 and PAF antagonists for clinical evaluation in asthma. Currently the drugs are available to conduct the clinical studies which should help to define the role of LTD_4 and PAF in the pathogenesis of asthma. The next one to two years should be extremely exciting as clinical studies investigate the usefulness of antagonists of these lipid mediators, either alone or in combination, in ameliorating the symptoms of asthma, especially chronic inflammation of airways and nonspecific airway hyperreactivity.

REFERENCES

1. R.C. Murphy, S. Hammarström, and B. Samuelsson, Leukotriene C: A slow reacting substance from murine mastocytoma cells, Proc. Natl. Acad. Sci. U.S.A., 76:4275 (1979).

2. B. Samuelsson, Leukotrienes: Mediators of immediate hypersensitivity reactions and inflammation, Science, 220:568 (1983).

3. H.R. Morris, G.W. Taylor, P.J. Piper, and J.R. Tippins, Slow reacting substance of anaphylaxis from guinea pig lung, Nature, 285:104 (1980).

4. C.H. Kellaway and E.R. Trethewie, The liberation of a slow reacting smooth muscle-stimulating substance in anaphylaxis, Q.J. Exp. Physiol. Cogn. Med. Sci., 30:121 (1940).

5. J. Benveniste, P.M. Henson, and C.G. Cochrane, Leukocyte dependent histamine release from rabbit platelets. The role of IgE and a platelet activating factor, J. Exp. Med., 136:1356 (1972).

6. C.A. Demopoulos, R.N. Pinkard, and D.J. Hanahan, Platelet activating factor. Evidence for 1-0-alkyl-2-acetyl-sn-glyceryl-3-phosphoryl-choline as the active component (a new class of lipid chemical mediators), J. Biol. Chem., 254:9355 (1979).

7. J. Benveniste, J.P. LeCouedic, J. Polonsky, and M. Tence, Structural analysis of purified platelet activating factor by lipases, Nature, 269:170 (1977).

8. C.L. Swendsen, J.M. Ellis, F.H. Chilton III, J.T. O'Flaherty, and R.L. Wykle, 1-0-alkyl-2-acyl-sn-glycero-3-phosphocholine: a novel

source of arachidonic acid in neutrophils stimulated by calcium ionophore A23187, <u>Biochem. Biophys. Res. Commun.</u>, 113:72 (1983).

9. J.H. Musser, A.F. Kreft, and A.J. Lewis, New developments concerning leukotriene antagonists: A review, <u>Agents Actions</u>, 18:332 (1986).

10. J.H. Fleisch, L.E. Rinkema, C.A. Whitesitt, and W.S. Marshall, Development of cysteinyl leukotriene receptor antagonists, <u>Advances in Inflammation Research</u>, 12:173 (1988).

11. C.D. Perchonock, T.J. Torphy, and S. Mong, Peptidoleukotrienes: Pathophysiology, receptor biology and receptor antagonists, <u>Drugs of the Future</u>, 12:871 (1987).

12. P. Braquet, P.E. Chabrier, and J.M. Mencia-Huerta, The promise of PAF-acether antagonists, <u>Advances in Inflammation Research</u>, 12:135 (1988).

13. P.J. Barnes, K.F. Chung, and C.P. Page, Platelet-activating factor as a mediator of allergic disease, <u>J. Allergy Clin. Immunol.</u>, 81:919 (1988).

14. K.F. Chung and P.J. Barnes, PAF Antagonists: Their potential therapeutic role in asthma, <u>Drugs</u>, 35:93 (1988).

15. J. Augstein, J.B. Farmer, T.B. Lee, P. Sheard, and M.L. Tattersall, Selective inhibitor of slow reacting substance of anaphylaxis, <u>Nature New Biol.</u>, 245:215 (1973).

16. R.A. Appleton, J.R. Bantick, T.R. Chamberlain, D.N. Hardern, T.B. Lee, and A.D. Pratt, Antagonists of slow reacting substance of anaphylaxis. Synthesis of a series of chrome-2-carboxylic acids, <u>J. Med. Chem.</u>, 20:371 (1977).

17. P. Sheard, M.C. Holroyde, A.M. Ghelani, J.R. Bantick, and T.B. Lee, Antagonists of SRS-A and leukotrienes, in "Leukotrienes and Other Lipoxygenase Products", B. Samuelsson and R. Paoletti (eds.): Raven Press, New York (1982), pp. 229-235.

18. R.D. Krell, R. Osborn, L. Vickery, K. Falcone, M. O'Donnell, J. Gleason, C. Kinzig, and D. Bryan, Contraction of isolated airway smooth muscle by synthetic leukotrienes C_4 and D_4, <u>Prostaglandins</u> 22:387 (1981).

19. J.H. Fleisch, L.E. Rinkema, K.D. Haisch, D. Swanson-Bean, T. Goodson, P.P.K. Ho, and W.S. Marshall, LY171883, 1-<2-hydroxy-3-propyl-4-<4-(1-H-tetrazol-5-yl) butoxy>phenyl>ethanone, an orally active leukotriene D_4 antagonist, <u>J. Pharmacol. Exp. Ther.</u>, 233:148 (1985).

20. G.W. Carnathan, J.H. Sanner, J.M. Thompson, C.M. Prusa, and M. Miyano, Antagonism of the in vivo and in vitro effects of leukotriene D_4 by SC-39070 in guinea pigs, <u>Agents Actions</u>, 20:124 (1987).

21. M. O'Donnell, A.F. Welton, H. Crowley, D. Brown, R. Garippa, N. Cohen, G. Weber, B. Banner, and R.J. Lopresti, Pharmacological profile of Ro 23-3544, a new aerosol active leukotriene receptor antagonists, Advances in Prostaglandin, Thromboxane and Leukotriene Research, 17:519 (1987).

22. T.R. Jones, Y. Guindon, E. Champion, L. Charette, R.N. Dehaven, D. Denis, D. Ethier, A.W. Ford-Hutchinson, R. Fortin, R. Frenette, J.Y. Gauthier, R. Hamel, P. Masson, A. Maycock, C. McFarlane, H. Piechuta, S.S. Pong, J. Rokach, C. Yoakim, and R.N. Young, L-648,051: An aerosol active leukotriene D_4 receptor antagonist, Advances in Prostaglandin, Thromboxane and Leukotriene Research, 17: 1012 (1987).

23. R.N. Young, T.R. Jones, J.G. Atkinson, P. Bélanger, E. Champion, D. Denis, R.N. Dehaven, A.W. Ford-Hutchinson, R. Fortin, R. Frenette, J.Y. Gauthier, J. Gillard, Y. Guindon, M. Kakushima, P. Masson, A. Maycock, C.S. McFarlane, H. Piechuta, S.S. Pong, J. Rokach, H. Williams, C. Yoakim, and R. Zamboli, Novel arylthio-and arylsulfonylpropyl oxyacetophenones: Design and synthesis of L-648,051 and L-649,923, potent antagonists of leukotriene D_4, Advances in Prosta- glandin, Thromboxane and Leukotriene Research, 17: 544 (1987).

24. R.G. Van Inwegen, A. Khandwala, R. Gordon, P. Sonnino, S. Coutts, and S. Jolly, REV 5901: An orally effective peptidoleukotriene antagonist, detailed biochemical/pharmacological profile, J. Pharmacol. Exp. Ther., 241:117 (1987).

25. J.M. Hand, J.H. Musser, A.F. Kreft, S. Schwalm, I. Englebach, M. Auen, M. Skowronek, and J.Y. Chang, Wy-48,252 (1,1,1-trifluoro-N-[3-(2-quinolinylmethoxy) phenyl] methanesulfonamide): A selective orally active leukotriene antagonist, The Pharmacologist, 29:174 (1987).

26. L. Charette, T.R. Jones, E. Champion, P. Masson, A.W. Ford-Hutchinson, R. Dehaven, S.S. Pong, M. Belley, R. Frenette, J.Y. Gauthier, S. Leger, J. Rokach, H. Williams, R.N. Young, and R. Zamboni, In vitro pharmacology of L-660,711, a new LTD_4 receptor antagonist, Fed. Proc., 2:A1264 (1988).

27. T.R. Jones, M. Belley, E. Champion, L. Charette, R. Dehaven, A.W. Ford-Hutchinson, R. Frenette, J.Y. Gauthier, S. Leger, C.S. McFarlane, P. Masson, H. Piechuta, S.S. Pong, J. Rokach, H. Williams, R.N. Young, and R. Zamboni, Pharmacology of L-660,711, a potent selective, orally active LTD_4 receptor antagonist, Am. Rev. Respir. Dis., 137:A427 (1988).

28. P. Masson, T.R. Jones, L. Charette, E. Champion, C.S. McFarlane, H. Piechuta, A.W. Ford-Hutchinson, M. Belley, R. Dehaven, R. Frenette, J.Y. Gauthier, S. Leger, S.S. Pong, J. Rokach, H. Williams, R.N. Young, and R. Zamboni, In vivo pharmacology of L-660,711, a potent and selective leukotriene antagonist, Fed. Proc., 2:A1265 (1988).

29. G.W. Carnathan, D. Sweeney, J. Travis, and R.G. Van Inwegen, The effect of RG 12525 on leukotriene D_4-mediated pulmonary responses in guinea pigs, Inflammation Research Association, Fourth International Conference: A67 (1988).

30. J.G. Gleason, R.F. Hall, C.D. Perchonock, K.F. Erhard, J.S. Frazee, T.W. Ku, K. Kondrad, M.E. McCarthy, S. Mong, S.T. Crooke, G. Chi-Russo, M.A. Wasserman, T.J. Torphy, R.M. Muccitelli, D.W. Hay, S.S. Tucker, and L. Vickery-Clark, High-affinity leukotriene receptor antagonists. Synthesis and pharmacological characterization of 2-Hydroxy-3-[(2-carboxyethyl)thio]-3-[2-(8-phenyloctyl) phenyl] propanoic acid, J. Med. Chem., 30:959 (1987).

31. D.W.P. Hay, R.M. Muccitelli, S.S. Tucker, L.M. Vickery-Clark, K.A. Wilson, J.G. Gleason, R.F. Hall, M.A. Wasserman, and T.J. Torphy, Pharmacologic profile of SK&F 104353: A novel, potent and selective peptidoleukotriene receptor antagonist in guinea pig and human airways, J. Pharmacol. Exp. Ther., 243:474 (1987).

32. D.W. Snyder, R.E. Giles, R.A. Keith, Y.K. Yee, and R.D. Krell, In vitro pharmacology of ICI 198,615: A novel, potent and selective peptide leukotriene antagonist, J. Pharmacol. Exp. Ther., 243:548 (1987).

33. C. Buckner, J. Fedyna, R. Krell, J. Robertson, R. Keith, V. Matassa, F. Brown, P. Bernstein, Y. Yee, J. Will, R. Fishleder, R. Saban, B. Hesp, and R. Giles, Antagonism by ICI 204,219 of leukotriene receptors in guinea pig and human airways, Fed. Proc., 2:A1264 (1988).

34. T. Obata, F. Nambu, T. Kitagawa, H. Terashima, M. Toda, T. Okegawa, and A. Kawasaki, ONO-1078: An antagonist of leukotrienes, "Advances in Prostaglandin, Thromboxane and Leukotriene Research", 17:540 (1987).

35. N. Barnes, P.J. Piper, and J. Costello, The effect of an oral leukotriene antagonist L-649,923 on histamine and leukotriene D_4-induced bronchoconstriction in normal man, J. Allergy Clin. Immunol., 79:816 (1987).

36. J. Biollaz, E. Stahl, J.Y. Hsieh, L. Distlerath, A. Jaeger, P. Leuenberger, and J.L. Schelling, Tolerability and pharmacokinetics of L-648,051, a leukotriene antagonist, in healthy volunteers, Eur. J. Clin. Pharmacol., 33:603 (1988).

37. G.D. Phillips, P. Raggerty, C. Robinson, and S.T. Holgate, Dose-related antagonism of leukotriene D_4-induced bronchoconstriction by p.o. administration of LY-171883 in nonasthmatic subjects, <u>J. Pharmacol. Exp. Ther.</u>, 246:732 (1988).

38. N. Barnes, J. Evans, J. Zakrzewski, P. Piper, and J. Costello, Pharmacology and physiology of leukotriene and their antagonists, <u>Ann. N. Y. Acad. Sci.</u>, 524:369 (1988).

39. J.M. Evans, N.C. Barnes, J.T. Zabrzewski, H.P. Glenny, P.J. Piper, and J.F. Costello, The activity of an inhaled leukotriene (LT) antagonist (SKF 104,353-Z_2) on LTD_4-induced bronchoconstriction in normal man, <u>Br. J. Clin. Pharmacol.</u>, 26:P61 (1988).

40. J.R. Britton, S.P. Hanley, and A.E. Tattersfield, The effect of an oral leukotriene D_4 antagonist L-649,923 on the response to inhaled antigen in asthma, <u>J. Allergy Clin. Immunol.</u>, 79:811 (1987).

41. E. Israel, E.F. Juniper, M.M. Morris, A.R. Dowell, F.E. Hargreave, and J.M. Drazen, A leukotriene D_4 (LTD_4) receptor antagonist, LY171883, reduces the bronchoconstriction induced by cold air challenge in asthmatics: a randomized, double-blind, placebo controlled trial, <u>Am. Rev. Respir. Dis.</u>, 137:A27 (1988).

42. J.H. Fleisch, M.L. Cloud, and W.S. Marshall, A brief reveiw of preclinical and clinical studies with LY171883 and some comments on newer cysteinyl leukotriene receptor antagonists, <u>Ann. N. Y. Acad. Sci.</u>, 524:356 (1988).

43. P.N. Mathur, J.T. Callaghan, N.A. Farid, and A.J. Sylvester, The prevention of allergen induced late asthmatic response by LY171883 a leukotriene antagonist, <u>Clin. Res.</u>, 34:580A (1986).

44. Z.-I. Tereshita, S. Tsushima, Y. Yoshioka, H. Nomura, Y. Inada, and K. Nishikawa, CV-3988 - a specific antagonist of platelet activating factor (PAF), <u>Life Sci.</u>, 32:1975 (1983).

45. Z.-I. Terashita, Y. Imura, and K. Nishikawa, Inhibition by CV-3988 of the binding of [^{3}H]-platelet activating factor (PAF) to the platelet, <u>Biochem. Pharmacol.</u>, 34:1491 (1985).

46. Z.-I. Terashita, Y. Imura, M. Takatani, S. Tsushima, and K. Nishikawa, CV-6209, a highly potent antagonist of platelet activating factor in vitro and in vivo, <u>J. Pharmacol. Exp. Ther.</u>, 242:263 (1987).

47. V. Lagente, S. Desquand, P. Hadvary, M. Cirino, A. Lellouch-Tubiana, J. Lefort and B.B. Vargaftig, Interference of the PAF antagonist Ro 19-3704 with PAF and antigen-induced bronchoconstriction in the guinea-pig, <u>Br. J. Pharmacol.</u>, 94:27 (1988).

48. D.A. Handley, R.C. Anderson, and R.N. Saunders, Inhibition by SRI

63-072 and SRI 63-119 of PAF-acether and immune complex effects in the guinea pig, Eur. J. Pharmacol., 141:409 (1987).

49. V. Lamant, G. Mauco, P. Braquet, H. Chap, and L. Douste-Blazy, Inhibition of the metabolism of platelet activating factor (PAF-acether) by three specific antagonists from Ginkgo biloba, Biochem. Pharmacol., 36:2749 (1987).

50. B.F. Omini, G. Rossoni, and P. Braquet, Protection by two ginkgolides, BN-52020 and BN-52021, against guinea-pig lung anaphy-laxis, Pharmacol. Res. Commun., 18:775 (1986).

51. T.Y. Shen, S.B. Hwang, M.N. Chang, T.W. Doebber, M.H. Lam, M.S. Wu, and X. Wang, The isolation and characterization of kadsurenone from haifenteng (Piper futokadsura) as an orally active specific receptor antagonist of platelet-activating factor, Int. J. Tissue React., 7:339 (1985).

52. S.-B. Hwang, M.-H. Lam, T. Biftu, T.R. Beattie, and T.-Y. Shen, Trans-2,5-Bis-(3,4,5-trimethoxyphenyl) tetrahydrofuran. An orally active specific and competitive receptor antagonist of platelet activating factor, J. Biol. Chem., 260:15639 (1985).

53. S.-B. Hwang, M.-H. Lam, A.W. Alberts, R.L. Bugianesi, J.C. Chabala, and M.M. Ponpipom, Biochemical and pharmacological characterization of L-659,989: an extremely potent, selective and competitive recep-tor antagonist of platelet-activating factor, J. Pharmacol. Exp. Ther., 246:534 (1988).

54. R.N. Saunders, R.G. Van Valen, M.K. Melden, W.J. Houlihan, and D.A. Handley, Pharmacology of the PAF antagonist SDZ 64-142, Fed. Proc., 2:A412 (1988).

55. J. Casals-Stenzel, Triazolodiazepines are potent antagonists of platelet activating factor (PAF) in vitro and in vivo, Naunyn Schmiedebergs Arch. Pharmacol., 335:351 (1987).

56. H. Mikashima, S. Takehara, Y. Muramoto, T. Khomaru, M. Terasawa, T. Tahara, and Y. Maruyama, An antagonistic activity of etizolam on platelet-activating factor (PAF). In vitro effects on platelet aggregation and PAF receptor binding, Jpn. J. Pharmacol., 44:387 (1987).

57. J. Casals-Stenzel, G. Muacevic, and K.-H. Weber, Pharmacological actions of WEB 2086, a new specific antagonist of platelet activat-ing factor, J. Pharmacol. Exp. Ther., 241:974 (1987).

58. G. Muacevic, W. Stransky, and K.H. Weber, Antagonism of PAF-induced bronchoconstriction and intrathoracic accumulation of platelets in the guinea pig by the hetrazepines WEB 2170 and STY 2108, Naunyn Schmiedebergs Arch. Pharmacol., 337[Suppl.]:R88 (1988).

59. H. Heuer, Activity of the hetrazepines WEB 2170 and STY 2108, two new and potent PAF-antagonists on PAF-induced changes in vitro and endotoxin or PAF-induced hypotension in the rat, Naunyn Schmiedebergs. Arch. Pharmacol., 337[Suppl.]:R70 (1988).

60. M. O'Donnell, H. Crowley, B. Yaremko and A. Welton, Pharmacological Profile of Ro 24-0238, a novel compound with dual actions: PAF receptor antagonism and thromboxane A_2 synthase inhibition, Am. Rev. Respir. Dis., in press (1989).

61. J. Lefort, P. Sedivy, S. Desquand, J. Randon, E. Coëffier, I. Maridonneau-Parini, A. Floch, J. Benveniste and B.B. Vargaftig, Pharmacological profile of 48740 R.P., a PAF-acether antagonist, Eur. J. Pharmacol., 150:257 (1988).

62. J. Arnout, A. van Hecken, I. deLepeleire, Y. Miyamoto, I. Holmes, P. deSchepper, and J. Vermylen, Effectiveness and tolerability of CV-3988, a selective PAF antagonist, after intravenous administration to man, Br. J. Clin. Pharmacol., 25:445-451 (1988).

63. W.S. Adamus, H. Heuer, C.J. Meade, E.R. Kempe, and H.M. Brecht, Effect of intravenous or inhalative WEB 2086 on ex vivo platelet activating factor induced platelet aggregation in man, Prostaglandins, 35:797 (1988).

64. W.S. Adamus, H. Heuer, C.J. Meade, and H.M. Brecht, Effect of peroral WEB 2086 on ex vivo platelet activating factor induced platelet aggregation in man, Prostaglandins, 35:836 (1988).

65. J.L. Pinquier, P. Sedivy, R. Bruno, F. Gaisne, A. Opriou, F. Bompart, D. deLauture, G. Strauch, and J. Grégoire, Tolerance study, pharmacokinetics and ex vivo PAF-induced platelet aggregation after repeated oral doses of 48740 RP in normal volunteers, Prostaglandins, 35:837 (1988).

66. P. Guinot, P. Braquet, J. Duchier, and A. Cournot, Inhibition of PAF-acether induced weal and flare reaction in man by a specific PAF antagonist, Prostaglandins, 32:160 (1986).

67. K.F. Chung, M. McCusker, C.P. Page, G. Dent, Ph. Guinot, and P.J. Barnes, Effect of a ginkgolide mixture (BN 52063) in antagonising skin and platelet responses to platelet activating factor in man, Lancet, 1:248 (1987).

68. P. Guinot, C. Brambilla, J. Duchier, P. Braquet, B. Bonvoisin, and A. Cournot, Effect of BN 52063, a specific PAF-acether antagonist, on bronchial provocation test to allergens in asthmatic patients. A preliminary study, Prostaglandins, 34:723 (1987).

69. D.W.P. Hay, R.M. Muccitelli, L.M. Vickery-Clark, K.A. Wilson, L. Bailey, S.S. Tucker, L.P. Yodis, R.D. Eckardt, J.F. Newton, J.M.

Smallheer, M.E. McCarthy, J.G. Gleason, M.A. Wasserman, and T.J. Torphy, Pharmacological profile of SKF S-106203, a novel leukotriene (LT) receptor antagonist, in guinea-pig airways, The Pharmacologist, 30:A96 (1988).

$9\alpha,11\beta$-PROSTAGLANDIN F_2: A NEW PROSTANOID, THAT INHIBITS PLATELET AGGREGATION AND CONSTRICTS BLOOD VESSELS

Xiao Rong He, Charles Polsen and Patrick Y-K. Wong

Departments of Pharmacology, New York Medical College
Valhalla, New York 10595

INTRODUCTION

Nugteren and Hazelhof (1)were the first to report the formation of PGD_2 from endoperoxides (PGG_2 and PGH_2). Subsequently, PGD_2 was found to be one of the major products of arachidonic acid cascade in many tissue and cell types (2). Since then the transformation of PGH_2 to PGD_2 has been demonstrated in brain homogenates (3,4) and neuroblastoma cells (5). The enzyme PGD_2 synthetase, which catalyzed the conversion of PGH_2 to PGD_2, has been purified to homogeneity and clearly distinguished from that of glutathione-S-transferase(6). It has been reported that PGD_2 is released by platelets during aggregation (7) and was found to be a potent inhibitor of platelet aggregation, with a potency only less than that of prostacyclin (PGI_2) and its stable biologically active metabolite, 6-keto-PGE_1 (8,9). The metabolism of prostaglandin D_2 in the monkey has been reported by Ellis et al. (10), who found that more than two-thirds of the PGD_2 metabolites have the cyclopentane 1,3-diol ring structure ($PGF_{2\alpha}$). These workers postulated the existence of an enzyme 11-ketoreductase which may have converted the infused PGD_2 to $PGF_{2\alpha}$ before it was further degraded by 15-hydroxyprostaglandin dehydrogenase and β-oxidation. Subsequently, Wong (11) and Wantanabe et al. (12) independently reported the isolation and purification of the enzyme 11-ketoreductase from the rabbit liver and rat lung. Recently, Liston and Roberts (13) reported that the transformation of PGD_2 in human subjects was similar to that found in the monkey. This biotransformation is catalyzed primarily by 11-ketoreductase, reducing PGD_2 to various F-type (1,3-diol ring structure) metabolites with a stereochemistry different from that of $PGF_{2\alpha}$ ($9\alpha,11\beta,15$-L trihydroxyprosta-5-cis,13-transdienoic acid). Furthermore, the same group characterized F-type metabolite generated by human liver in the presence of NADPH as a cofactor and named this new metabolite as $9\alpha,11\beta$-PGF_2 (13). In this chapter we report the metabolic fate of exogenous [^{3}H]PGD_2 in the isolated perfused rabbit liver. Using a recirculating system (two passes), we identified the new prostanoid $9\alpha,11\beta$-PGF_2 as the major product. Structural elucidation of this new prostanoid was accomplished by gas chromatography/mass spectrometry and chemical methods. The biological activity profile of $9\alpha,11\beta$-PGF_2 was found to be different from PGD_2 and $PGF_{2\alpha}$. It is an inhibitor of platelet aggregation and contracts canine coronary artery strips. Thus, the metabolic transformation of PGD_2 to $9\alpha,11\beta\text{-}PGF_2$ represents a potential pathway for the generation of a biologically active prostanoid in the hepatic circulation.

EXPERIMENTAL PROCEDURES

Male New Zealand rabbits were anesthetized with ketamine hydro-chloride (50 mg/kg) intramuscularly. After midline laparotomy, the liver was exposed, the lieno-gastric vein was tied off, and the portal vein was cannulated. The liver was flushed with Tyrode's solution, removed from the animal, and placed in a humidified and thermostatically controlled chamber. The liver was perfused through the portal vein with oxygenated Tyrode's solution, ($37^{\circ}C$) at a rate of 10 ml/min using a Watson-Marlow roller pump, as previously described (14). $[^3H]PGD_2$ ($8\mu Ci/7.4\ \mu M$) in 100 μl of absolute ethanol was injected into the portal cannula over 3 min. Effluents were collected during administration and thereafter for an additional 20 min. After recirculating twice the final perfusate was collected in a 500-ml Erlenmeyer flask and immersed in an ice bath.

Extraction and Purification

The perfusate was acidified with 1N formic acid to pH 3.5 and extracted three times with an equal volume of ethyl acetate. Extracts were combined and evaporated to dryness under N_2. The crude extract was then dissolved in 2 ml. of 15% EtOH and loaded onto a C-18 Sep-Pak cartridge for further purification as described previously by Powell (15). The methyl formate fraction which contained over 90 ± 1.2% of the radioactivity recovered from the perfusate was dried under a stream of N_2. The residue was redissolved in 100 μl of acetone and separated on a TLC plate (Brinkman, 2.5 mm x 25 cm) comigrating with authentic PGD_2, PGE_2, and $PGF_{2\alpha}$ standards. The TLC plate was developed twice with the organic phase of isooctane/ethyl acetate/acetic acid/water (25:55:10:55, v/v). Radioactive products were detected on a Packard radiochromatogram scanner, Model 7201. Radioactive zones comigrating with authentic standards were scraped from the TLC plate and extracted three times with methanol.

High Performance Liquid Chromatography

The materials recovered from TLC plates were dried under N_2 and then separated using an ODS ultrasphere C18 column (5μm, 10 mm x 25 cm, Beckman Instruments) with a solvent system of $CH_3CN:H_2O$ (35:65, v/v), pH 2.95, at a flow rate of 1 ml/min. Simultaneously, the radioactive fractions were collected every minute with an on-line fraction collector. Radioactivity of each fraction was assessed by liquid scintillation counting.

Gas Chromatography-Mass Spectrometry (GC-MS)

The substances recovered after RP-HPLC purification were dried under N_2. A portion of the resultant lipid extract was methyl-esterified with diazomethane in ether:methanol (9:1) and subsequently treated with methoxyamine HCl in pyridine (5mg/ml). Finally, the oxime esters were converted to trimethylsilyl (Me_3Si) esters by treatment with bistrimethylsilyl trifluoroacetamide to form methyloxime trimethylsilyl derivatives before analysis with GC-MS. Portions of the residue were also converted to the Me_3Si ester derivatives with bistrimethylsilyl trifluoroacetamide containing 1% trimethylchlorosilane. The reagent was

removed by evaporation under a stream of N_2 and the residue was
dissolved in a small aliquot of hexane before injection. GC-MS analysis
was carried out with a HP5895-B mass spectrometer. The 6-foot
Chromosorb (HP) column with 1% SE-30 was kept at 210°C, the flow at 40
ml/min, the injector temperature at 260°C, and the ion source at
200°C. Electron energy was 70 eV.

Bioassay

HPLC fractions corresponding to $9\alpha,11\beta$-PGF$_2$ were collected
and dried under N_2 for bioassay. The residue was resuspended in a
small volume of 0.9% saline and tested for musculotropic activity on
Krebs superfused canine coronary arteries.

Platelet Aggregation: Platelet aggregation studies were performed with
0.5-ml aliquots of platelet rich plasma (PRP) kept at 37°C and stirred
at 1200 rpm in a dual-channel Payton aggregation module and transcribed
on a linear recorder (Payton Associates, Buffalo, NY). The
concentration of $9\alpha,11\beta$-PGF$_2$, needed to inhibit platelet
aggregation was determined for each batch of PRP. This dose was used
throughout the experiments to inhibit aggregation induced by ADP
(3-10μM) and by thrombin (0.8-1.0 unit /ml). $9\alpha,11\beta$-PGF$_2$
was stored in dry acetone (1mg/ml) at -25°C and diluted with saline
before use.

RESULTS AND DISCUSSION

Figure 1A shows a typical radiochromatogram scan of a radioactive
product extracted from rabbit liver perfusate (N =4) . Two major
radioactive products (zone I and II) were detected. Zone I (R_F =
0.43) migrated ahead of authentic PGF$_{2\alpha}$ standard (R_F = 0.38),
and zone II (R_F = 0.77). Zones I an II represent 41 $\pm$ 1.6% and 54 $\pm$
1.4% of the recovered radioactivity, respectively. RP-HPLC purification
of the material in zone I revealed one major radioactive peak, compound
"A" (retention time 10.2 min), which eluted earlier than PGF$_{2\alpha}$
standard (retention time similar to that of authentic PGD$_2$ standard
(15.0 min).

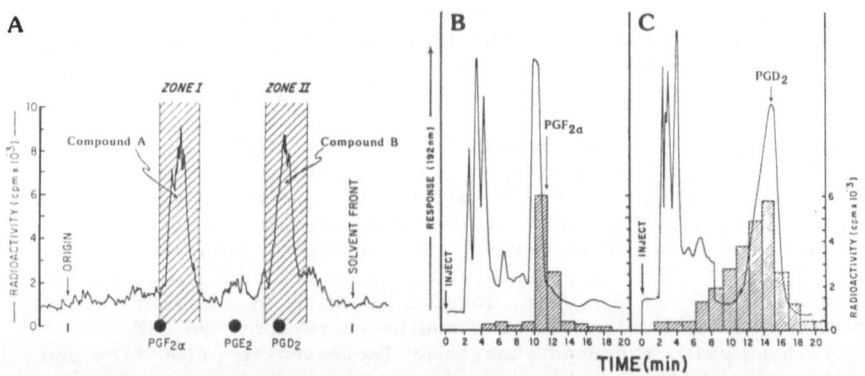

Fig. 1. Radiochromatograph scan and HPLC analysis of radioactive
products from rabbit liver after infusions of [^{3}H]PGD$_2$-A, the
perfusate was acidified with 1 N HCl to pH 3.5 and extracted three times
with equal volumes of ethyl acetate. The ethyl acetate fraction was
vacuum-evaporated to dryness. The residue was redissolved in 100 μl
of acetone, applied to a thin-layer chromatographic plate, and developed
(continued)

Gas chromotography analysis of compound A gave a C-value of 24.8. The mass spectrum of the methyl ester Me_3Si derivative of compound A showed the major fragment ions at m/z 584 [M^+], 569 [M - 15], 513 [M - 71], 494 [M -90], 423 [M -(90 + 71)], 333 [M -(2 x 90 + 71)], 307 [423 - 116], 217 [307 - 90], 191 base peak [$Me_3SiO=CH-OSiMe_3$], 173 [M - ($Me_3SiO^+=CH-C_{16}-C_{20}$)], 147, and 129. The mass spectrum was identical to that reported for the Me_3Si derivative of 9,11,15-tri-hydroxyprosta-5,13-dienoic acid (13). Further structural confirmation was provided by the failure of compound A to react with n-butylboronic acid to form n-butylboronic ester (16). This experiment suggests that compound A contains 1,3-trans-hydroxy groups at C-9 and C-11. Assuming the stereochemistry of the α-hydroxy group of PGD_2 is invariant during passage through the liver, the additional hydroxy at C-11 should be in the B position. Thus, compound A should be 9α, 11β,15-L-trihydroxyprosta-5-cis,13-trans-dienoic acid, (9α, 11β-PGF_2). Compound B (Fig. 1C), purified by HPLC, was subsequently identified by GC/MS to be PGD_2. In addition, incubation of [^{3}H]PGD_2 with purified 11-ketoreductase from rabbit liver also resulted in the generation of [^{3}H]9_α,11_β-PGF_2. However, under similar conditions incubation of [^{3}H]PGH_2 with 11-ketoreductase failed to produce any detectable amount of [^{3}H]9_α,11_β-PGF_2.

These data suggest a selective synthetic route for this compound, that is, exclusive conversion via the 11-ketoreductase from PGD_2 (Fig. 3.).

When testing for biological activity, 9_α,11_β-PGF_2 inhibited ADP (6 to 10 μM) induced platelet aggregation in a dose-dependent manner (Fig.4, A and B) (N = 3). 9_α,11_β-PGF_2 also disaggregated clumped platelets dose-dependently (Fig. 4C). The antiaggregatory activity of 9_α,11_β-PGF_2 was approximately 40-fold less than its parent compound, PGD_2, while isomer $PGF_{2\alpha}$ had no effect on platelet aggregation (Fig. 4D). Vascular smooth muscle contractile activity was determined by superfused canine coronary artery strips, which responded differently to 9_α,11_β-PGF_2, U46619 (epoxy - methano analog of PGH_2) PGD_2,and $PGF_{2\alpha}$. Both PGD_2 and $PGF_{2\alpha}$ at doses about 30 times higher than that of 9_α,11_β-PGF_2, elicited only slight contractile response in this tissue (Fig. 2E). To further define the biological activity of 9α,11β-PGF_2, with respect to kidney function, renal clearance studies were conducted in anesthetized male Sprague - Dawley rats. An abrupt and pronounced increases in urine flow and sodium excretion were observed upon administration of 9α,$11\beta PGF_2$ at a dose of 7.5 μg/min. Intravenous infusion of highlypurified 9α, 11β-PGF_2 (2,5 μg/min, n=9) elevated urine flow (28$\pm$6 μl/min, P>.05), urinary sodium/potassium (0.96$\pm$0.31, P<.05), hematocrit (0.5$\pm$0.3, volumes/100 ml, P <.05) and urinary sodium excretion (2.3$\pm$1.0 μEq/min). Similar responses but of greater magnitude were obtained with $PGF_{2\alpha}$ (2.5 μg/min). Glomerular filtration rate (GFR) and mean arterial pressure (MAP) were unaffected. In contrast, PGD_2 (2.5 μg/min) lowered MAP with concomitant reductions in GFR, urine flow and sodium excretion. 9α,11β-PGF_2 (2.5 μg,/min) produced consistent increases in urine flow and excretion of sodium and chloride in rats treated with meclofenamate, 2

---

twice with isooctane/ethyl acetate/acetic acid/water (25:55:10:50, v/v). Radioactive zones were identified by comparison with authentic standards. B and C, RP-HPLC chromatography of zone I and zone II recovered from TLC plates. UV absorption was monitored at 192 nm and radioactivity was assessed by liquid scintillation counting.

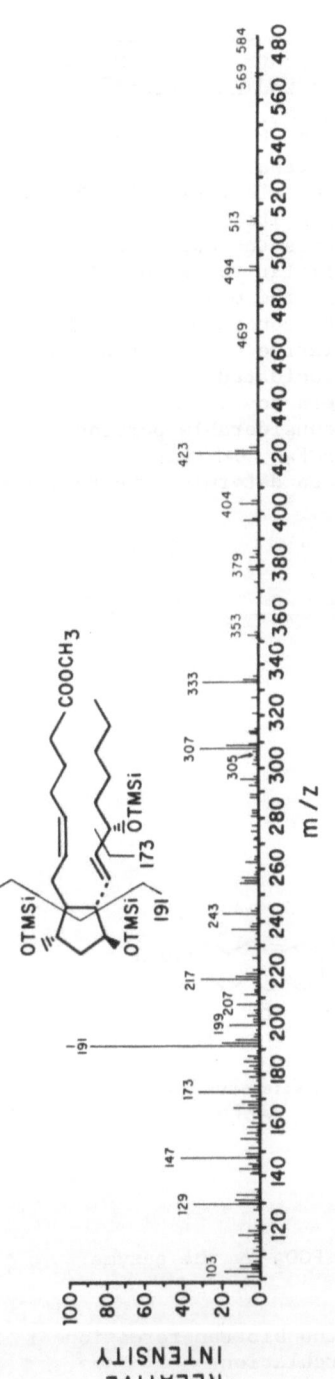

Fig. 2. Mass spectrum of the methyl ester trimethylsilyl derivatives of compound A (9α, 11β-PGF₂). OTMSi, methyl ester trimethylsilyl ester.

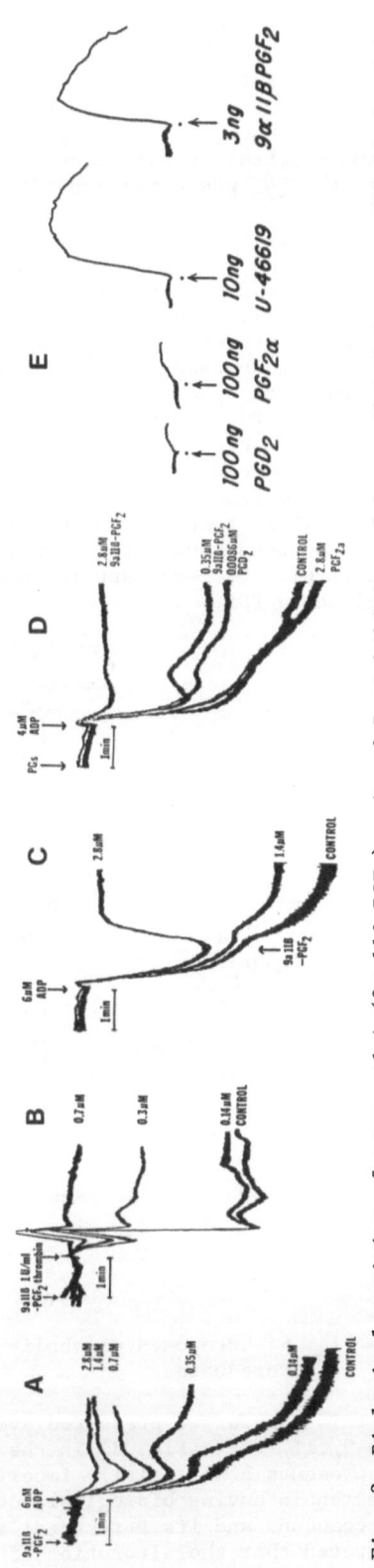

Fig. 3. Biological activity of compound A (9α,11β-PGF₂). A and B, inhibition of human platelet aggregation induced by ADP (4 μM) and thrombin (1.0 unit/ml), respectively. C, disaggregatory activity of 9α,11β-PGF₂. D, comparison of antiaggregatory activity of 9α,11β-PGF₂, PGF₂α and PGD₂. E, contractile activity of 9α,11β-PGF₂ on canine coronary artery strip compared with PGF₂α, PGD₂ and U-46619.

mg/kg/hr i.v., indicating that these responses were not dependent on endogenous PG synthesis (17). These results show that $9\alpha,11\beta$-PGF$_2$ and PGF$_{2\alpha}$ promotes the excretion of sodium and water via a mechanism not involved in the elevation of GFR or MAP. The changes noted in these experiments and the ability of these F series PGs to be formed in vivo suggest that they may play a role in the regulation of water and electrolyte excretion in the rat. In contrast to PGD$_2$, we found that PGF$_{2\alpha}$ possesses considerable diuretic and natriuretic activity in the absence of increases in GFR and MAP. These observations in the rat, are consistent with the findings of Zook and Strandhoy (18) who reported that PGF$_{2\alpha}$ infused into the canine renal artery increased water and electrolyte excretion without altering MAP, GFR or renal blood flow. Thus, $9\alpha.11\beta$-PGF$_2$ differs from its biological PG precursor, PGD$_2$, in that it promotes the excretion of salt and water whereas its renal effects are similar to, albeit less potent, than its epimer, PGF$_{2\alpha}$. Since, PGF$_{2\alpha}$ is the major immunoreactive PG in rat urine, especially under conditions of high sodium (19) and high potassium intake (20), relative contribution of $9\alpha,11\beta$-PGF$_2$ to renal PG levels remains to be elucidated. However, as $9\alpha,11\beta$-PGF$_2$ crossreacts with antisera to PGF$_{2\alpha}$ (21) it is tempting to speculate that a considerable portion of this immunoreactive material may be $9\alpha,11\beta$-PGF$_2$. In this context it will be important in future studies to determine the relative level of these PGs.

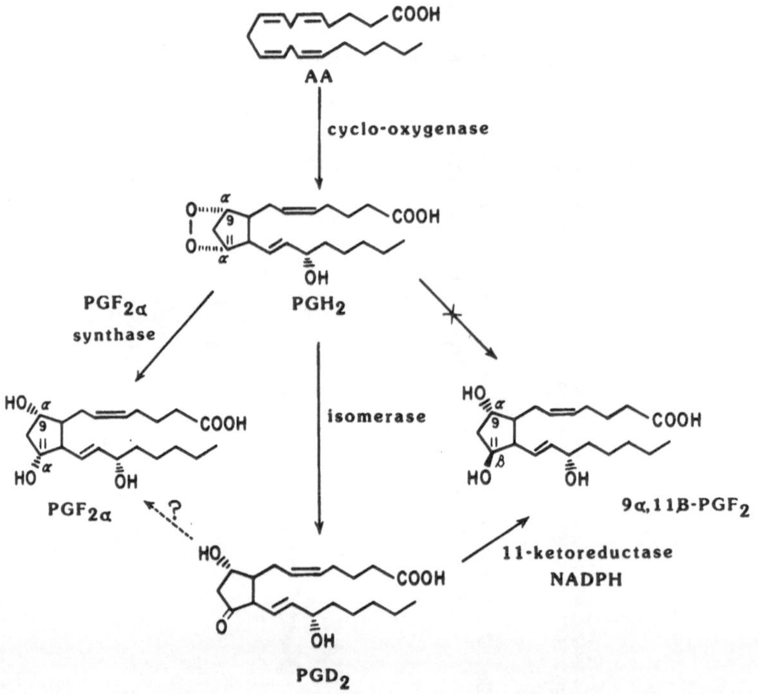

Fig. 4 - Proposed metabolic pathway of PGD$_2$ by the enzyme 11-ketoreductase

In this chapter we presented evidence for the biotransformation of PGD$_2$ to $9_\alpha,11_\beta$-PGF$_2$ (Fig. 3) in the hepatic circulation. This represents a potentially important pathway for the generation of a new prostanoid having biological activities distinct from those of its parent compound and its structural isomer, PGF$_{2\alpha}$. We also demonstrated that the alteration of the hydroxy group at C-11, of PGF$_{2\alpha}$ and $9_\alpha11_\beta$PGF$_2$ from an α and β position respectively, resulted in a change in antiaggregatory and musculotropic activities and renal function of this prostanoid. The formation of $9\alpha,11\beta$-PGF_2 and $PGF_{2\alpha}$ in vivo and the changes noted in these experiments suggest that these F series PGs may play a role in the regulation of water and electrolyte excretion in the rat. The physiological significance of this 11-ketoreductase metabolic pathway and the participation of $9_\alpha,11_\beta$-PGF_2 in cardiovascular system and in various diseased state remains to be defined.

REFERENCES

1. D.H. Nugteren and E. Hazelhof, Isolation and properties of intermediates in prostaglandin biosynthesis, Biochim. Biophys. Acta 326:448-461 (1973).
2. B. Samuelsson, M. Goldyne, E. Granstome, M. Hamberg, S. Hammarstrom and C. Malmsten, Prostaglandins and thromboxanes, Ann. Rev. Biochem. 47:997-1029 (1978).
3. M. Abdel-Halim, M. Hamberg, B. Sjoquist and E. Anggard, Identification of prostaglandin D_2 as a major prostaglandin in homogenates of rat brain, Prostaglandins 14:633-643 (1977).
4. F.F. Sun, J.P. Chapman and J.C. McGuire, Metabolism of prostaglandin endoperoxide in animal tissues, Prostaglandins 14:1055-1074 (1977).
5. T. Shimizu, N. Mizuro, T.Amano and O. Hayaishi, Prostaglandin D_2, a neuromodulator, Proc. Natl. Acad. Sci. U.S.A. 76:6231-6234 (1979).
6. E. Christ-Hazelhof and D.H. Nugteren, Purification and characterization of prostaglandin endoperoxide D-isomerase, a cytoplasmic, glutathione-requiring enzyme, Biochim. Biophys. Acta 572:43-51 (1979).
7. O. Oelz, R. Oelz, H.R. Knapp, B.J. Sweetman and J.A. Oates, Biosynthesis of prostagladnin D_2. 1. Formation of prostaglandin D_2 by human platelets, Prostaglandins 13:225-234 (1977).
8. G. DiMinno, M.J. Silver and G. DeGaetano, Prostaglandins as inhibitors of human platelet aggregation, Brit. J. Haemat. 43:637-647 (1979).
9. P.Y-K Wong, J.C. McGiff, F.F. Sun and W.H. Lee, 6-keto-prostaglandin E_1 inhibits the aggregation of human platelets, Europ. J. Pharmacol. 60:245-248 (1979).
10. C.K. Ellis, M.D. Smigel, J.A. Oates, O. Adz and B.J. Sweetman, Metabolism of prostaglandin D_2 in the monkey, J. Biol. Chem. 254:4152-4163 (1979).
11. P.Y-K Wong, Purification and partial characterization of prostaglandin D_2 11-keto-reductase in rabbit liver, Biochim. Biophys. Acta 659:169-178 (1981).
12. K. Watanabe, T. Shimiza and O. Hayaishi, Enzymatic conversion of prostaglandin D_2 to $F_{2\alpha}$ in the rat lung, Biochem. Int. 2:603-610 (1981).
13. T.E. Liston and L.J. Roberts II, Transformation of prostagladnin D_2 to $9\alpha,11\beta$-(15S)-trihydroxy-prosta-(5Z,13E)-dien-1-oic acid ($9\alpha,11\beta$-prostaglandin F_2): a unique biologically active prostaglandin produced enzymatically in vivo in humans, Proc. Natl. Acad. Sci. U.S.A. 82:6030-6034 (1985).
14. P.Y-K Wong, K.U. Malik, D.M. Desiderio, J.C. McGiff and F.F. Sun, Hepatic metabolism of prostacyclin (PGI_2) in the rabbit: formation of a potent novel inhibitor of platelet aggregation, Biochim. Biophys. Res. Commun. 93:486-494 (1980).
15. W.L. Powell, Rapid extraction of oxygenated metabolites of arachidonic acid from biological samples using octadecylsilyl silica, Prostaglandins 20:947-957 (1980).
16. C. Pace-Asciak and L.S. Wolfe, N-butylboronate derivatives of the F prostaglandins. Resolution of prostagladnins of the E and F series

by gas-liquid chromatography, J. Chromatogr. 56:129-135 (1971).

17. C.T. Stier, J. Roberts II and P.Y-K Wong, Renal response to 9α,11β-prostaglandin F_2 in the rat, J. Pharmacol. Exp. Therap. 243:487-491 (1987).

18. T.E. Zook and J.W. Strandhoy, Mechanisms of the natriuretic and diuretic effects of prostaglandin $F_{2\alpha}$, J. Pharmacol. Exp. Ther., 217:674-680 (1981).

19. D.F. Wendelborn, K. Seibert and J. Robert II, Isomeric prostaglandin F_2 compounds arising from prostaglandin D_2: a family of icosanoids produced in vivo in humans, Proc. Natl. Acad. Sci. U.S.A. 85:304-308 (1988).

20. A. Nasjletti, A. Erman, L.M. Cagen, D.P. Brooks, J.T. Crofton, L. Share and P.G. Baer, High potassium intake selectively increases urinary $PGF_{2\alpha}$ excretion in the rat, Am. J. Physiol. 248:F382-388 (1985).

STENOSIS AND VASCULAR DAMAGE AS AN EXPERIMENTAL MODEL OF ARTERIAL THROM-

BOSIS: A ROLE FOR PROSTANOIDS

Marco Prosdocimi

Fidia Research Laboratories
Via Ponte della Fabbrica, 3/A
35031 Abano Terme, Italy

INTRODUCTION

Arachidonic acid, a membrane bound fatty acid, is released following a variety of stimuli. Upon release the fatty acid undergoes a
series of reactions which may yield prostanoids. Prostanoids are potent
agents capable of eliciting profound effects within their immediate
environment. One such effect, the formation of an arterial thrombus, is
regulated by the interaction of the endothelium and subendothelium of
the blood vessel wall with platelets and white blood cells (de Gaetano
et al., 1986; Dejana, 1987; Prosdocimi et al., 1988a). Once activated,
platelets may aggregate to generate the thrombus, often formed in
patients with coronary atherosclerosis. This process may, in turn, lead
to an active phase of unstable angina or to a myocardial infarction (see
for review Fuster et al., 1988). In addition, it has been suggested that
the thrombotic process plays a major role in provoking cerebral and
peripheral ischemic pathology (Folts, 1980; Born et al., 1983; Kistler
et al., 1984; Fitzgerald et al. 1984; Hess et al., 1985). Thus, the
study of prostanoids in arterial thrombosis is an area of intensive
investigation. This article will focus on the role of two arachidonate
metabolites, prostacyclin and thromboxane, and the application of an
experimental model of arterial thrombosis induced by vessel wall damage
and flow alterations.

Several years ago, Folts et al. (1976) reported that a critical
stenosis of canine coronary artery, produced by a plastic cylinder
surrounding the vessel, causes cyclical variations of blood flow (CBFV).
Using the obstructive cylinder, blood flow may progressively drop to
zero, after which it may be restored by gently shaking the occluder, or
it may suddenly and spontaneously restore itself (Fig. 1). These original observations were subsequently confirmed by several groups working
in canine coronary artery (Uchida et al., 1980; Aiken et al., 1981; Bush
et al., 1984 a,b; Tada et al., 1984; Bolli et al., 1985; Prosdocimi et
al., 1985 a,b), in porcine coronary artery (Nichols et al., 1986), and
in other experimental systems (see below).

Degree of stenosis and extent of endothelial damage regulate the
appearance of CBFV. CBFV may cause myocardial ischemia with increased
lactate production (Prosdocimi et al., 1985a), ECG abnormalities
(Folts et al., 1976) and a reduced threshold for ventricular fibrilla-

tion (Kowey et al., 1983). The prominent role of platelets as the cause of vascular occlusion is suggested by angiographic examination (Folts et al., 1982), by the prevention of CBFV and occlusion by drugs which inhibit platelet activation (see below) and by the presence of a platelet thrombus at the site of stenosis in post mortem examination (Folts et al., 1976; Bush et al., 1984b; Ashton et al., 1986). In this experimental system the efficacy of a drug in preventing the formation of a thrombus can be estimated by observing its effect on CBFV: in other words, if CBFV are reduced or abolished one can assume that the drug under examination has reduced in vivo platelet aggregation, platelet interaction with the vessel wall or both. On the other hand, a "weak" general activation of platelets, like that obtained with epinephrine administration, may result in a more pronounced formation of the thrombus as indicated by more frequent and ample CBFV (Bertha and Folts, 1984).

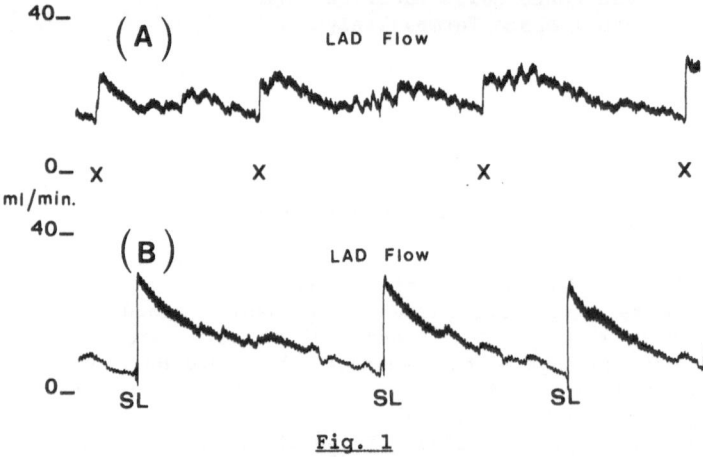

Fig. 1

Typical tracings of coronary blood flow in stenotized arteries in different experiments. Blood flow restoration occurred spontaneously (X) in one experiment (A), was induced by sliding the occluder (SL) in the other (B).

Many different agents have been studied in this experimental particular model and some of the relevant findings are summarized below. Acetylsalicylic acid (ASA) and other cyclooxygenase inhibitors are active anti-thombotics which may reduce or prevent CBFV. However, the degree of stenosis determines whether compounds of this class will be active in all animals tested (Folts et al., 1976) or only in some of them (Aiken et al., 1981; Prosdocimi et al., 1985b; Weselchouch et al. 1987). Moreover, simultaneous administration of epinephrine greatly reduces ASA efficacy (Folts and Rowe, 1988). Prostacyclin (PGI$_2$), whether infused locally or systemically, totally abolishs CBFV, though its action is of short duration (Aiken et al., 1981; Machleidt et al., 1985; Prosdocimi et al., 1985a). Other agents proven to be very effective anti-thrombotics are 5HT$_2$ receptor antagonists, especially ketanserin (Bush et al., 1984a, Busch 1987), and a monoclonal antibody against platelet glycoprotein IIb-IIIa (Coller et al., 1986).

Vasodilating agents like nitroglycerin, and papaverine, as well as dipyridamole and heparin are not effective (Folts et al., 1976; Bolli et al., 1985; Weselcouch et al., 1987), indicating that vasospasm and coagulation activation should not be considered major causes of vascular occlusion in this experimental model.

Several compounds of differing chemical structures have been developed as selective thromboxane (TX) synthase inhibitors. These compounds appear to be extremely active in preventing CBFV, regardless of the degree of stenosis (Uchida and Murao 1981; Aiken et al., 1981; Bush et al., 1984b). It is well known that ex vivo platelet aggregation is inhibited more by ASA than by TX synthase inhibitors; however, in this model, TX synthase inhibitors are much more effective than ASA in preventing CBFV. One might speculate that ASA should be used at low dose, in order to spare vascular prostacyclin synthesis. Although this is an interesting point, the "selectivity" of ASA is much more easily attained by oral route than by the intravenous route utilized in this model (Cerletti et al., 1986a), not allowing for a definitive response. Moreover, the fact that ASA efficacy is reduced when platelets are "primed" by epinephrine (Folts and Rowe, 1988) or when the thrombogenic challenge is increased by a more severe stenosis, suggests that its inefficacy might be due to insufficient platelet suppression. If so, it would be difficult to explain the powerful action of TX synthase inhibitors.

Indeed, there are several reasons to think that the efficacy of TX synthase inhibitors is due to their effect on platelet-vessel wall interaction, at least in canine models of arterial thrombosis. These reasons can be summarized as follows: i) in a dog model of arterial thrombosis the efficacy of TX synthase inhibitors is proportional to their stimulation of prostacyclin (Simpsom et al., 1986) ii) the efficacy of TX synthase inhibitors in reducing CBFV is greatly reduced if vessel cyclooxygenase is blocked (Uchida and Murao, 1981; Aiken et al., 1981) iii) despite the presence of coronary stenosis, dogs with high levels of 6-keto-PGF$_{1alpha}$ in the coronary sinus do not show CBFV (Tada et al., 1984).

It has been suggested that endoperoxides produced by platelets may be used to produce other prostanoids by the platelets themselves or by the vessel wall, particularly after TX synthase blockade (Marcus et al., 1980; Cerletti et al., 1986b; Papp et al., 1986). As an hypothesis, this kind of mechanism might explain the clear-cut reduction of CBFV observed by several authors with TX synthase. A question then arises: what is the relevance of this experimental model to a drug clinical response? Indeed there is no clear evidence that TX synthase inhibitors are clinically effective anti-thrombotic agents. A detailed discussion on this point is beyond the scope of this paper; however, it should be stressed that all the data here discussed were obtained during acute experiments with a single administration, while clinical trials on thombosis must rely on repeated chronic administration and much different end points.

Another drug which was found to be effective in preventing CBFV without decreasing vascular prostacyclin production is an experimental agent named AD$_6$. This compound decreases coronary CBFV but does not reduce the elevated 6-keto-PGF$_{1alpha}$ levels that can be found in cardiac venous blood during CBFV (Prosdocimi et al., 1985b). As this agent inhibits platelet aggregation (Galli et al., 1980; Prosdocimi et al., 1986; Zanetti et al., 1986) and may increase prostacyclin release from the vessel wall (Dejana et al., 1982; Petroni et al., 1985), its efficacy points out again the important role of platelet and vascular prostanoids in the formation of thrombotic occlusion in this particular experimental model.

It now seems appropriate to consider how different authors examined the synthesis of prostanoids within their experimental systems. In our experiments, we measured 6-keto-PGF$_{1alpha}$ and TXB$_2$ levels in the great cardiac vein after the left arterial descending coronary artery (LAD) was stenotized, taking the greatest care to avoid in vitro synthesis of TX (Prosdocimi et al., 1985a,b). Others have measured arterial plasma levels of the same prostanoids by cannulating the artery beyond the stenosis (Bush et al., 1984b). Tada et al. (1984), compared dogs with stenosis and no CBFV, to dogs with CBFV, and obtained plasma samples from the coronary sinus to estimate 6-keto-PGF$_{1alpha}$ and TXB$_2$. Using continuous electrical stimulus to induce the coronary thrombosis, Fitzgerald et al. (1987), in a chronic canine model, measured the urinary excretion of the stable end products of PGI$_2$ and TXA$_2$. Despite the differences in methodology, it appears that PGI$_2$ synthesis is increased in coronary circulation and can be estimated by local sampling. On the other hand, despite its clear role in promoting CBFV, an increased synthesis of TXA$_2$ might not be detected depending on the site of sampling and the method used. In any case, if one considers also the data obtained during complete coronary occlusion (Prosdocimi et al., 1988b), it is clear that a reduction of coronary blood flow increases PGI$_2$ release, a fact that should be considered in the evaluation of drugs to be used during ischemia.

An interesting extension of these findings is the possibility that the same mechanism, i.e., platelet activation induced by a stenotic damaged artery, may cause vascular occlusion in different arteries. It has been shown that carotid arteries may show CBFV after stenosis (Folts 1980; Coller et al., 1986); and we have recently characterized this phenomenon in dog femoral arteries (Prosdocimi et al., in press). Indeed it was found that the femoral preparation is quite similar to the coronary preparation in terms of CBFV appearance and of response to pharmacological intervention. Likewise, ASA prevented CBFV in 2/3 of the experiments, while PGI$_2$ or a TX synthase inhibitor were effective in every instance.

In vessels other than the coronary artery, endothelial damage in a site of reduced blood flow may trigger platelet aggregation and arterial occlusion, a process which can be reduced by drugs. Since platelet involvement in ischemic pathology of peripheral organs is not as well understood as that of coronary ischemic disease, these findings outline the possibility of extending to other areas what was found for the heart. From the data obtained in experimental models of arterial thrombosis, it appears that arachidonate metabolites in the platelets and the vessel wall may affect vascular occlusion. Data from clinical studies also show that pharmacological intervention in platelet activation may have important consequences for patients. Thus a challenge for the future will be to further expand our knowledge of the role of prostanoids, in order to develop pharmacological agents aimed at preventing thrombosis.

ACKNOWLEDGEMENTS

I wish to thank Barbara Corey for editorial assistance in preparing this manuscript.

REFERENCES

Aiken, J.W., Shebuski, R.J., Miller, O.V., and Gorman, R.R., 1981, Endogenous prostacyclin contributes to the efficacy of a thromboxane synthetase inhibitor for preventing coronary artery thrombosis, J. Pharmacol. Exp. Ther., 219:299.

Ashton, J.H., Schmitz, J.M., Campbell, W.B., Ogletree, M.L., Raheja, S., Taylor, A.L., Fitzgerald, C., Buja, L.M. and Willerson, J.T., 1986, Inhibition of cyclic flow variations in stenosed canine coronary arteries by thromboxane A$_2$/prostaglandin H$_2$ receptor antagonists, Circulations Res., 59:568.

Bertha, B.G., and Folts, J.D., 1984, Inhibition of epinephrine-exacerbated coronary thrombus formation by prostacyclin in the dog, J. Lab. Clin. Med., 103:204.

Bolli, R., Brandon, T.A., Mace, M.L., and Weilbaecher, D.G., 1985, Influence of alpha-adrenergic blockade on platelet mediated thrombosis in stenosed canine coronary arteries, Cardiovasc. Res., 19:146.

Born, G.V.R., Görög, P., and Begent, N.A., 1983, The biologic background to some therapeutic uses of aspirin, Am. J. Med., 14:2.

Bush, L.R., Campbell, W.B., Kern, K., Tilton, G.D., Apprill, P., Ashton, J., Schmitz, J., Buja, L.M., and Willerson, J.T., 1984a, The effects of alpha$_2$-adrenergic and serotoninergic antagonists on cyclic blood flow alterations in stenosed canine coronary arteries, Circ. Res., 55:642.

Bush, L.R., Campbell, W.B., Buja, L.M., Tilton, G.D., and Willerson, J. T., 1984b, Effects of the selective thromboxane synthetase inhibitor dazoxiben on variations in cyclic blood flow in stenosed canine coronary arteries, Circulation, 69:1161.

Bush, L.R., 1987, Effects of the serotonin antagonists, cyproheptadine, ketanserin and mianserin, on cyclic flow reductions in stenosed canine coronary arteries, J. Pharmacol. Exp. Ther., 240:674.

Cerletti, C., Gambino, M.C., Garattini, S., and de Gaetano, G., 1986a, Biochemical selectivity of oral versus intravenous aspirin in rats. Inhibition by oral aspirin of cyclooxygenase activity in platelets and presystemic but not systemic vessels, J. Clin. Invest., 78:323.

Cerletti, C., Minoldo, S., Bucchi, F., Del Maschio, A., and de Gaetano, G., 1986b, Requirement of ADP for arachidonic acid-induced platelet aggregation: studies with selective thromboxane-synthase inhibitors, Biochem. Pharmacol., 35:1201.

Coller, B.S., Folts, J.D., Scudder L.E., and Smith, S.R., 1986, Antithrombotic effect of a monoclonal antibody to the platelet glycoprotein IIb/IIIa receptor in an experimental animal model, Blood, 68:783.

De Gaetano, G., Cerletti, C., Dejana, E., and Vermylen, J., 1986, Current issues in thrombosis prevention with antiplatelet drugs, Drugs, 31:517.

Dejana, E., de Castellarnau, C., Balconi, G., Rotilio, D., Pietra, A., and de Gaetano, G., 1982, AD$_6$, a coronary dilating agent, stimulates PGI2 production in rat aorta ex vivo and in human endothelial cells in culture, Pharmacol. Res. Commun., 14:719.

Dejana, E., 1987, Endothelium, vessel injury and thrombosis, Haematologica, 72:89.

Fitzgerald, D.J., Smith, B., Pedersen, A.K., and Brash, A.L., 1984, Increased prostacyclin biosynthesis in patients with severe atherosclerosis and platelet activation, N. Engl. J. Med., 310:1065.

Fitzgerald, D.J., Wright, F., and Fitzgerald, G.A., 1987, Platelet-dependent reocclusion following coronary thrombolysis with tissue plasminogen activator. Clin. Res., 35:278A (Abstr.).

Folts, J.D., Crowell, E.D., and Rowe, G.G., 1976, Platelet aggregation in partially obstructed vessels and its elimination with aspirin, Circulation, 54:365.

Folts, J.D., 1980, Platelet aggregation in stenosed coronary or cerebral arteries: A mechanism for sudden death?, Wisc. Med. J., 79:24.

Folts, J.D., Gallagher, K., and Rowe, G.G., 1982, Blood flow reductions in stenosed canine coronary arteries: vasospasm or platelet aggregation? $\underline{Circulation.}$, 65:248.

Folts, J.D., and Rowe, G.G., 1988, Epinephrine potentiation of in vivo stimuli reverses aspirin inhibition of platelet thrombus formation in stenosed canine coronary arteries, $\underline{Thromb.\ Res.}$, 50:507.

Fuster, V., Badimon, L., Cohen, M., Ambrose, A., Badimon, J.J., and Chesebro, J., Insights into the pathogenesis of acute ischemic syndromes, $\underline{Circulation}$, 77:1213.

Galli, C., Agradi, E., Petroni, A., and Socini, A., 1980, effects of 8-monochloro-3-beta-diethylaminoethyl-4-methyl-7-ethoxy carbonyl methoxy coumarin (AD_6) on aggregation, arachidonic acid metabolism and thomboxane B_2 formation in human platelets, $\underline{Pharmacol.\ Res.\ Commun.}$, 12:329.

Hess, H., Mietaschk, A., and Deichsel, G., 1985, Drug-induced inhibition of platelet function delays progression of peripheral occlusive arterial disease, $\underline{Lancet}$, 1:415.

Kistler, J.P., Ropper, A.H., and Heros, R.C., 1984, Therapy of ischemic cerebral vascular disease due to atherothrombosis, $\underline{N.\ Engl.\ J.\ Med.}$, 31:27.

Kowey, P.R., Verrier, R.L., Lown, B., and Handin, R.I., 1983, Influence of intracoronary platelet aggregation on ventricular electrical properties during partial coronary artery stenosis, $\underline{Am.\ J.\ Cardiol.}$, 51:596.

Machleidt, C., Rose P., Mittmann, U., and Thomae K., 1985, Prevention of coronary platelet aggregation with a phosphodiesterase inhibitor RX-RA 69, $\underline{Throm.\ Res.}$, 37:595.

Marcus, A.J., Weksler, B.B., Jaffe, E.A., and Broekman, M.J., 1980, Synthesis of prostacyclin from platelet-derived endoperoxides by cultured human endothelial cells, $\underline{J.\ Clin.\ Invest.}$, 66:979.

Nichols, T.C., Bellinger, D.A., Johnson, T.A., Lamb, M.A., and Griggs, T.R., 1986, Von Willebrand's disease prevents occlusive thrombosis in stenosed and injured porcine coronary arteries, $\underline{Circ.\ Res.}$, 59:15.

Papp, A.C., Crowe, L., Pettigrew, L.C., and Wu, K.K., 1986, Production of eicosanoids by deendothelialized rabbit aorta: interaction between platelets and vascular wall in the synthesis of prostacyclin, $\underline{Thromb.\ Res.}$, 42:549.

Petroni, A., Socini, A., Blasevich, M., Borghi, A., Galli C., Differential effects of various vasoactive drugs on basal and stimulated levels of TXB_2 and $6\text{-ketoPGF}_{1alpha}$ in rat brain, $\underline{Prostaglandins}$, 29:579.

Prosdocimi, M., Finesso, M., Gorio, A., Languino, L.R., Del Maschio, A., Castagnoli, M.N., de Gaetano, G., and Dejana, E., 1985a, Coronary and systemic 6-ketoprostaglandin F_{1alpha} and thromboxane B_2 during myocardial ischemia in dog, $\underline{Am.\ J.\ Physiol.}$, 248:H-493.

Prosdocimi, M., Finesso, M., Tessari, F., Gorio, A., Languino, L.R., de Gaetano, G., and Dejana, E., 1985b, Inhibition by AD_6 (8-monochloro-3-beta-diethylaminoethyl-4-methyl-7- ethoxycarbonylmethoxy coumarin) of platelet aggregation in dog stenosed coronary artery, $\underline{Thromb.\ Res.}$, 39:399.

Prosdocimi, M., Zatta, A., Gorio, A., Zanetti, A., and Dejana, E., 1986, Action of AD_6 (8-monochloro-3-beta-diethylaminoethyl-4-methyl-7- -ethoxycarbonylmethoxy coumarin) on human platelets in vitro, $\underline{Naunyn\text{-}Schmiedeberg's\ Arch.\ Pharmacol.}$, 332:305.

Prosdocimi, M., Finesso, M., and Dejana, E., 1988a, A critical approach to the study of new agents for the prevention of arterial thrombosis: a comment, $\underline{Pharmacol.\ Res.\ Commun.}$, 20:1.

Prosdocimi, M., Finesso, M., Banzatto, N., Zanetti, A., de Gaetano, G., and Dejana, E., 1988b, Prostacyclin release in the coronary circulation during sustained stimulation in in vitro and in vivo experimental systems, $\underline{Thromb.\ Haemost.}$, 59:180.

Prosdocimi, M., Zatta, A., and Finesso, M., Stenosis and vascular damage as a cause of thrombosis in the dog femoral artery, Naunyn-Schmiedeberg's Arch. Pharmacol., in press.

Simpson, J.P., Smith, B.C., Rosenthal, G., and Lucchesi, R.B., 1986, Reduction in the incidence of thrombosis by the thromboxane synthetase inhibitor CGS 13080 in a canine model of coronary artery injury, J. Pharmacol. Exp. Ther., 238:497.

Tada, M., Esumi, K., Yamagishi, M., Kuzuya, T., Matsuda, H., Abe, H., Uchida, Y., and Murao, S., 1984, Reduction of prostacyclin synthesis as a possible cause of transient flow reduction in a partially constricted canine coronary artery, J. Mol. Cell Cardiol., 16:1137.

Uchida, Y., Yoshimoto, N., and Murao, S., 1980, Angiographic changes in the coronary artery associated with cyclical reductions of coronary blood pressure, JPN Circ. J., 44:163.

Uchida, Y., and Murao, S., 1981, Effects of thromboxane synthetase inhibitors on cyclical reduction of coronary blood flow in dogs, JPN Heart J., 22:971.

Weselcouch, O.E., Humphrey, W.R., and Aiken, J.W., 1987, Effects of low doses of aspirin and dipyridamole on platelet aggregation in the dog coronary artery, J. Pharmacol. Exp. Ther., 240:37.

Zanetti, A., Zatta, A., Prosdocimi, M., and Dejana, E., The effect of AD_6 (8-monochloro-3-beta-diethylamino-ethyl-4-methyl-7-ethoxycarbonylmethoxy coumarin) on washed human platelet aggregation induced by platelet activating factor (PAF) and epinephrine, Europ. J. Pharmacol., 128:119.

RENAL AND PLATELET EICOSANOIDS IN CHRONIC GLOMERULAR DISEASE

Carlo Patrono

Department of Pharmacology
Catholic University School of Medicine, Rome, Italy

INTRODUCTION

Eicosanoid is the generic term which refers to lipoxygenase and cyclooxygenase products of arachidonate metabolism. Prostaglandins (PG) and the other eicosanoids are autacoids which do not have a circulating, endocrine function but rather act in a paracrine or autocrine manner affecting cells close to or at the site of PG synthesis[1]. Nonsteroidal anti-inflammatory drugs (NSAD) inhibit either irreversibly (aspirin) or reversibly the cyclooxygenase enzyme which converts arachidonate to the PG-endoperoxides. Presently, no similar inhibitory agents are clinically available which inhibit the lipoxygenase enzymes converting arachidonate to leukotrienes and monohydroxy fatty acids. Although glucocorticoids can limit substrate availability through the induction of a recently characterized phospholipase A_2-inhibitory protein named lipocortin, their in vivo effects on endogenous PG production are rather inconsistent.

LOCALIZATION OF RENAL PROSTAGLANDIN SYNTHESIS

Eicosanoid synthesis in the kidney is localized to specific sites and is not uniformly present throughout the nephron[1]. Since the initial discovery of PG synthesis in the renal medulla, it has been recognized that the medullary tissue synthesizes greater amounts of PGs than the cortex. It is generally accepted that the regional heterogeneity of arachidonate metabolism, as well as the lack of vascular communications between the medulla and the cortex, dictate that PGs synthesized in the cortex (glomeruli and vasculature) regulate cortical function and PGs synthesized in the medulla (collecting tubule and medullary interstitial cells) regulate medullary function.[1] Table 1 summarizes the principal sites of PG synthesis in the kidney, the major PGs produced at each site, and their principal actions. Assessment of PG synthesis by different components of the nephron is based on immunofluorescent microscopy, separation of glomeruli and nephron segments with measurement of PG synthesis or by cell cultures of specific components of the nephron with measurements of eicosanoid turnover.[1,2] Some species variation exists and the majority of data are based on studies of rat, rabbit, and human kidney. In the cortex, the major sites of PG synthesis include arteries, arterioles and the glomerulus. The proximal tubule and the loop of Henle show little cyclooxygenase activity, but may convert arachidonate to several epoxygenase derivatives.[2] The large amounts of PGE_2 produced by the renal medulla primarily derive from the substantial biosynthetic activity of collecting tubule and interstitial cells. Eicosanoids synthesized within the kidney are either degraded in the kidney, by enzymes acting on the $\Delta 13,14$ double bond and on the hydroxyl group at C-15, or are removed from the kidney in the lymphatic and venous drainage or by excretion into the urine.[1]

Table 1. Principal renal sites of prostaglandin synthesis and major actions.

Site	Eicosanoid	Action
Vasculature	PGI_2	Vasodilation
Glomerulus	PGI_2, PGE_2 TXA_2	Maintain GFR Reduce GFR*
Collecting tubule	PGE_2, $PGF_{2\alpha}$	Enhance excretion of NaCl and water
Medullary interstitial cells	PGE_2	Vasodilation and natriuresis-diuresis

* TXA_2 reduces GFR in pathophysiologic situations such as glomerulonephritis, transplant rejection, and ureteral obstruction.

Reproduced from Patrono and Dunn, Kidney Int 1987; 32:1-12, (ref. 3) with permission.

ASSESSMENT OF GLOMERULAR EICOSANOID BIOSYNTHESIS

Largely indirect evidence supports the notion that the urinary excretion of primary unmetabolized eicosanoids, including TXB_2, may represent a fraction of intrarenal eicosanoid production.[3] The evidence concerning urinary TXB_2, as obtained in humans, derives from infusion studies of exogenous TXB_2 in healthy subjects,[4] from the investigation of patients with lupus nephritis[5] and from pharmacologic studies of selective and non-selective cyclooxygenase inhibitors in health and disease.[3] These human studies have measured the urinary excretion of TXB_2 and 2,3-dinor-TXB_2, a major derivative of the ß-oxidation pathway of systemic TXB_2 metabolism, and have demonstrated a dissociation of their excretory pattern possibly suggestive of a renal vs extra-renal origin. No information of similar nature is available in animal studies, even though measurements of urinary TXB_2 have been used extensively in rat and murine models of glomerular disease. Thus, the inference made in the latter studies that urinary TXB_2 may reflect intrarenal TXA_2 production is largely speculative and not supported by the appropriate experimental evidence.

Measurement of ex vivo glomerular TXB_2 production in response to added substrate or other stimuli, represents a capacity-related index conceptually similar to the measurement of serum TXB_2 i.e. platelet TXB_2 production in response to endogenously formed thrombin.[6] These measurements have been used extensively to monitor disease-associated changes in glomerular PG-endoperoxide metabolism. The relationship of enhanced glomerular TXB_2 production, as detected ex vivo, to the actual rate of TXA_2 biosynthesis in vivo remains, however, to be defined. Perhaps more importantly than a quantitative assessment, measurement of eicosanoid production in isolated glomeruli may provide useful information on qualitative differences in disease-related expression of PG-endoperoxide metabolism, possibly reflecting changes in the cellular source(s) of a particular eicosanoid (e.g. TXA_2) or the biochemical cooperation between resident and infiltrating cells.

URINARY PROSTAGLANDIN AND THROMBOXANE B_2 EXCRETION IN CHRONIC GLOMERULAR DISEASE

A number of studies have addressed the issue of urinary PGE_2 excretion in chronic renal disease (reviewed in ref. 7). With the exception of patients with severe renal failure (inulin clearance less than 25 ml per minute) in whom the excretion rate of PGE_2 was profoundly diminished[7] and patients with systemic lupus erythematosus (SLE) in whom urinary PGE_2 excretion was moderately increased,[8] most patients with mild to moderate renal failure were described as having normal excretory rates.[7] The inclusion of male patients in some of these studies is a potentially confounding factor, in view of the highly variable and unpredictable origin (i.e. renal versus seminal) of PGE_2 in male urine.[9]

In a study of 20 healthy women and 16 female patients with biopsy-diagnosed chronic glomerulonephritis (creatinine clearance: 110±5 and 91±19 ml/minute/1.73 m^2 respectively; mean±SD), Ciabattoni et al.[10] found that control subjects and patients excreted PGE_2 at almost identical rates, i.e. 7.6±2.7 versus 7.4±2.4 ng per hour. Although urinary PGE_2 excretion was significantly increased in a group of 23 female patients with SLE nephritis, only eight patients (six with active renal lesions) had urinary PGE_2 excretion in excess of two standard deviations of the normal mean.[5] In most of these studies, the urinary excretion of PGE_2 did not correlate with any of the measured parameters of cortical or medullary function to a statistically significant extent, in either patients or control subjects. An entirely novel finding of Ciabattoni et al.[10] was the demonstration of a significantly reduced excretion of 6-keto-$PGF_{1\alpha}$ in female patients with chronic glomerular disease, including SLE nephropathy. In SLE patients with active renal lesions, the reduction was greater than 50 percent,[5] i.e. similar to that which is inducible by the administration of a relatively high dose of aspirin in healthy women.[11] In these patients, the urinary excretion of 6-keto-$PGF_{1\alpha}$ showed a statistically significant positive correlation with both the glomerular filtration rate and renal blood flow.[5] That such a biochemical change is not a consequence of a chronic immune disease process is indicated by the finding of a normal excretion rate of 6-keto-$PGF_{1\alpha}$ in a group of 25 age-matched female patients with rheumatoid arthritis (Ciabattoni, Caruso, and Patrono, unpublished observations). Although the reduced excretion of the PGI_2 hydration product in chronic glomerular disease may have reflected a reduced glomerular mass available for PGI_2 synthesis, this appears to be unlikely inasmuch as TXB_2, the second most abundant cyclooxygenase product in human glomeruli, was excreted at a normal rate or at an accelerated rate under the same circumstances.[5]

Urinary TXB_2 excretion is markedly enhanced in SLE patients but not in patients with other forms of chronic glomerular disease.[5] Moreover, patients with active renal lesions differ significantly from those with inactive lesions by having a two-fold higher TXB_2 excretion rate.[5] A non-platelet intrarenal source of enhanced TXA_2 production was suggested by the unaltered ex vivo and in vivo indices of platelet TXB_2 production.[5] Interestingly, the ex vivo renal synthesis of TXB_2 is also increased in the MRL-lpr and NZBxW mice with spontaneous lupus nephritis.[12] As in the human disease, a platelet source of increased intrarenal TXB_2 production could be excluded on the basis of inhibitor studies.[12] Glomerular mesangial cells and monocytes were indicated as the most likely sources of TXA_2 synthesis.[12] A cellular source allowing the interaction of TXA_2 with mesangial receptors is consistent with our finding of a statistically significant inverse correlation between urinary TXB_2 and glomerular filtration rate.[5] The mechanism(s) responsible for enhanced glomerular TXA_2 production in lupus nephritis remain entirely speculative.[5,12] Although such biochemical alteration might contribute to deteriorating renal function in SLE nephropathy, the precise role of enhanced intrarenal TXA_2 production remains to be assessed by specific receptor antagonists or tissue-selective synthesis inhibitors (see below).

RENAL PROSTAGLANDIN SYNTHESIS INHIBITION IN MAN

Pharmacologic inhibition of renal PG synthesis is thought to be reflected by a variably reduced excretion of primary unmetabolized PGs. Most, if not all, widely used NSAD have been tested for their acute and/or chronic effects on urinary PG excretion. These include indomethacin, ibuprofen, naproxen, aspirin, fenoprofen, diclofenac, sulindac, piroxicam and flurbiprofen[3]. Their effects have been characterized in healthy subjects as well as in patients with renal, hepatic, rheumatic and cardiovascular disease. Some generalizations can be drawn from the results of such studies[3]: a) with the possible exception of sulindac (see below), all of these NSAD have been shown to reduce urinary PG excretion by at least 50% when used at full antiinflammatory dosage; a maximal reduction in the range of 60 to 80% has been described with the vast majority of these agents, although no detailed dose-response studies have been carried out to allow a quantitative assessment of relative potencies; b) such a maximal suppression of renal PG synthesis can be shown to occur within 24 to 48 hours of treatment, and is fully reversible within 48 to 72 hours after drug withdrawal, depending upon pharmacokinetics of the individual agent; c) the apparent reduction in urinary PG excretion following a given cyclooxygenase inhibitor is not substantially modified by disease processes affecting renal or hepatic function, although the latter can obviously alter the pharmacokinetics of some NSAD; d) despite early reports of partial attenuation of NSAD-induced biochemical and functional changes during continued drug administration, such a phenomenon has not been confirmed in controlled studies.

Eighteen studies of sulindac administration in health and disease have been reviewed recently[3]. The following points have emerged from such a critical overview: 1) when given to human subjects at the recommended therapeutic dose of 400 mg/day, sulindac does not appear to influence cortical sites of renal cyclooxygenase activity, as reflected by urinary 6-keto-$PGF_{1\alpha}$, with the possible exception of patients with cirrhosis and ascites; 2) under the same circumstances, the drug may affect medullary sites of cyclooxygenase activity, as reflected by urinary PGE_2, in approximately one third of the cases thus far evaluated; 3) the drug does appear to blunt i.v. furosemide-induced PGE_2 release; 4) the mechanism(s) underlying these peculiar features of sulindac is largely unknown, although likely related to its redox pro-drug nature[3].

A different mechanism is responsible for the selective sparing of renal cyclooxygenase activity by low-dose aspirin.[13] The mechanism underlying this selectivity is probably related to a different rate of recovery of cyclooxygenase activity in glomeruli versus platelets, following irreversible acetylation of the enzyme, and possibly to a different aspirin "sensitivity" of glomerular cyclooxygenase. The finding of a normal pattern of furosemide-induced renin release and urinary 6-keto-$PGF_{1\alpha}$ excretion after three to four weeks of low-dose (0.45 mg/kg/day) aspirin treatment in healthy subjects[13] indicates that renal PGI_2-producing cells are readily activatable at a time of virtually complete suppression of platelet cyclooxygenase activity. Thus, low-dose aspirin represents an ideal pharmacologic tool to investigate the role of intraglomerular platelet activation in the progression of chronic glomerular disease without the risk inherent to higher conventional dosage which might compromise PG-dependent renal function.

THE EFFECTS OF PROSTAGLANDINS AND CYCLOOXYGENASE INHIBITORS ON RENAL FUNCTION

Renal function is not critically dependent upon the integrity of PG synthesis, at least under ordinary circumstances.[1,3] Inhibition of PG synthesis in normal animals and humans does not induce a significant decline of renal function. It is probable that basal, endogenous PG synthesis does contribute to control of renal vascular resistance, glomerular filtration and salt excretion in healthy subjects, but administration of NSAD does not alter renal function since other regulatory mechanisms (adrenergic tone, renin secretion, dopamine, adenosine) are uncompromised and can compensate for the inhibition of PG-synthesis.[3]

In animals under anesthesia, especially after laparotomy, acute inhibition of PG synthesis reduces renal blood flow substantially, although glomerular filtration rate is largely unaffected. Different responses of anesthetized surgically-stressed dogs and conscious animals to the acute inhibition of PG synthesis are partially attributable to the effects of anesthesia and surgery on major vasoconstrictor hormones, especially angiotensin II, vasopressin, and catecholamines. In experimental and clinical circumstances, in which the vasoconstrictor hormones are increased, renal PG synthesis is augmented and renal function becomes "PG-dependent". Infusion of angiotensin II, vasopressin or norepinephrine into the renal artery stimulates renal PG synthesis measured either as secretion into renal venous blood or excretion into the urine. In vitro studies have confirmed that angiotensin and vasopressin stimulate vasodilatory PG release in glomerular mesangial and epithelial cells, and renal medullary interstitial cells.[3] Pretreatment with NSAD potentiated the renal vasoconstriction induced by angiotensin II, α-adrenergic nerve stimulation, and norepinephrine or α-adrenergic drugs. These experiments reinforce the belief that the vasoconstrictor substances stimulated cortical PGE_2 and PGI_2 which modulated the constrictor action of angiotensin or norepinephrine.[3] The major clinical circumstances in which vasoconstrictor hormones increase to maintain cardiovascular homeostasis include extracellular volume depletion, congestive heart failure, nephrotic syndrome and hepatic disease.[3]

Diseases such as atherosclerotic cardiovascular disease and chronic glomerular disease (including lupus nephritis) may reduce renal PGE_2 or

PGI$_2$ and thereby enhance the susceptibility to NSAD despite normal levels of constrictor hormones.[10] Figure 1 summarizes the hypothesis[3] about the modulating effect of renal PGE$_2$ and PGI$_2$ on the intrarenal constrictor action of angiotensin II, vasopressin, and norepinephrine. According to this hypothesis, drug- and/or disease-induced suppression of cortical PG synthesis is associated with a lower threshold for the contractile response of the glomerular mesangium and arterioles to a variety of agonists. This simplified scheme does not include the important possibility that glomerular and vascular PGE$_2$ and PGI$_2$ may antagonize the renal effects of diverse contractile compounds, such as platelet-activating factor, TXA$_2$, leukotriene C$_4$-D$_4$, and other vasoconstrictor agents.

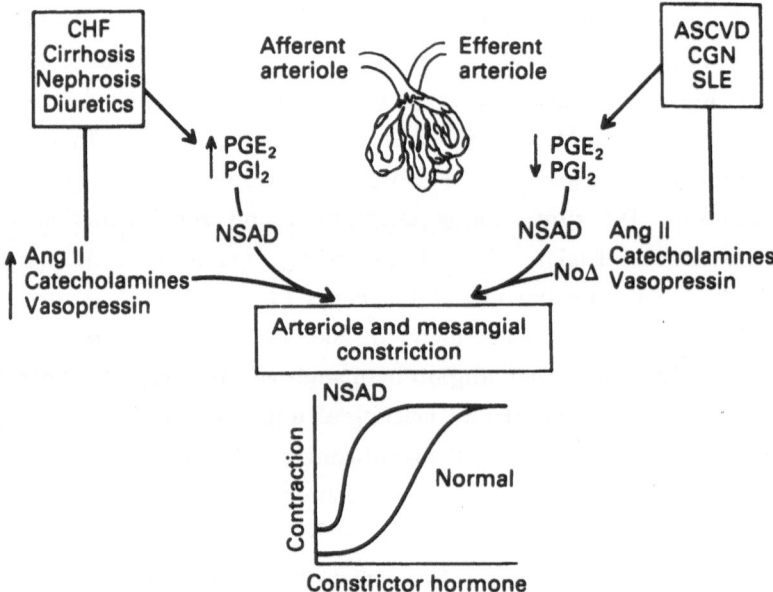

Fig. 1. Scheme depicting the balance between vasoconstriction and vasodilation existing in the pre- and post-glomerular circulation, and the glomerular mesangium. Abbreviations include: arteriosclerotic cardiovascular disease (ASCVD); chronic glomerulonephritis (CGN); systemic lupus erythematous (SLE); congestive heart failure (CHF); angiotensin II (ANG II); nonsteroidal antiinflammatory drugs (NSAD). The graph schematically depicts the enhanced arteriolar and mesangial contraction to constrictor hormones after inhibition of prostaglandin synthesis.

PLATELET AND/OR GLOMERULAR EICOSANOID INHIBITION IN CHRONIC GLOMERULAR DISEASE

In many renal diseases, loss of renal function correlates with evidence on biopsy of the deposition of fibrin and, less obviously, platelets in glomerular arteries and arterioles.[14] It has been argued by Kincaid-Smith[14] that in many glomerular diseases, progression is the result of thrombosis and the hyalinization of glomerular thrombi or their organization by myointimal proliferation in arteries. A critical viewpoint has been put forth by Border,[15] suggesting that activation of the coagulation system is merely an epiphenomenon of glomerular injury.

Platelets are potential sources of a number of mediators possibly affecting immune-complex deposition, capillary permeability, mesangial function, and glomerular hemodynamics. Moreover, platelets contain at least two mitogens - epidermal growth factor and platelet-derived growth factor - and a number of potentially chemotactic factors (reviewed in ref. 16). In a manner similar to their proposed contribution to atherosclerotic lesions,[16] platelets might contribute to glomerular lesions, e.g. by inducing proliferation of mesangial cells with an increase of the mesangium as is seen in membranoproliferative glomerulonephritis.[17] The experimental and clinical evidence supporting the involvement of platelets in mediating or amplifying glomerular injury has been reviewed by Cameron.[18] Platelets and/or platelet-related antigens can be found within the glomeruli of patients with glomerulonephritis.[18] Moreover, platelet survival can be shortened and the intraplatelet concentration of serotonin can be reduced.[18]

With the notable exception of platelets from nephrotic patients, which synthesize more TXB_2 when challenged _ex vivo_ possibly as a result of hypoalbuminemia,[19] platelets obtained from patients with different forms of chronic glomerular disease do not differ from normal platelets in terms of maximal capacity to produce TXB_2 in response to thrombin.[5] However, no information is available on _in vivo_ platelet TXB_2 production except for SLE patients, in whom we have described[5] a normal excretion rate of 2,3-dinor-TXB_2. Interestingly, glomerular thrombi occur frequently in SLE (in 50 percent of biopsies with diffuse and focal proliferative glomerulonephritis) and appear to represent a singularly important factor in predicting whether glomerulosclerosis subsequently develops.[20]

To test the hypothesis that the vasoconstrictor and mesangial contractile actions of TXA_2 might influence glomerular hemodynamics in lupus nephritis, Pierucci et al.[21] examined the short-term functional effects of a selective thromboxane receptor antagonist, BM 13,177, and of low-dose aspirin in two separate randomized, placebo-controlled studies. Forty-eight hour continuous infusion of BM 13,177 in 10 patients was associated with a statistically significant increase of inulin and para-aminohippurate clearances by 24 ± 12 and $26 \pm 13\%$ respectively, and with a doubling of bleeding time.[21] These hemodynamic changes were associated with a significant increase in sodium excretion, with no change in arterial blood pressure. Single oral doses of aspirin in the range 25 to 200 mg caused a dose-dependent irreversible inhibition of platelet TXB_2 production, with a pattern substantially similar to that previously described in healthy subjects.[13] Repeated b.i.d. dosing with 20 mg aspirin for 4 weeks caused a selective, cumulative inhibition of platelet cyclo-oxygenase activity and a doubling of bleeding time. Neither time- nor treatment-related differences were detected in urinary TXB_2 and 6-keto-$PGF_{1\alpha}$ excretion and inulin clearance, in 10 patients.[21] These findings would suggest that, in lupus nephritis, impairment of renal function is, at least in part, hemodynamically mediated and reversible. Moreover, platelets do not represent a major source of intraglomerular TXA_2 synthesis and action. Whether the short-term changes in renal function associated with thromboxane antagonism can translate into long-term benefits in terms of progression of lupus nephritis remains to be determined.

In contrast to other areas of human disease, such as coronary artery disease, where a role for local platelet activation can be strongly argued for on the basis of inhibitor trials,[22] the case for glomerular thrombosis playing an important role in the development of glomerular sclerosis and progressive renal disease remains to be proved in humans. The results of trials employing a combination of anticoagulants, steroids, cytotoxic drugs, and dipyridamole[15,17] are difficult to interpret in trying to understand the contribution, if any, of each individual agent. In a recent prospective, randomized, double-blind trial,[23] 40 patients with type I membranoproliferative glomerulonephritis were treated with dipyridamole (75 mg three times daily) and aspirin (325 mg three times daily) or with placebo for as long as 84 months, with masked conditions of the trial ending after one year of treatment. Efficacy analysis revealed that aspirin and dipyridamole significantly decreased the rate of decline of renal function and the development of end stage renal failure. However, if in addition to loss of renal function, complications of treatment were also designated as failures, then the difference between the two groups was not statistically significant. Moreover, no difference between the groups was noted with regard to proteinuria. Perhaps the most impressive results are related to the follow-up of these patients. Thus, nine of the 19 patients who were originally assigned to the placebo group aquired end-stage renal disease, on average 33 months after entry into the study. In the active treatment group, only three of the 21 patients acquired end-stage renal disease, on average 62 months after entry into the study. It should be pointed out that data from 20 percent of the patients entered into the trial were not analysed for various reasons,[23] thus preventing an intention-to-treat analysis. The mechanism(s) underlying the apparent beneficial effect of this combined treatment is probably related to suppression of TXA_2-related platelet function by aspirin. Any effect on glomerular cyclooxygenase activity is likely to have influenced glomerular eicosanoid production only partially and non-selectively with negative consequences, if any, on glomerular hemodynamics. The contribution of dipyridamole to the observed effects of the combination cannot be derived from this study. In a recent prospective trial,[24] 47 patients with type I membranoproliferative glomerulonephritis were randomly assigned to treatment with a combination of cyclophosphamide, coumadin, and dipyridamole (100 mg four times daily) or to no specific therapy for 18 months. Actuarial survival, progression of the renal disease, and proteinuria did not differ between the two groups to any statistically significant extent.[24]

That platelet activation and intraglomerular thrombosis may have a broader role in the development of glomerulosclerosis is suggested by the study of Purkerson et al.[25] in rats with subtotal renal ablation. Long-term oral administration of OKY 1581, a selective TX-synthase inhibitor, in rats with a remnant kidney increased renal blood flow and glomerular filtration rate, decreased protein excretion, lowered blood pressure, and improved renal histology.[25] Unfortunately, the use of a rather large dose of the inhibitor (20 mg/kg twice daily) precludes the possibility of distinguishing the effects resulting from inhibition of platelet TX-synthase from those resulting from inhibition of the glomerular enzyme. Of particular interest was the finding that despite the increase in hyperfiltration and hyperperfusion seen with the administration of OKY 1581, there was amelioration of the renal disease in this model.[25]

It should also be mentioned that in the studies of Purkerson et al.,[25,26] most of the maneuvers designed to decrease the progressive glomerulosclerosis also resulted in marked decreases in arterial blood pressure. These included OKY-1581, aspirin when given alone in low doses (5 mg/kg) or in combination with dipyridamole (50 and 10 mg/kg, respectively), heparin, coumadin and a combination of antihypertensive drugs. The following sequence of events has been suggested by these Investigators:[26] reduced renal mass causing vasodilation of arterioles in residual glomeruli would lead to hyperperfusion and intraglomerular hypertension. The latter will result in mechanical damage of the endothelium of glomerular capillaries followed by platelet aggregation, intraglomerular thrombosis and release of factors which may produce hyperplasia and hypertrophy of medium and small arterioles and subsequent sclerosis of the tissue.

Conflicting results have been obtained by Zoja et al.,[27] showing that selective inhibition of platelet TXB_2 generation by aspirin (a loading dose of 100 mg/kg followed by 15 mg/kg daily) failed to protect rats with reduced renal mass from the development of progressive glomerular sclerosis. These Investigators have argued that the beneficial results obtained by Purkerson et al.[25] with a selective TX-synthase inhibitor might be attributed to an effect on TXA_2 synthesis by resident glomerular cells (not inhibited by aspirin) or to lowering of systemic blood pressure.[27]

The Milan normotensive rat strain (MNS) is characterized by a genetically determined, age-related glomerular sclerosis accompanied by heavy proteinuria and deterioration of renal function.[28] Increased glomerular production of TXB_2 has been described in this model of spontaneous glomerular damage not associated with systemic hypertension[29] Long-term administration of FCE 22178, a selective TX-synthase inhibitor, reduced proteinuria, preserved renal function and improved renal histology with no significant change in systemic blood pressure.[30] These results would support the contention that selective inhibition of intraglomerular TXA_2 production per se is responsible for the prevention of progressive glomerular damage irrespective of changes in arterial blood pressure.

Whether intraglomerular platelet activation and/or enhanced TXA_2 production by glomerular mesangial and epithelial cells is the primary target of FCE 22178 remains to be determined. This drug inhibits TXB_2 production in isolated MNS glomeruli at significanty lower concentrations than in whole blood from the same animals,[31] a finding at variance with previous results obtained with dazoxiben[32] and other imidazole-analogue TX-synthase inhibitors. Thus, "tissue-selective" inhibitors, such as FCE 22178, may help to clarify the relative contribution of glomerular vis-a-vis platelet TX-synthase in the progression of glomerulosclerosis and may provide new therapeutic strategies in TXA_2-dependent loss of renal function.

ACKNOWLEDGEMENT

We wish to thank Maria Luisa Bonanomi for expert editorial assistance.

REFERENCES

1.   M.J. Dunn, Renal prostaglandins, in: "Renal endocrinology", M.J. Dunn ed., Williams and Wilkins, Baltimore (1983).

2.   D. Schlondorff, Renal prostaglandin synthesis: sites of production and specific actions of prostaglandins, Am. J. Med. 81:1 (1986).

3.   C. Patrono, and M.J Dunn, The clinical significance of inhibition of renal prostaglandin synthesis, Kidney Int. 32:1 (1987).

4.   C. Patrono, G. Ciabattoni, F. Pugliese, A. Pierucci, I.A. Blair, and G.A. FitzGerald, Estimated rate of thromboxane secretion into the circulation of normal man, J. Clin. Invest. 77:590 (1986).

5.   C. Patrono, G. Ciabattoni, G. Remuzzi, E. Gotti, S. Bombardieri, O. Di Munno, G. Tartarelli, G.A. Cinotti, B.M. Simonetti, and A. Pierucci, Functional significance of renal prostacyclin and thromboxane A_2 production in patients with systemic lupus erythematosus. J. Clin. Invest. 76:1011 (1985).

6.   C. Patrono, G. Ciabattoni, E. Pinca, F. Pugliese, G. Castrucci, A. De Salvo, M.A. Satta, and B.A. Peskar, Low-dose aspirin and inhibition of thromboxane B_2 production in healthy subjects, Thromb. Res. 17:317 (1980).

7.   M. Lebel, and J.H. Grose, Abnormal renal prostaglandin production during the evolution of chronic nephropathy. Am. J. Nephrol. 6:96 (1986).

8. R.P. Kimberly, J.R. Gill jr, R.E. Bowden, H.R. Keiser, and P.H. Plotz, Elevated urinary prostaglandins and the effects of aspirin on renal function in lupus erythematosus. Ann. Intern. Med. 89:336 (1978).

9. C. Patrono, A. Wennmalm, G. Ciabattoni, J. Nowak, F. Pugliese, and G.A. Cinotti, Evidence for an extrarenal origin of urinary prostaglandin E_2 in healthy men, Prostaglandins 18:623 (1979).

10. G. Ciabattoni, G.A. Cinotti, A. Pierucci, B. M. Simonetti, M. Manzi, F. Pugliese, P. Barsotti, G. Pecci, F. Taggi, and C. Patrono, Effects of sulindac and ibuprofen in patients with chronic glomerular disease. Evidence for the dependence of renal function on prostacyclin, N. Engl. J. Med. 310:279 (1984).

11. I.W. Reimann, E. Golbs, C. Fischer, and J.C. Frolich, Influence of intravenous acetylsalicylic acid and sodium salicylate on human renal function and lithium clearance, Eur. J. Clin. Pharmacol. 29:435 (1985).

12. V.E. Kelley, S. Sneve, and S. Musinski, Increased renal thromboxane production in murine lupus nephritis, J. Clin. Invest. 77:252 (1986).

13. P. Patrignani, P. Filabozzi, and C. Patrono, Selective cumulative inhibition of platelet thromboxane production by low-dose aspirin in healthy subjects, J. Clin. Invest. 69:1366 (1982).

14. P. Kincaid-Smith, Anticoagulants are of value in the treatment of renal disese, Am. J. Kidney Dis. 3:299 (1984).

15. W.A. Border, Anticoagulants are of little value in the treatment of renal disease, Am. J. Kidney Dis. 3:308 (1984).

16. R. Ross, The pathogenesis of atherosclerosis. An update, N. Engl. J. Med. 314:488 (1986).

17. J.P. Hayslett, Role of platelets in glomerulonephritis, N. Engl. J. Med. 310:1457 (1984).

18. J.S. Cameron, Platelets in glomerular disease, Ann. Rev. Med. 35:175 (1984).

19. G. Remuzzi, G. Mecca, D. Marchesi, M. Livio, G. De Gaetano, M.B. Donati, and M.J. Silver, Platelet hyperaggregability and the nephrotic syndrome, Thromb. Res. 16:345 (1979).

20. K.S. Kant, V.E. Pollak, M.A. Weiss, H.I. Glueck, M.A. Miller, and E.V. Hesse, Glomerular thrombosis in systemic lupus erythematosus: prevalence and significance, Medicine, 60:71 (1981).

21. A. Pierucci, B.M. Simonetti, G. Pecci, G. Mavrikakis, S. Feriozzi, G.A. Cinotti, P. Patrignani, G. Ciabattoni, and C. Patrono,

Thromboxane antagonism improves renal function in lupus
nephritis, N. Engl. J. Med. (in press).

22. C. Patrono, Aspirin for the prevention of coronary thrombosis:
current facts and perspectives, Eur. Heart J. 7:454 (1986).

23. J.V. Donadio, C.F. Anderson, J.C. Mitchell, K.E. Holley, D.M.
Ilstrup, V. Fuster, and J.H. Chesebro, Membranoproliferative
glomerulonephritis. A prospective clinical trial of platel-
et-inhibitor therapy, N. Engl. J. Med. 310:1421 (1984).

24. D.C. Cattran, C.J. Cardella, J.M. Roscoe, R.C. Charron, P.C.
Rance, S.M. Ritchie, and P.N. Corey, Results of a controlled
drug trial in membranoproliferative glomerulonephritis, Kidney
Int. 27:436 (1985).

25. M.L. Purkerson, J.H. Joist, J. Yates, A. Valdes, A. Morrison, and
S. Klahr, Inhibition of thromboxane synthesis ameliorates the
progressive kidney disease of rats with subtotal renal ablation,
Proc. Natl. Acad. Sci. USA. 82:193 (1985).

26. M.L. Purkerson, J.H. Joist, J. Yates, and S. Klahr, Role of
hypertension and coagulation in the progressive glomerulopathy
of rats with subtotal renal ablation, Mineral Electrolyte Metab.
13:370 (1987).

27. C. Zoja, A. Benigni, M. Livio, A. Bergamelli, S. Orisio, M.
Abbate, T. Bertani, and G. Remuzzi, Selective inhibition of
platelet thromboxane generation with low-dose aspirin does not
protect rats with reduced renal mass from the development of
progressive disease, Submitted for publication.

28. A. Brandis, G. Bianchi, E. Reale, U. Helmechen, and K. Kunn,
Age-dependent glomerulosclerosis and proteinuria occurring in
rats of the Milan normotensive strain and not in rats of the Milan
hypertensive strain, J. Lab. Invest. 55:234 (1986).

29. F. Pugliese, P. Menè, and G.A. Cinotti, Glomerular prostaglandin
and thromboxane synthesis in normotensive and hypertensive
rats of the Milan strain before and after development of
hypertension, J. Hypertension 4(suppl 3):S391 (1984).

30. P. Salvati, C. Ferti, L. Duzzi, R. Ferrario, N. Perico, G.
Remuzzi, and G. Bianchi, Effect of thromboxane synthase
inhibitor on age-dependent glomerulosclerosis in Milan
normotensive rats [Abstract], 10th International Congress of
Nephrology, London (1987).

31. P. Salvati, F. Pugliese, C. Ferti, L. Pierucci, R. Ferrario, and
C. Patrono, Selective inhibition of glomerular thromboxane-

synthase in rat models of progressive glomerulosclerosis,
[Abstract], Kidney Int. (in press).

32. P. Patrignani, P. Filabozzi, F. Catella, F. Pugliese, and C.
Patrono, Differential effects of dazoxiben, a selective thromboxane-synthase inhibitor, on platelet and renal prostaglandin
endoperoxide metabolism, J. Pharmacol. Exp. Ther. 228:472
(1984).

ROLE OF LEUKOTRIENES IN EXPERIMENTAL GASTRIC ULCERATION

B.M. Peskar, E. Bacha and P. Nowak

Department of Experimental Clinical Medicine
Ruhr-University of Bochum
Bochum, FRG

INTRODUCTION

Gastric mucosal damage induced by topical irritants such as ethanol, strong acid or strong base are preceded by severe disturbances of the gastric mucosal microcirculation resulting in a decrease in mucosal blood flow, vascular stasis, marked engorgement of microvessels and leakage of plasma proteins and blood cells.[1,2] Gastroprotective compounds such as prostaglandins (PG) prevent the microcirculatory changes caused by the irritants.[1,2] The cysteinyl leukotrienes (LT) LTC4 and LTD4 infused into the arterial supply of the rat stomach cause a rapid and marked decrease in vascular flow rate.[3,4] Furthermore, LTC4, but not LTD4, has been found to induce sluggish blood flow and stasis in the rat gastric submucosal microcirculation closely resembling the effects of topical irritants.[5] Finally, both LTC4 and LTD4, although not ulcerogenic themselves, potentiate the noxious effects of gastric irritants.[6,7]

EFFECT OF ULCEROGENS ON RAT GASTRIC MUCOSAL LEUKOTRIENE FORMATION

Fragments of rat gastric mucosa incubated in vitro release large amounts of the cyclooxygenase-derived products 6-keto-PGF1α, PGE2 and thromboxane B2 and smaller amounts of cysteinyl-LT and LTB4 into the medium. Oral instillation of ethanol results in a dose-dependent increase in the mucosal release of cysteinyl-LT (Fig. 1) and LTB4 (data not shown), during a subsequent in vitro incubation, while release of cyclooxygenase-derived products of arachidonate metabolism such as PGE2 (Fig. 1) or the vasoconstricting and pro-ulcerogenic thromboxane,[8] is not affected by ethanol. High pressure liquid chromatography revealed that the cysteinyl-LT released from fragments of rat gastric mucosa during incubation in vitro under basal conditions as well as after ethanol challenge consist practically exclusively of LTC4.[8] Stimulation of gastric mucosal LTC4 formation was not found with other topical irritants. Thus, oral instillation of hypertonic solution (25% NaCl), strong acid (0.6 N HCl) or strong base (0.2 N NaOH) caused severe damage to the gastric mucosa, but did not stimulate mucosal release of

137

LTC4 during the subsequent in vitro incubation. This indicates that the increased LTC4 formation observed after ethanol exposure of the gastric mucosa is not the consequence of tissue damage or lesion production.

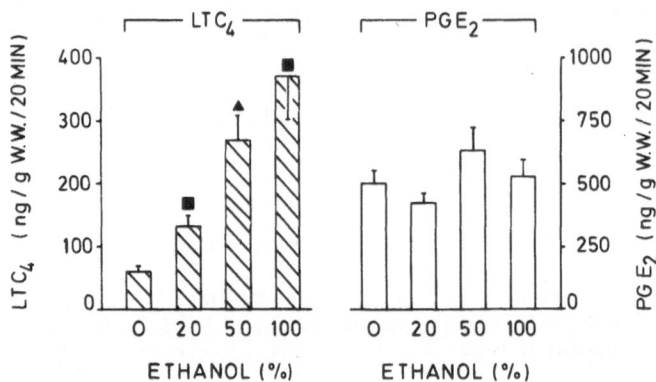

Fig. 1.   Release of LTC4 and PGE2 from fragments of rat gastric corpus mucosa incubated ex vivo 5 min after oral administration of 1.5 ml water or ethanol (20, 50 or 100%). Results show the mean ± SEM of 8 rats per group. ■ $p < 0.05$, ▲ $p < 0.001$ compared to 0% ethanol.

A great number of gastroprotective compounds prevent the stimulatory action of ethanol on rat gastric mucosal LTC4 formation. Thus, the sulfhydryl-containing agent cysteamine and the sulfhydryl-blocking compound diethyl maleate inhibit the stimulatory action of ethanol on rat gastric mucosal LTC4 formation closely parallel to their protective activity (Fig. 2). A similar correlation between gastroprotection and inhibition of mucosal LTC4 formation was found with other sulfhydryl-modulating agents as well as various metals.[10] In doses that practically abolished mucosal leukotriene formation most of these agents inhibited biosynthesis of prostaglandins indicating that inhibition of gastric leukotriene generation does not shift arachidonate metabolism to the cyclooxygenase pathway. This finding also indicates that the gastroprotection induced by agents that modulate gastric mucosal sulfhydryl levels is not mediated by increased formation of protective prostaglandins.

Sodium salicylate differs from other non-steroidal antiinflammatory drugs by its lack of gastrointestinal toxicity. Sodium salicylate was even found to protect against the necrotizing action of ethanol.[11,12] Similar to the effects of sylfhydryl-modulating agents sodium salicylate dose-dependently inhibits the increase in rat gastric mucosal LTC4 formation caused by ethanol exposure.[12] The inhibitory effect on LTC4 formation (ID50 40 mg/kg) parallels the protective activity (ID50 12 mg/kg) of the drug. Sodium salicylate does not inhibit gastric leukotriene formation in rats not challenged with ethanol indicating that the drug is not a 5-lipoxygenase enzyme inhibitor.[12] It remains to be investigated at which step in the chain of events leading to the stimulation of LTC4 formation by ethanol the interference of sodium salicylate and other protective drugs with inhibitory action on leukotriene formation

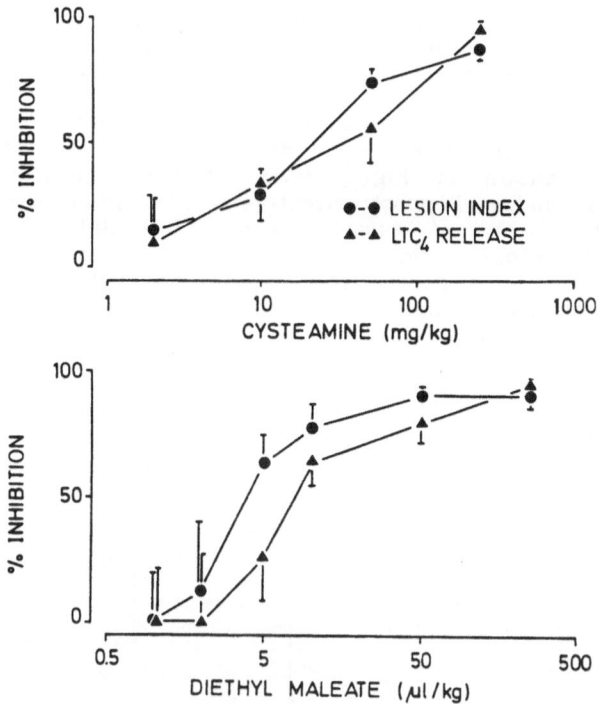

Fig. 2.   Effect of oral treatment with cysteamine or diethyl
maleate on ethanol-induced gastric mucosal lesion
formation and LTC4 release. 1.5 ml ethanol was given
30 min after drug treatment. Rats were killed 5 min
later. Results are expressed as % inhibition (mean ±
SEM, n = 6 per group) compared to vehicle-treated
rats. Data derived from Lange et al. (ref. 9).

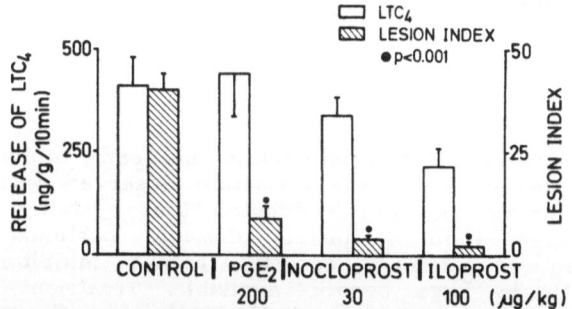

Fig. 3.   Effect of various prostaglandins on gastric mucosal
damage and LTC4 release in rats challenged with ethanol. 1.5 ml ethanol was given intragastrically 30
min after oral treatment with PGE2, nocloprost or
iloprost. Mucosal damage and release of LTC4 from mucosal fragments incubated ex vivo was determined as
described elsewhere.[8] Data represent the mean ± SEM
of 6 experiments per group.

occurs. The elucidation of the mechanism underlying this interference is of particular interest as it may represent a basic principle involved in the gastroprotection induced by certain drugs.

Naturally occurring prostaglandins and synthetic prostaglandin analogs are among the compounds exhibiting most marked gastroprotection. As shown in Fig. 3 PGE_2, the PGE_2 analog nocloprost and the PGI_2 analog iloprost effectively prevented the necrotizing action of ethanol on rat gastric mucosa, but did not significantly affect the stimulatory action of the irritant on mucosal LTC_4 formation. This further supports the concept that the increase in mucosal LTC_4 formation elicited by ethanol is not related to the tissue damage as it occurs despite full protection.

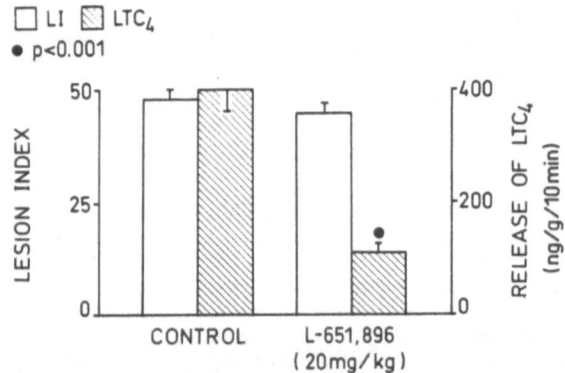

Fig. 4. Effect of L-651,896 on gastric mucosal damage and LTC_4 release in ethanol-treated rats. 1.5 ml ethanol were given intragastrically 30 min after oral treatment with L-651,896. 5 min later mucosal damage was evaluated and release of LTC_4 by gastric mucosal fragments was determined as decribed elsewhere.[8] Values represent the mean ± SEM of 6 experiments per group.

From the close interrelationship between inhibition of gastric mucosal damage and LTC_4 formation observed with certain gastroprotective drugs we have suggested that cysteinyl-LT may contribute to ethanol-induced gastric damage, particularly via their marked vasoactive actions. Recently, potent inhibitors of leukotriene biosynthesis have become available. Treatment of rats with the 5-lipoxygenase inhibitor L-651,896[13] significantly inhibited rat gastric mucosal LTC_4 formation after ethanol challenge, but did not protect against mucosal damage (Fig. 4). Lack of gastroprotective action of 5-lipoxygenase inhibitors in rats has also been reported by Wallace et al.[14] and Boughton-Smith and Whittle.[15] From these results one has to conclude that despite the pro-ulcerogenic effects of exogenous cysteinyl-LT, the marked increase in gastric mucosal LTC_4 formation elicited by ethanol is not causally related to its vascular actions and necrotizing effect.

Table 1. Effect of PAF on maximal flow reduction and maximal release of cysteinyl-LT in the isolated perfused rat stomach.

	Basal	PAF (ng)		
		3	16	50
	(22)	(8)	(6)	(7)
Flow reduction (%)	–	53±3	72±3	84±6
Cys-LT release (ng/min)	<0.18 ±0.01	0.3 ±0.08*	1.2 ±0.2**	3.0 ±0.5**

Maximal flow reduction expressed as % of basal flow (3.1 ± 0.1 ml/min) was determined 3 min, maximal LT release 2 min after bolus injection of 3, 16 or 50 ng PAF. Values represent the mean ± SEM of (n) experiments. ** $p < 0.001$, * $p < 0.05$ compared to basal leukotriene release. Methods used have been described elsewhere.[8]

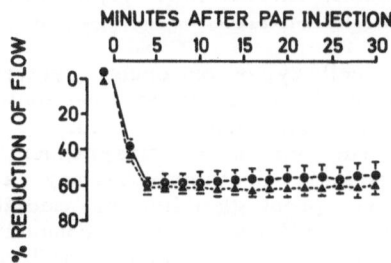

Fig. 5. Effect of L-651,896 on PAF-induced flow reduction in the isolated perfused rat stomach. The gastric vasculature was perfused via an intraaortic canula and the perfusate was collected from the portal vein. Infusion of L-651,896 (1×10^{-5} M) was started 8 min before bolus injection of 3 ng PAF and lasted throughout the experiment. Values are expressed as the mean ± SEM of % reduction of flow compared to basal values (3.3 ± 0.2 ml /min). ● PAF, ▲ PAF in the presence of L-651,896.

ROLE OF CYSTEINYL LEUKOTRIENES IN PLATELET ACTIVATING FACTOR-INDUCED GASTRIC FLOW REDUCTION

Platelet activating factor (PAF) has been described to be a potent gastric ulcerogen[16] and to cause ischemic bowel necrosis[17] in the rat. PAF injection results in marked flow reduction in the isolated perfused rat small intestine which was suggested to be mediated by release of endogenous LTC_4.[18] In the rat stomach perfused via the vasculature in situ bolus injections of PAF (3–50 ng) dose-dependently increased the release of cysteinyl-LT (consisting of a mixture of LTC_4, LTD_4 and LTE_4) into the perfusate. Simultaneously, flow rates through the gastric vasculature were markedly reduced (Table 1). Infusion of the 5-lipoxygenase inhibitor L-651,896 (1×10^{-5} M) reduced the peak release of cysteinyl-LT caused by bolus injection of 3 ng PAF from 862 ± 161 pg/min to 251 ± 296 pg/min ($p < 0.05$, $n = 5$) but did not affect the PAF-induced flow reduction (Fig. 5). Similarly, infusions of nordihydroguaiaretic acid in concentrations that significantly inhibited the stimulatory actions of PAF on release of cysteinyl-LT had no effect on the flow reduction caused by PAF.[3] Furthermore, the PAF-induced flow reduction was not counteracted by the cysteinyl-LT receptor antagonist FPL 55712, although the flow reduction caused by infusion of exogenous LTC_4 in concentrations 300 times higher than those released by PAF was completely antagonized.[3] On the other hand, both flow reduction and increase in cysteinyl-LT release by PAF injection was dose-dependently attenuated by the PAF receptor antagonist BN 52021.[3] These data demonstrate that PAF has a stimulatory action on cysteinyl-LT in the vascularly perfused rat stomach. Despite the pronounced vasoconstrictor action of exogenous cysteinyl-LT[3] these arachidonate metabolites do not, however, mediate the decrease in rat gastric vascular flow caused by PAF.

EFFECT OF NON-STEROIDAL ANTIINFLAMMATORY DRUGS ON GASTRIC MUCOSAL LEUKOTRIENE FORMATION

In a number of cell types or organ systems inhibition of the cyclooxygenase pathway of arachidonate metabolism is paralleled by increased formation of leukotrienes. If this effect also occurs in the gastric mucosa the enhanced biosynthesis of vasoconstricting and potentially ulcerogenic cysteinyl-LT may add to the reduced formation of protective prostaglandins in mediating the gastrotoxicity of non-steroidal antiinflammatory compounds. In rats oral treatment with indomethacin or aspirin inhibited release of both cyclooxygenase products and LTC_4 from gastric mucosal fragments incubated ex vivo.[12] There was, however, a shift in the balance between protective prostaglandins and potentially ulcerogenic LTC_4 since the inhibitory action of indomethacin and aspirin was more pronounced on formation of cyclooxygenase-derived than on 5-lipoxygenase-derived products. As, however, pretreatment of rats with the potent leukotriene biosynthesis inhibitor L-663,536[19] did not protect against indomethacin- or aspirin-induced lesions, this shift in balance is obviously not involved in the pathogenesis of the gastrotoxicity caused by non-steroidal antiinflammatory compounds.

ACKNOWLEDGEMENTS

Nocloprost and iloprost were kindly provided by Dr. W. Losert, Schering Co., Berlin, FRG. L-651,896 was a gift from Dr. A. W. Ford-Hutchinson, Merck-Frosst Co., Pointe-Claire, Dorval, Canada. BN 52021 was a gift from Dr. P. Braquet, Institute Henri Beaufour, Le Plessis Robinson, France.

REFERENCES

1. P. H. Guth, G. Paulsen, and H. Nagata, Histologic and microcirculatory changes in alcohol-induced gastric lesions in the rat: effect of prostaglandin cytoprotection, <u>Gastroenterology</u> 87:1083 (1984).
2. G. Pihan, D. Majzoubi, C. Haudenschild, J. S. Trier, and S. Szabo, Early microcirculytory stasis in acute gastric mucosal injury in the rat and prevention by 16,16-dimethyl prostaglandin E_2 or sodium thiosuslfate, <u>Gastroenterology</u> 91:1415 (1986).
3. A. Dembinska-Kiec, B. A. Peskar, M. K. Müller, and B. M. Peskar, The effect of platelet-activating factor on flow rate and eicosanoid release in the isolated perfused rat gastric vascular bed. <u>Prostaglandins</u>, in press.
4. B. M. Peskar, Cysteinyl leukotrienes in experimental ulcers in rats, <u>in:</u> Leukotrienes and Prostanoids in Health and Disease, U. Zor, Z. Naor, A. Danon, eds., Karger, Basel, in press.
5. B. J. R. Whittle, N. Oren-Wolman, and P. H. Guth, Gastric vasoconstrictor actions of leukotriene C4, PGF_{2a}, and thromboxane mimetic U-46619 on rat submucosal microcirculation in vivo. <u>Am. J. Physiol.</u> 248:580 (1985).
6. G. Pihan, C. Rogers, and S. Szabo, Vascular injury in acute gastric mucosal damage. Mediatory role of leukotrienes. <u>Dig. Dis. Sci.</u> 33:625 (1988).
7. S. J. Konturek, T. Brzozowski, D. Drozdowicz, and G. Beck, Role of leukotrienes in acute gastric lesions induced by ethanol, taurocholate, aspirin, platelet-activating factor and stress in rats. <u>Dig. Dis. Sci.</u> 33: 806 (1988).
8. B. M. Peskar, K. Lange, U. Hoppe, et al: Ethanol stimulates formation of leukotriene C4 in rat gastric mucosa. <u>Prostaglandins</u> 31:283 (1986).
9. K. Lange, B. A. Peskar, and B. M. Peskar, Stimulation of rat gastric mucosal leukotriene C4 formation by ethanol and effect of gastric protective drugs, <u>Adv. Prostaglandin, Thromboxane, and Leukotriene Res</u>. 17:299, (1987).
10. B. M. Peskar and K. Lange, Role of leukotriene C4 in gastric protection by sulfhydryl-modulating agents and metals in the rat. <u>Gastroenterology</u> 92:1573 (1987).
11. A. Robert, Gastric cytoprotection by sodium salicylate, <u>Prostaglandins</u> 21 (Suppl.):139 (1981).
12. B. M. Peskar, U. Hoppe, K. Lange, and B. M. Peskar, Effects of non-steroidal anti-inflammatory drugs on rat gastric mucosal leukotriene C4 and prostanoid release: relation to ethanol-induced injury. <u>Br. J. Pharmacol.</u> 93:937(1988).
13. R. J. Bonney, K. Hand,E. E. Opas, B. Olson, A. Dollob, L. W. Argenbright, and J. L. Humes, L-651,896, a novel dual inhibitor of prostaglandin and leukotriene synthesis that posesses potent topical anti-inflammatory and analgesic activity. <u>Clin. Res.</u> 34: 739A (1986).
14. J. L. Wallace, P. L. Beck, and G. P. Morris: Is there a role for leukotrienes as mediators of ethanol-induced gastric mucosal damage? <u>Am. J. Physiol.</u>245:G117(1988).
15. N. K. Boughton-Smith and B. J. R. Whittle, Failure of the inhibition of rat gastric mucosal 5-lipoxygenase by novel acetohydroxamic acids to prevent ethanol-induced damage. <u>Br. J. Pharmac.</u> 95:155 (1988).

16. A. C. Rosam, J. L. Wallace, and B. J. R. Whittle, Potent ulcerogenic actions of platelet-activating factor on the stomach. <u>Nature</u> 319:54(1986).

17. F. Gonzalez-Crussi and W. Hsueh, Experimental model of ischemic bowel necrosis. The role of platelet-activating factor and endotoxin. <u>Am.J. Pathol.</u> 112:127 (1983).

18. W. Hsueh, F. Gonzalez-Crussi, and J. L. Arroyave, Release of leukotriene C4 by isolated, perfused rat small intestine in response to platelet-activating factor. <u>J. Clin. Invest.</u> 78: 108 (1986).

19. J. Gillard, A. W. Ford-Hutchinson, C. Chan, S. Charleson, D. Denis, A. Foster, R. Fortion, S. Leger, C. S. McFarlane, H. Morton, H. Piechuta, D. Riendau, C. A. Rouzer, J. Rokach, and R. Young, L-663,536 (3-[3-(4-chlorobenzyl)-3-t-butyl-thio-5-isopropylindol-2-yl]-2,2-dimethylpropanoic acid) a novel, orally active leukotriene biosynthesis inhibitor, <u>Can. Physiol. Pharmacol.</u>, in press.

ROLE OF LEUKOTRIENES IN INFLAMMATORY BOWEL DISEASE

B.M. Peskar,[1] K.M. Müller,[2] M. Arndt[3] and F. Pelster[3]

[1]Dept. of Experimental Clinical Medicine and [2]Dept. of Pathology, Bergmannsheil Hospital, Ruhr-University of Bochum, and [3]Dept. of Surgery, University of Münster, FRG

INTRODUCTION

Ulcerative colitis and Crohn's disease are characterized by severe mucosal inflammation and mucosal ulceration. As the initiating event of both diseases is not known the aim of drug treatment is to prevent the amplification and/or maintenance of the inflammatory reaction. Development of effective drugs is hampered by the fact that it is not known which chemical mediator/s are responsible for the mucosal inflammation in these patients. Various agents including peptides, vasoactive amines and lipid-derived mediators have been found to elicit the typical reactions found at sites of inflammation such as vasodilation, plasma leakage, activation of inflammatory cells or tissue damage. During an inflammatory event increased formation of several pro-inflammatory agents occurs which may act in concert. Experimental and clinical work is necessary to establish whether inhibition of biosynthesis or action of a certain pro-inflammatory mediator does indeed prevent or reduce symptoms in a given inflammatory disorder.

PROSTAGLANDINS AND LEUKOTRIENES IN INFLAMMATORY BOWEL DISEASE

During recent years search for anti-inflammatory drugs has mainly concentrated on compounds that inhibit prostaglandin (PG) formation. Prostaglandins are derived from polyunsaturated C_{20}-fatty acids by the activity of the enzym cyclooxygenase. Prostaglandins, particularly PGE_2, exert potent pro-inflammatory actions due to their vasodilating properties, their sensitizing action on nociceptors and their potentiating effect on the actions of other pro-inflammatory mediators such as histamine and bradykinin (for review see ref. 1). Increased formation of prostaglandins is found in various inflammatory conditions (for review see ref. 1). Furthermore, non-steroidal anti-inflammatory compounds which inhibit cyclooxygenase and reduce prostaglandin formation[2] inhibit the development of inflammatory reactions, particularly hyperemia, pain and edema formation, in a variety of inflammatory disorders. This type of drugs also offers prompt relief from symptoms in patients with certain inflammatory disease states such as rheumatoid arthritis or degenerative joint disease. Likewise, inflamed mucosa of patients with active ulcerative colitis or Crohn's disease has an increased capacity to synthezise prostaglandins during incubation in vitro (for review see ref. 3). Furthermore, increased amounts of prostaglandins are released into the gut lumen of these patients and intestinal prostaglandin formation correlates well with disease activity.[4] In addition to their potent pro-inflammatory actions prostaglandins stimulate intestinal secretion of fluid and electrolytes, induce diarrhoe, increase mucus production and contract gastrointestinal smooth muscle (for review see ref. 3). It has, therefore, been suggested that prostaglandins contribute significantly to mucosal inflammation and symptoms in inflammatory bowel disease patients. However, contrary to other inflammatory disorders, cyclooxygenase inhibitors such as indomethacin[5] or flurbiprofen[6] are of no benefit in the treatment of acute attacks in patients with inflammatory bowel disease. Treatment with these drugs has even been found to worsen clinical symptoms in some patients and to deteriorate certain functions of the intestinal mucosa e.g. absorption of electrolytes or mucosal potential difference.[5,6] Increased mucosal prostaglandin formation in patients with inflammatory bowel disease thus seems to be an epiphenomenon rather than a crucial pathogenetic event.

Metabolism of arachidonic acid via the 5-lipoxygenase pathway results in formation of products some of which have pronounced pro-inflammatory actions. Leukotriene (LT)B$_4$ is a potent chemoattractant and induces aggregation and degranulation of leukocytes (for review see ref. 7). The cysteinyl-LT LTC$_4$, LTD$_4$ and LTE$_4$ promote plasma leakage, increase mucus production, contract gastrointestinal smooth muscle (for review see ref. 8) and stimulate intestinal secretory processes.[9] Sharon and Stenson[10] first reported that inflamed mucosa of patients with ulcerative colitis or Crohn's disease synthesizes significantly more LTB$_4$ than normal colonic mucosa. Similarly, mucosa of these patients exhibits a marked increase in the release of cysteinyl-LT (Fig. 1).

EFFECT OF ANTI-INFLAMMATORY DRUGS ON THE HUMAN COLONIC LEUKOTRIENE SYSTEM

In patients with ulcerative colitis sulphasalazine has been found to be an effective treatment both in mild to moderate clinical attacks and as maintenance therapy to reduce the risk of relaps. Sulphasalazine is also beneficial in the treatment of active Crohn's colitis. In the colon sulphasalazine is broken down by bacterial enzymes liberating 5-aminosalicylic acid and sulphapyridine. While sulphapyridine is rapidly absorbed, most of the 5-aminosalicylic acid remains in the gut lumen. 5-aminosalicylic acid, but not sulphapyridine, has therapeutic efficacy comparable to sulphasalazine in patients with inflammatory bowel disease (for review see ref. 11). Human colonic epithelial cells rapidly acetylate 5-aminosalicylic acid which can be measured in plasma and urine in the acetylated form.[12] This raises the possibility that at least part of the therapeutic efficacy of 5-aminosalicylic acid is due to the metabolite acetyl-5-aminosalicylic acid. Topical 4-aminosalicylic acid which differs from 5-aminosalicylic acid by the position of the amino-group has a therapeutic efficacy comparable to 5-aminosalicylic acid in the treatment of mild to moderate colitis.[13]

Recent studies have shown that sulphasalazine inhibits formation of 5-hydroxyeicosatetraenoic acid and LTB$_4$ by human polymorphonuc-

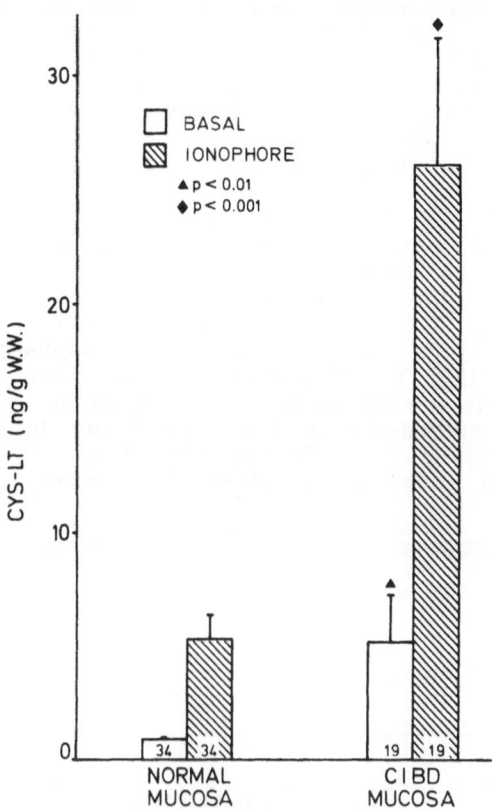

Fig. 1. Release of cysteinyl-LT from normal mucosa and mucosa
of patients with chronic inflammatory bowel disease.
Two rectal biopsy specimens were obtained by endos-
copy from patients with ulcerative colitis or Crohn's
disease (CIBD) or patients without rectal disease.
All specimens of CIBD mucosa showed severe inflammation as revealed by histology. Mucosal specimens were
incubated in modified Tyrode solution at 37°C for 20
min (basal release) and thereafter for 20 min in the
presence of ionophore A23187 (5 μg/ml). Release of
cysteinyl-LT (consisting of a mixture of LTC$_4$, LTD$_4$
and LTE$_4$ as shown by HPLC analysis) into the medium
was quantitated using radioimmunoassay. Values represent the mean ± SEM of (N) experiments.

lear cells.[14] 5-aminosalicylic acid inhibited formation of 5-hydroxyeicosatetraenoic acid, but not LTB₄, while sulphapyridine was practically inactive.[14] Sulphasalazine also inhibited formation of LTB₄ and various lipoxygenase-derived hydroxy fatty acids by human colonic mucosa.[10] 5-aminosalicylic acid, however, was described to be a selective cyclooxygenase inhibitor in human[15] and rat[16] colonic mucosa. Studies from our laboratory revealed that both sulphasalazine and 5-aminosalicylic acid dose-dependently inhibit release of LTB₄ and cysteinyl-LT from normal colonic mucosa (obtained from patients operated for colonic cancer) and inflamed mucosa (obtained from patients operated for active Crohn's disease).[17,18] Sulphasalazine was about ten times more effective than its metabolite. Inhibition of intestinal formation of LTB₄ and cysteinyl-LT was also found by 4-aminosalicylic acid and acetyl-5-aminosalicylic acid (Fig. 2).

Sulphasalazine and the various salicylates differ, however, in their actions on colonic release of PGE₂. While 5-aminosalicylic acid and 4-aminosalicylic acid (1–15 mmol/l each) effectively reduced formation of the cyclooxygenase product, acetyl-5-aminosalicylic acid had only minor effects and sulphasalazine increased release of PGE₂ (Fig. 2). Sulphasalazine has been shown to have complex effects on the enzymes of prostaglandin synthesis and degradation. Thus, sulphasalazine has been found to increase as well as inhibit the activity of PGE₂ synthetase[20] and to inhibit prostaglandin degrading enzymes[21] prepared from human colonic mucosa.

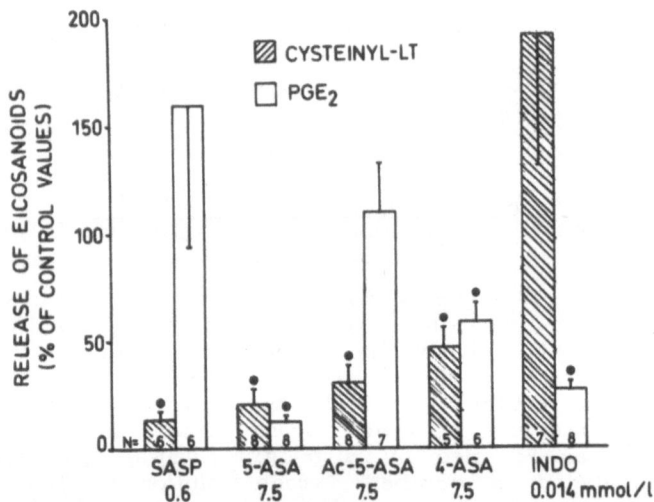

Fig. 2. Effect of anti-inflammtory drugs on the release of cysteinyl-LT and PGE₂ from human colonic mucosa. Fragments of colonic mucosa obtained from patients undergoing surgery for colonic cancer were incubated in the absence (controls) or presense of drugs at 37°C for 20 min. Release of cysteinyl-LT was stimulated by ionophore A23187 (5 μg/ml). Values are given as percentage release of the corresponding control values and are expressed as mean ± SEM of (N) experiments. ● p at least < 0.05 compared to control incubations in the absence of drugs, as calculated using Student's t-test for paired values. Data derived from Peskar and Coersmeier (ref. 19).

These multiple actions which are readily influenced by the experimental conditions used may explain the high variability of the effects of sulphasalazine on the prostaglandin system described in the literature. The finding that inhibition of human colonic mucosal leukotriene formation is observed with all salicylate drugs known to be of benefit in the treatment of patients with inflammatory bowel disease, while inhibition of prostaglandin formation is observed with some compounds, but not others, may suggest that leukotrienes are more relevant mediators than prostaglandins in this type of intestinal inflammation. This concept is supported by the finding that indomethacin which is clinically ineffective selectively inhibits human colonic prostaglandin formation (IC_{50} for PGE_2 1 µmol/l) without reducing formation of leukotrienes (Fig. 2). However, inhibion of colonic leukotriene formation in vitro is not only found with drugs which have anti-inflammatory activity in inflammatory bowel disease patients. Thus, sulphapyridine, the inactive carrier moiety of the sulphasalazine molecule, also inhibited formation of cysteinyl-LT by human colonic mucosa in vitro (Fig. 2). The inhibitory action of sulphapyridine on release of cysteinyl-LT (IC_{50} 1.4 mmol/l) is comparable to that of 5-aminosalicylic acid (IC_{50} 3.7 mmol/l). It remains to be investigated whether the lack of therapeutic efficacy of sulphapyridine is due to the specific pharmacokinetic properties of the drug which, contrary to 5-aminosalicylic acid, is rapidly absorbed and not retained in the gut lumen. In this context it may be of interest that sulphapyridine inhibits also release of cysteinyl-LT from human synovial tissue in vitro.[22] In contrast to inflammatory bowel disease patients, sulphapyridine has been found to be the active moiety of sulphasalazine when the drug is used in the treatment of patients with rheumatoid arthritis.[23]

The concentrations necessary to inhibit human colonic leukotriene formation in vitro by the various salicylates are in the millimolar range. Such concentrations are indeed reached in the gut lumen of patients treated with sulphasalazine or orally active 5-aminosalicylic acid drugs.[24] Nevertheless, such high concentrations may not accumulate continuously in all patients, particularly when severe diarrhoea is present. This could possibly explain that not all patients respond favourably to salicylate therapy. Recently, a number of selective 5-lipoxygenase inhibitors with an inhibitory action on leukotriene formation several orders of magnitude more potent than that of the salicylates have been developped. If leukotrienes are indeed pathogenetically relevant mediators of mucosal inflammation in patients with inflammatory bowel disease, such potent and selective 5-lipoxygenase inhibitors should be considerably more effective than conventional treatment with salicylates. Clinical trials with this type of drugs are necessary to define the role of leukotrienes and other 5-lipoxygenase-derived products in the pathogenesis of mucosal inflammation in patients with ulcerative colitis and Crohn's disease and to show whether effects on the intestinal leukotriene system contribute to the mechanism of action of sulphasalazine, 5-aminosalicylic acid and 4-aminosalicylic acid.

ACKNOWLEDGEMENTS

This work was supported by the Deutsche Forschungsgemeinschaft (grant Pe 215/6-1).

REFERENCES

1. G. A. Higgs, S. Moncada, and J. R. Vane, Eicosanoids in inflammation, Ann. Clin. Res. 16:287 (1984).
2. J. R. Vane, Inhibition of prostaglandin synthesis as a mechanism of action for the aspirin-like drugs, Nature 231:232 (1971).
3. D. S. Rampton and C. J. Hawkey, Prostglandins and ulcerative colitis, Gut 25:1399 (1984).
4. K. Lauritsen, L. S. Laursen, K. Bukhave, and J. Rask-Madsen, Effects of topical 5-aminosalicylic acid and prednisolone on prostaglandin E_2 and leukotriene B_4 levels determined by equilibrium in vivo dialysis of rectum in relapsing ulcerative colitis, Gastroenterology 91:837 (1986).
5. T. Gilat, J. Ratan, P. Rosen, and J. Peled, Prostaglandins and ulcerative colitis, Gastroenterology 77:1083 (1979).
6. D. S. Rampton and G. E. Sladen, Prostaglandin synthesis inhibitors in ulcerative colitis: Flurbiprofen compared with convential treatment, Prostaglandins 21:417 (1981).
7. M. A. Bray, Leukotrienes in inflammation, Agents Actions 19:87 (1986).
8. P. J. Piper, Formation and actions of leukotrienes, Physiol. Rev. 64:744 (1984).
9. P. L. Smith, D. P. Montzka, G. P. McCafferty, M. A. Wassermann, and J. D. Fondacaro, Effect of sulfidopeptide leukotrienes D_4 and E_4 on ileal ion transport in vitro in the rat and rabbit, Am. J. Physiol. 255:G175 (1988).
10. P. Sharon and W. F. Stenson, Enhanced synthesis of leukotriene B_4 by colonic mucosa in inflammatory bowel disease, Gastroenterology 86:453 (1984).
11. C. J. Hawkey and A. B. Hawthorne, Medical treatment of ulcerative colitis: scoring the advances, Gut 29:1298 (1988).
12. A. Ireland, J. D. Priddle, and D. P. Jewell, Acetylation of 5-aminosalicylic acid by human colonic epithelial cells, Gastroenterology 90:1471 (1986).
13. M. Campieri, G. A. Lanfranchi, F. Bertoni, C. Brignola, M. R. Minguzzi, and G. Labo, A double-blind clinical trial to compare the effects of 4-aminosalicylic acid to 5-aminosalicylic acid in topical treatment of ulcerative colitis, Digestion 29:204 (1984).
14. W. F. Stenson and E. Lobos, Sulfasalazine inhibits the synthesis of chemotactic lipids by neutrophils, J. Clin. Invest. 69:494 (1982).
15. N. K. Boughton-Smith, C. J. Hawkey, and B. J. R. Whittle, Biosynthesis of lipoxygenase and cyclo-oxygenase products from (^{14}C)-arachidonic acid by human colonic mucosa, Gut 94:65 (1983).
16. P. Sharon and W. F. Stenson, Metabolism of arachidonic acid in acetic acid colitis in rats. Similarity to human inflammatory bowel disease, Gastroenterology 88:55 (1985).
17. K. W. Dreyling, U. Hoppe, B. A. Peskar, K. Schaarschmidt and B. M. Peskar, Leukotrienes in Crohn's disease: Effect of sulfasalazine and 5-aminosalicylic acid, Adv. Prostaglandins, Thromboxane and Leukotriene Res. 17:339 (1987).
18. B. M. Peskar, K. W. Dreyling, B. May, K. Schaarschmidt, and H. Goebell, Possible mode of action of 5-aminosalicylic acid, Dig. Dis. Sci. 32:51S (1987).

19. B. M. Peskar and Ch. Coersmeier, Effect of anti-inflammatory drugs on human colonic leukotriene formation, in: "Inlammatory Bowel Diseases - Basic Research and Clinical Implications" H. Goebell, B. M. Peskar, H. Malchow, eds., pp.153, MTP Press Ltd., Lancaster, (1988).

20. T. Schlenker and B. M. Peskar, Dual effect of sulphasalazine on colonic prostaglandin synthetase, Lancet 2:815 (1981).

21. B. M. Peskar, T. Schlenker, and H. Weiler, Effect of sulphasalazine (SASP) and 5-aminosalicylic acid (5-ASA) on the human colonic prostaglandin system, Gut A444 (1982).

22. H. R. Wittenberg, K. Kleemeyer, U. Hoppe, B. M. Peskar, and B. A. Peskar, Release of eicosanoids from human synovial tissue and the effect of anti-inflammatory drugs, in: "Prostaglandins in Clinical Research" H. Sinzinger and K. Schrör, eds., pp.277, Alan R. Liss, New York (1987).

23. T. Pullar, J. A. Hunter, and H. A. Capell, Which component of sulphasalazine is active in rheumatoid arthritis? Br. Med. J. 290:1535 (1985).

24. K. Lauritsen, J. Hansen, M. Ryde, and J. Rask-Madsen, Colonic azodisalicylate metabolism determined by in vivo dialysis in healthy volunteers and patients with ulcerative colitis, Gastroenterology 86:1496 (1984).

GASTRIC CYTOPROTECTION

G.P. Velo, G. Cavallini; G. Brocco; P.G. Orlandi;
and L. Franco

▲Istituto di Farmacologia and Clinica Medica
△University of Verona, Divisione di Medicina
Ospedale S. Camillo, Trento, Italy

KEYWORDS/ABSTRACT: cytoprotection / prostaglandins / cytoprotective drugs/ carbenoxolone / NSAIDs / prostaglandin E_2 analogues.

Prostaglandins play an important role in maintaining the integrity of the gastrointestinal mucosa. Clinical evidence indicates that synthetic analogues of PGs are effective in the prevention and treatment of peptic ulcers. A number of drugs such as carbenoxolone sulglicotide used in peptic ulcer therapy appears to exert a benefical effect by increasing endogenous PGs. The phenomenon, called "cytoprotection", may be connected to the stimulation both mucus and bicarbonate secretion and may have a trophic effect on gastric mucosa. Non steroidal anti-inflammatory drugs, which block the biosynthesis of PGs, provide indirect information on the importance of local PG formation as regards the maintenance of gastrointestinal mucosal integrity.

Experimental ulceration by a variety of noxious agents can be prevented by prostaglandins (PGs). Robert et al. (1) have shown that pretreatment with several different prostaglandins protected the rat gastric mucosa against macroscopic damage caused by acid, ethanol, bile acids and hypertonic saline. "Cytoprotection" is the term used by Jacobson et al. (2) and Robert (3) to describe this mucosal protective action, which occurred in the rat at doses much lower than those necessary for gastric antisecretory activity. All tested prostaglandins, except thromboxanes, have a cytoprotective effect.

The presence of mild irritants in gastric contents, such as 10%-25% ethanol, 0,05-0,075 M NaOH, 2%-5% NaCl, 0.1-0.35 N HCl macroscopically leads to a reduction in mucosal injury caused by subsequent exposure to necrotizing concentrations of these agents (4-6). Since some works have demonstrated that mild irritants can stimolate the formation and release of PGs by the gastric mucosa (4, 6, 7), it has been proposed that "adaptive cytoprotection" is due to stimulation of endogenous prostaglandin synthesis (4).

"Adaptive cytoprotection" studies are, however, discordant; there are doubts about whether this process is dependent on prostaglandin synthesis (8). Mild irritants, that are protective, like 20% alcohol, have not always been shown to stimulate endogenous prostaglandin synthesis in experimental animals (9). At present there are no similar experiences for man. For this reason we have decided to study in our own laboratory the effect of 20% and 40% ethanol, in acute administration, on gastric PGE_2 release in man with and without previous chronic alcohol exposure. The results indicate that 20% ethanol did not modify the release of PGE_2 either in non alcoholic patients or in chronic alcoholics (Tab. 1).

TAB. 1. Gastric juice PGE_2 output after saline and 20% ethanol in non alcoholic patients and chronic alcoholics. (M ± SD)
** P < 0.01 vs. non alcoholic patients.

SUBJECT	N	AFTER SALINE ng/30'	AFTER 20% ETHANOL ng/30'
NON ALCHOLIC PATIENTS	10	35.3 ± 10.9	37.8 ± 12.4
CHRONIC ALCOHOLICS	11	112.0 ± 70.5 **	105.9 ± 84.0 **

On the other hand 40% ethanol significantly increased PGE_2 release in control patients but not in chronic alcoholics (Table 2).

TAB. 2. Gastric juice PGE_2 output after saline and 40% ethanol in non alcoholic patients and chronic alcoholics. (M ± SD)
* P < 0.05 vs. non alcoholic patients
** P < 0.01 vs. saline

SUBJECT	N.	AFTER SALINE ng/30'	AFTER 40% ETHANOL ng/30'
NON ALCOHOLIC PATIENTS	8	38.84 ± 10.40 **	85.18 ± 33.95
CHRONIC ALCOHOLICS	10	79.94 ± 52.89 *	87.84 ± 45.83

The PGE$_2$ levels were always significantly higher in chronic alcoholics versus control patients. The results indicate that only 40%, but not 20% ethanol, is irritant for human gastric mucosa and can increase endogenous PGE$_2$. Increased PGE$_2$ basal values in chronic alcoholics could explain the lack of further release after acute alcohol administration.

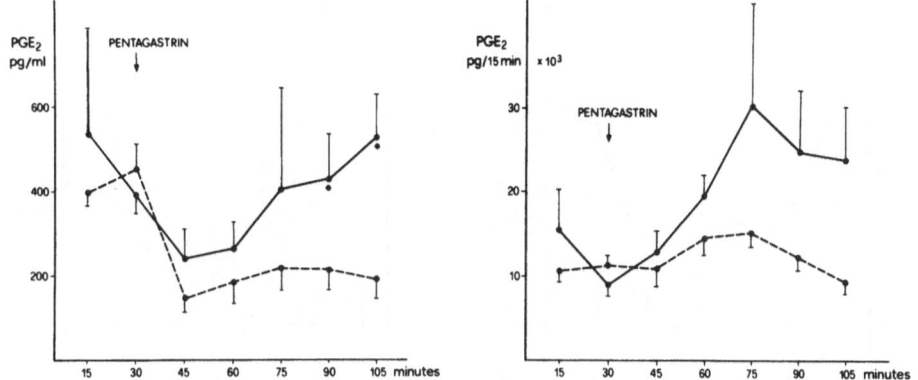

FIG. 1.   Concentration and output of PGE$_2$ in gastric juice before (broken lines) and after (solid lines) carbenoxolone (M ± SE). *P<0.05
A similar behaviour is evident after ISF 2715 (Fig.2).

CYTOPROTECTIVE DRUGS

A number of drugs used in peptic ulcer therapy, such as carbenoxolone, sulglicotide etc., are considered to be cytoprotective drugs. Recent studies have shown that carbenoxolone and its derivative ISF 2715, which has a lower aldosterone-like activity, may act, at least partly, through the prostaglandin system. It has been reported that these drugs inhibit the degradation of endogenous PGs by blocking the metabolizing enzymes, thus causing increased tissue and gastric juice levels of PGs (10-14). We have evaluated in healthy volunteers the effect of carbenoxolone and its derivative, ISF 2715, both orally administered, on the gastric PG system. Both concentration and output of PGE$_2$ in gastric juice tend to increase after carbenoxolone (Fig. 1).

Szabo et al. reported that certain compounds containing sulphydryl groups like dimercaprol, cysteamine and penicillamine were protective against ethanol induced damage in rats (16). Protection by N-acetyl-cystein against indomethacin-induced gastric erosions has been demonstrated suggesting that the PG biosynthesis is required for their protective action (17).

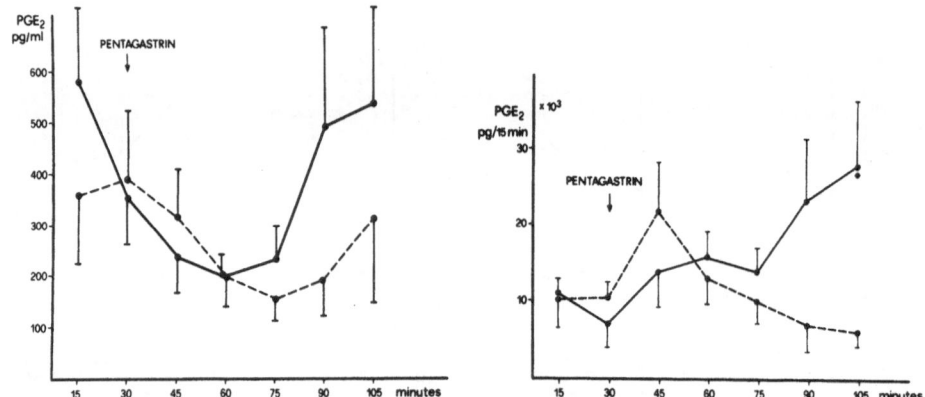

FIG. 2. Concentration and output of PGE$_2$ in gastric juice before (broken lines) and after (solid lines) ISF 2715 (M ± SE). * p < 0.05
A similar effect of sucralfate and sulglycotide was associated with increased prostaglandin levels (15).

EXOGENOUS PROSTAGLANDINS

Vane demostrated that indomethacin and aspirin (18), and other Authors later that non-steroidal anti-inflammatory drugs (NSAIDs) are potent blockers of cyclooxygenase, the enzyme involved in the first step of arachidonic acid conversion into PGs. The most common side effects of NSAIDs are the various forms of gastric complaints. The capacity of NSAIDs to block PG biosynthesis has been associated with the anti-inflammatory properties of such drugs and with their damaging effect on the gastrointestinal mucosa (19). Such depletion would exert a negative cytoprotective effect, according to which the gastric mucosa becomes sensitive to its acid content and can be damaged.

This provides indirect information on the importance of local PG formation for the maintenance of gastrointestinal mucosa integrity. Although the exact relationship between the damaging effects of these anti-inflammatory compounds and tissue levels of PGs needs further study and clarification, it is generally thought that an endogenous PG deficiency is at least partially responsible for the injury produced by these agents (20,21). Pretreatment with exogenous PGs concomitantly with or prior to the administration of NSAIDs can prevent such injury (22 - 24). However the mechanisms by which prostaglandins afford mucosal protection are unclear. Among the hypotheses for which there is some evidence are the following: a) strengthening of the gastric mucosal barrier with a reduction in H^+ back-diffusion (25); b) stimulation of the secretion of gastric mucus (26-28); c) increase in gastric and duodenal bicarbonate secretion (29): d) maintenance of mucosal blood flow (30-32). Since PGs have been demonstrated to prevent gastrointestinal mucosal damage and since they are naturally occurring compounds, it is quite natural that one of the major areas for their potential clinical utility is the healing of gastric and duodenal ulcers.

Several PGs of the E type are being developed for the treatment of gastric and duodenal ulcer. The number of double-blind clinical trials is increasing. In all of the controlled studies prostaglandin E_2 and synthetic analogues such as arbaprostil (15 [R]-15 methyl PGE_2), misoprostol (a synthetic PGE_1 methyl analogue), enprostil (a syntetic dehydro PGE_2 derivative), trimoprostil (11R, 16,16-trimethyl PGE_2), rioprostil (16-methyl-16-hydroxy alcohol analogue of PGE_1), and some others, were significantly more effective than placebo (33-36).

Further knowledge of these protective mechanisms of PGs in different tissues has great importance in the interpretation of the role of PGs in modulating gastrointestinal function and integrity, and should contribute to an understanding of the pathogenesis of various diseases.

REFERENCES

1. A. Robert, J. E. Nezamis, C. Lancaster, A. J. Hanchar, Cytoprotection by prostaglandins in rats: prevention of gastric necrosis produced by alcohol, HCl, NaOH, hypertonic Na Cl and thermal injury, Gastroenterology, 77:433 (1979).
2. E. D. Jacobson, T. K. Chandhury, W.J. Thompson, Mechanism of gastric mucosal cytoprotection by prostaglandins, Gastroenterology, 70:897 (1976).
3. A. Robert, Cytoprotection by prostaglandins, Gastroenterology, 77:761 (1979).
4. A. Robert, J. E. Nezamis, C. Lancaster, J. P. Davies, S. O. Field, A. J. Hanchar, Mild irritants provent gastric necrosis through "adaptive cytoprotection" mediated by prostaglandins, Am. J. Physiol., 245:113 (1983).

5. T. K. Chandhury, A. Robert, Prevention by mild irritants of gastric necrosis produced in rats by sodium taurocholate, <u>Dig. Dis. Sci.</u>, 25:830 (1980).

6. A. Robert, Cytoprotection and adapted cytoprotection, in: "Peptic ulcer disease: basic and clinical aspects", G. F. Melism, J. Boeve, J. J. Misiewiez, eds., Dordrecht, Boston, Lancaster, U.K. (1985).

7. S. J. Konturek, T. Brzozowsky, I. Piaztucki, T. Radecki, A. Dembinski, A. Dembinska, Role of locally generated prostaglandins in adaptive gastric cytoprotection, <u>Dig. Dis. Sci.</u>, 27:967 (1982).

8. C. J. Hawkey, D. S. Rampton, Prostaglandins and the gastrointestinal mucosa: Are they important in its function, disease, or treatment? <u>Gastroenterology</u>, 89:1162 (1985).

9. C. J. Hawkey, R. T. Kemp, R. P. Walt, N. K. Bhaskar, J. Davies, B. Filipowiez, Evidence that adaptative cytoprotection in rats is not mediated by prostaglandins, <u>Gastroenterology</u>, 94:948 (1988).

10. P. Minuz, G. Cavallini, G.P. Angelini, A. Lechi, G. Brocco, A. Riela, L. A. Scuro, G. P. Velo, Carbenoxolone and prostaglandin E_2 and F_2 gastric juice levels in man, <u>Pharmacol. Res. Commun.</u>, 16:875 (1984).

11. G. P. Velo, P. Minuz, A. Riela, G. Brocco, M. Degan, L. Franco, G. Cavallini, Gastric and systemic effects of carbenoxolone and its derivative ISF 2715 in humans, in: "Advances in Prostaglandin,Thromboxane and Leukotriene Research", B. Samuelsson, R. Paoletti, P. W. Ramwell, eds., Raven Press, New York (1987).

12. B. M. Peskar, A. Holland, B. A. Peskar, Effect of carbenoxolone on prostaglandin synthesis and degradation, <u>J. Pharm. Pharmac.</u>, 28:146 (1976).

13. B. M. Peskar, Effect of carbenoxolone on prostaglandin synthesizing and metabolizing enzymes and correlation with gastric mucosal carbenoxolone concentration, <u>Scand. J. Gastroent.</u>, 15:109 (1980).

14. J. Rask-Madsen, K. Bukhave, P. E. R. Madsen, C. Bekker, Effect of carbenoxolone on gastric prostaglandin E_2 levels in patients with peptic ulcer disease following vagal and pentagastrin stimulation, <u>Eur. J. Clin. Invest.</u>, 13:351 (1983).

15. R. Niada, M. Mantovani, G. Prino, C. Omini, F. Berti, Sulglycotide displays cytoprotective activity in rat gastric mucosa, <u>Int. J. Tiss. Reac.</u>, 3:285 (1983).

16. S. Szabo, J. S. Trier, P. W. Trankel, Sulfhydryl compounds may mediate gastric sytoprotection, <u>Science</u>, 214:200 (1981).

17. C. Johansson, S. Bergström, Prostaglandins and protection of the gastroduodenal mucosa, <u>Scand. J. Gastroenterol.</u>, 77:21 (1982).

18. J. R. Vane, Inhibition of prostaglandin synthesis as a mechanism of action for aspirin-like drugs, <u>Nature New Biol.</u>, 231:232 (1972).

19. S. I. Konturek, J. Piastucki, T. Brzozawski, T. Radecki, A. Dembinska-Kieć, A. Zmuda, R. Gryglewski, Role of prostaglandins in the formation of aspirin-induced gastric ulcers, Gastroenterology, 80:4 (1981).

20. T. A. Miller, Protective effects of prostaglandins against gastric mucosal damage: current knowledge and proposed mechanisms, Am. J. Phisiol., 245:601 (1983).

21. A. Robert, Prostaglandins and the gastrointestinal tract, in: "Physiology of the Gastrointestinal Tract", L. R. Johnson, ed., New York, Raven Press, 1047 (1981).

22. S. L. Kauffman, M. I. Grossman, Prostaglandin and cimetidine inhibit the formation of ulcers produced by parenteral salicylate, Gastroenterology, 75:1099 (1978).

23. C. Johansson, B. Kollberg, R. Nordemar, K. Samuelson, S. Bergström, Protective effect of prostaglandin E_2 in the gastrointestinal tract during indomethacin treatment of rheumatic disease, Gastroenterology, 78:479 (1980).

24. D. Y. Groham, N. M. Agrawal, S. H. Roth, Prevention of NSAID-induced gastric ulcer with misoprostol: multicentre, double-blind, placebo-controlled trial, Lancet, 3:1277 (1988).

25. F. Halter, W. H. Reinhart, H. R. Koelz, P. Meyrat, M. J. Leutze, O. Muller, 16-16 dimethyl prostaglandin E2 stimulates growth and maturation of rat gastric and small intestinal mucosa, Scand. J. Gastroenterol., 19:178 (1984).

26. M. Bickel, G. L. Kauffman, Gastric gel mucus thickness: effect of distention, 16,16-dimethyl prostaglandin E_2 and carbenoxolone, Gastroenterology, 80:770 (1981).

27. E. R. Lacy, Gastric mucosal resistence to a repeated ethanol insult, Scand. J. Gastroent., 20:110, 63 (1985).

28. A. E. Bell, L. A. Sellers, A. Allen, W. J. Cunliffe, E. R. Morris, S. B. Ross-Murphy, Properties of gastric and duodenal mucus: effect of proteolysis, disulfide reduction, bile, acid, ethanol, and hypertonicity on mucus gel structure, Gastroenterology, 88:269 (1985).

29. M. Feldman, Gastric bicarbonate secretion in humans. Effect of pentagastrin, bethaneed, and 11,16,16-trimethyl prostaglandin E2, J. Clin. Invest., 72:295 (1983).

30. W. G. Cloud, W. P. Ritchie, Evidence for cytoprotection of endogenous prostaglandins in gastric mucosa treated with bile acid, Surg. Forum, 33:150 (1982).

31. G. L. Kauffman, B. J. R. Whittle, Gastric vascular actions of prostanoids and the dual effect of arachidonic acid, Ann. J. Physiol., 242:682 (1982).

32. P. H. Guth, G. Paulsen, H. Nagate, Histologic and microcirculatory changes in alcohol-induced gastric lesions in the rat: effect of prostaglandin cytoprotection, Gastroenterology, 87:1083 (1984).

33. N. M. Agrawal, B. Saffouri, D. M. Kruss, D. A. Callison, E. Z. Dajani, Healing of benign gastric ulcer: a placebo-controlled comparison of two dosage regimens of misoprostol

a synthetic analog of prostaglandin E_1, <u>Dig. Dis. Sci.</u>, 30 (Suppl):1645 (1985).

34. A. P. Archambault, L. Holvorsen, S. P. Lee, Efficacy and safety of enprostil, a synthetic prostaglandin, and placebo in patients with duodenal ulcer, <u>Am. J. Gastroenterol.</u>, 79:828 (1984).

35. K. D. Bardhan, L. Whittaker, R. G. Hinchliffe, K. Cleur, K. Base, Trimoprostil vs cimetidine in duodenal ulcer, <u>Gut</u>, 25:A580 (1984).

36. H. G. Dammann, Th. A. Walter, P. Muller, B. Simon, Night-time rioprostil versus ranitidine in duodenal ulcer healing, <u>Lancet</u>, 1:335 (1986).

GASTRIC MUCOSAL DAMAGE BY NONSTEROIDAL ANTI-INFLAMMATORY DRUGS

A. Bennett and I.A. Tavares

Department of Surgery
King's College School of Medicine and Dentistry
The Rayne Institute
123 Coldharbour Lane
London SE5 9NU, UK

Gastric mucosal damage caused by nonsteroidal anti-inflammatory drugs (NSAIDs) is a major clinical problem, and it is therefore important to understand the mechanisms involved.   There are numerous complexities, including the fact that NSAIDs may have several actions besides inhibition of cyclo-oxygenase. However, even considering only the latter enzyme there will be inhibition of thromboxane synthesis as well as of the various PGs (some of which may have different actions); there may also be some diversion of substrate metabolism into leukotrienes and other fatty acid derivatives, although this is controversial.

The relationship between inhibition of prostaglandin (PG) synthesis and gastric mucosal damage is disputed. At one time, almost all of the emphasis by several investigators concentrated on this aspect, but it is now clear that some other factors are also important. Nevertheless, inhibition of PG formation by NSAIDs probably has a substantial role in causing mucosal damage. However, even with high doses of NSAIDs prostanoid synthesis is not completely blocked.

Most of the studies on the 'ulcerogenicity' of NSAIDs have been done using laboratory animals, but we have examined this problem by measuring the abilities of various NSAIDs to reduce PG and thromboxane formation by human isolated gastric mucosa. The first part of this chapter reviews our relevant published work, and then describes new results on other compounds.

Our previous experiments (Tavarés et al, 1987), obtained with a range of anti-inflammatory/analgesic drugs studied on specimens of human gastric mucosa removed at operation, found that the overall relative potencies for inhibiting the endogenous production of PGE, 6-keto-PGF$_{1\alpha}$ and thromboxane B$_2$ by mucosal pieces was generally: indomethacin = naproxen > ibuprofen > piroxicam; in contrast diflunisal, the prodrug sulindac, and the analgesic paracetamol usually had small or variable effects. This rank order was mainly similar to the inhibition of gastric microsomal PGE$_2$ formation from exogenous arachidonic acid, the relative potencies being: indomethacin > naproxen > ibuprofen = piroxicam = diflunisal; again sulindac and paracetamol had little or no effect.

The latter results fit with the fact that paracetamol is virtually devoid of anti-inflammatory activity or an ability to damage the gastric mucosa (Ivey et al, 1978) and that sulindac is a prodrug that acts only after conversion in the body to the active substance. However, the rank order of the abilities of NSAIDs to damage the gastric mucosa is contro- versial. A gastroscopic study in patients (Caruso and Bianchi Porro, 1980) found that the incidence of gastric ulceration plus erosion was: aspirin 50%, indomethacin 30%, naproxen 27%, ibuprofen 18%, sulindac 11%, and diflunisal 10%. Unfortunately there were relatively few patients, and many of the differences between the results were not statistically significant. Rainsford (1984) considered the relative damaging activity in man to be approximately: aspirin = indomethacin = piroxicam > ibuprofen = diflunisal > naproxen = sulindac > paracetamol. On the other hand, a recent analysis concludes that the abilities of many NSAIDs to damage the gastric mucosa cannot be clearly distinguished from each other on the basis of reported adverse drug reactions, except for ibuprofen which seems to be less irritant (CSM Update, 1986).

The amount of drug given per dose varies widely, and the recommended single doses of the substances in our published study differ by as much as 50-fold: paracetamol 1000 mg, ibuprofen 600 mg, diflunisal 500 mg, naproxen 250-500 mg, sulindac 200 mg, indomethacin 50 mg and piroxicam 20 mg. Assuming that our measurements of PG synthesis inhibition are relevant to gastric mucosal damage, it might at first seem logical that dose x potency would be the main determinant of the damage. However, our results indicate that this may not be true, at least with drugs that have a short of moderate half-life. When the potency for inhibition of prostanoid synthesis is multiplied by the dose, the ranking is: ibuprofen > naproxen > indomethacin > piroxicam > sulindac, diflunisal, paracetamol. Although paracetamol, and the prodrug sulindac in vitro, would be expected to be at the bottom of at the bottom of the scale, the position of ibuprofen at the top does not accord with clinical experience (Rainsford, 1984: CSM Update, 1986). Piroxicam too does not fit properly, because it can cause substantial damage (CSM update, 1986). Thus the ability to irritate the gastric mucosa generally may correlate somewhat better with our measurements of drug potency alone (the order is given earlier), rather than with potency x dose.

An explanation of this might be as follows. Acidic drugs are absorbed from the gastric lumen directly into the gastric mucosa, because drugs with appropriate pKa values are mainly unionised (and therefore more lipophilic) at low pH. Local tissue concentrations may be substantially greater than in plasma, and may approach the higher amounts used in the present experiments.   The drugs are retained intracellularly because they dissociate at the higher pH (Brune et al, 1977), so increasing the damage caused by NSAIDs. This process of drug distribution and intracellular retention also applies to acidic compounds that have entered the circulation after oral or parenteral administration.

The degree to which PG synthesis is inhibited after an NSAID is ingested depends on the amount and potency of the drug that penetrates the tissues after local absorption and from the blood stream.   NSAIDs are poorly soluble in water at acid pH, and some drug is therefore likely to be present as solid drug particles dispersed over the gastric mucosa. The total drug dose might therefore have little influence on the amount absorbed locally from a particle in contact with the surface, and if this is the case then drug potency may be the most important factor in determining the degree to which PG synthesis is inhibited at the site of gastric absorption.

The dose would clearly be important if most of the damage is caused by drug reaching the mucosa via the blood stream after gastrointestinal absorption. With systemically acting drug, the rate at which the circulating compound is metabolised is a particularly important additional factor. This may explain why piroxicam seems to cause more gastric damage than is predicted by our finding of a relatively low potency for inhibition of prostanoid synthesis; piroxicam differs from the other drugs in our study because of its particularly long half-life (about 24-36 hours), and a sustained block of cyclo-oxygenase might be particularly damaging if severe injury occurs only when PG synthesis is reduced below a critical level for a minimum period.   In support of this concept, PGs can exert biological effects that greatly outlast their destruction in the body, as shown by the hyperalgesia induced for several hours by PGE_2 injected into human skin (Ferreira, 1972). If mucosal protection by endogenous PGs formed prior to drug administration continues for some time after inhibition of PG synthesis has occurred, damage might be less with drugs whose half-life is sufficiently short to allow a return of gastric mucosal prostanoid synthesis towards normal between doses.

We hypothesised from these experiments that since NSAID potency seems to correlate somewhat better with gastric irritancy than does potency x dose, the damage to the stomach mucosa by NSAIDs with short or moderate half-lives might be due substantially (but not entirely) to local gastric absorption. This suggestion should be treated with caution, partly because Dearden and Nicholson (1984) concluded that although gastric irritancy in rats increases with anti-inflammatory potency, it decreases with potency when measured at the ED50 for anti-inflammatory activity. However, this correlation was strong only when 4/25 drugs were omitted, and Rainsford (1985), who has made several drug comparisons in rats, raised other criticisms. Furthermore, since the ranking of the recommended human dose is presumably similar to the ranking of the anti-inflammatory ED50 values, it might be expected from Dearden and Nicholson's conclusion that the more-potent drugs piroxicam and indometh-acin are least irritant in man; this clearly is not so.

The effect of cyclo-oxygenase inhibitors on gastric mucosal throm-boxane synthesis has generally received little attention. Thromboxane formation seems to be undesirable in the gastric mucosa (Kauffmann and Whittle, 1982), and thromboxane synthesis inhibitors can protect this tissue from damage (Konturek et al, 1983). In blocking cyclo-oxygenase, NSAIDs also reduce mucosal thromboxane synthesis, and this potentially beneficial effect might partly offset the damage due to block of PGE_2 and PGI_2 formation.

Implications of our hypotheses are that gastric mucosal damage may be less with drugs having (1) a low potency (in general, as well as on the gastric mucosal cyclo-oxygenase in particular), (2) poor gastric absorp-tion and local retention, (3) good solubility in gastric juice (to avoid particles in contact with the mucosa), (4) a short or moderate half-life, and (5) a strong inhibitory effect on thromboxane formation.

More recently, we have studied other drugs, including NSAIDs, on human gastric mucosa in vitro. These results are outlined below for the first time.

MATERIALS AND METHODS

Arachidonic acid, reduced glutathione, hydroquinone, haemoglobin and other chemicals were purchased from Sigma. Tritiated PGE_2, TXB_2 and 6-keto-$PGF_{1\alpha}$ were purchased from Amersham Radiochemical Centre. The immuno-logical cross-reactivities of the antisera used were: PGE antibody (Miles Laboratories), PGE_2 100%; PGE_1 100%; $PGF_{1\alpha}$ 0.35%; $PGF_{2\alpha}$ 0.5%; 15-keto-PGE_2 0.1%; PGD_2 0.04%; 6,15-diketo-$PGF_{1\alpha}$ <0.04%; 15-keto-$PGF_{1\alpha}$ <<0.04%; 13,14-dihydro-6-keto-$PGF_{1\alpha}$ <0.04%; 6-keto-$PGF_{1\alpha}$ 0.6%; TXB_2 <<0.04%. 6-keto-$PGF_{1\alpha}$ antibody (Wellcome Foundation): $PGF_{2\alpha}$ 0.84%; PGE_2 0.1%; TXB_2 0.02%. TXB_2 antibody (Wellcome Foundation): $PGF_{2\alpha}$ 0.11%; PGE_2 0.008%; 6-keto-$PGF_{1\alpha}$ 0.01%. LTC_4/ LTD_4 RIA kit (Amersham) LTC_4 100%; LTD_4 55.3%; LTE_4 8.6%; LTB_4 0.006%; PGs and TXB_2 <0.002%; 5, 12-di-HETE (6,8,10,14) 3.3%, 12-HETE 2.0%, PGs and TXB_2 <0.03%. Assay sensitivities were 10pg, and the intra-assay and inter-assay coefficients of variation were respectively 5-11% and 15-22% for the different eicosanoids.

Human gastric mucosa. Gastric tissues, taken at least 5 cm from any macroscopically detected lesions, were obtained from surgical specimens removed for benign or malignant disease. The mucosa/submucosa were cut off from the underlying muscle while the tissue was bathed in Krebs solution at room temperature, cut into pieces of 2-4 mm^2, washed with Krebs solution, and the excess fluid drained off.

Incubation of gastric mucosal pieces. Carefully weighed samples (50mg in the pirazolac experiments; 100mg in the acemetacin experiments) were pre-incubated in the presence of drugs, using concentrations of 0.1 (sometimes), 1, 10, and 100 μg or vehicle in 1 ml 0.1M tris-HCl buffer pH 7.4 0°C for 30 min. This pre-incubation fluid, containing any eicosanoids including those released by trauma, was discarded and replaced by 1 ml fresh incubation fluid (plus drugs or vehicle). After further incubation at 37°C for 30 min the fluid was removed following centrifugation, and stored at -20°C until measured in duplicate by radioimmunoassay using suitable dilutions of antisera and tritiated standards.

Microsomes. Using a Silverson homogeniser, 2g mucosa were homogen- ised for 30 sec at 0°C in 20 ml tris-HCl-EDTA buffer (0.1M:5mM, pH 8). The homogenate was centrifuged (10,000 x g, 15 min, 4°C), and the supernatant was removed and recentrifuged (100,000 x g, 60 min, 4°C) to give the microsomal pellet. This was rinsed and then resuspended in 4 ml tris-HCl-EDTA buffer (0.1M:1mM, pH 8). Aliquots of the microsomal suspension (100 μl) and cofactors (reduced gluthathione 50 μg, hydro- quinone 3.7 μg, and haemoglobin 3.3 μg in 100 μl) were pre-incubated for 15 min at 37°C in the absence or presence of drugs (1, 10, 100 μg in 700 μl). This was was followed by incubation with vehicle (RIA background control) or arachidonic acid (5 μg in 100μl to make a final volume of 1 ml) for a further 30 min at 37°C. After terminating the metabolic activ- ity with methanol/ formic acid (1 ml:10 μl) the products were extracted into diethyl ether (3 ml x 2) and evaporated to dryness. The extract was dissolved in tricene-buffered saline (1 ml, 0.1 M, pH 7.4) and stored at - 20°C until assayed.

The eicosanoid measurements are analysed statistically by Student's t-test for paired data (2-tailed tests).

RESULTS AND DISCUSSION

1. Pirazolac and dazoxiben

The NSAID pirazolac (Schering; 4-(p-chlorophenyl)-1-(p-flurophenyl)- pyrazole-3-acetic acid), in concentrations of 1-100 μg/ml, usually caused a concentration-related reduction in the amounts of PGE, 6-keto-PGF$_{1\alpha}$ and TXB$_2$ obtained from incubated human gastric mucosal pieces. It was about 100 times less effective on a weight basis than indomethacin which caused a reduction of about 90% with 1μg/ml. With the thromboxane synthase inhibitor dazoxiben, the amount of TXB$_2$ was greatly reduced, the effect being almost maximal (95%) at 1μg/ml, but in contrast the amounts of PGE and 6-keto-PGF$_{1\alpha}$ were up to 104% higher. These increases by dazoxiben are presumably due, at least in part, to diversion of substrate metabolism away from thromboxanes to PGs, but we cannot rule out other possibilities such as activation of cyclo-oxygenase, PGE/PGI synthases and/or phospholipase A_2.

In other experiments we examined the ability of pirazolac 1, 10 and 100μg/ml to inhibit the cyclo-oxygenase of human gastric mucosal microsomes as measured by the synthesis of PGE from added arachidonic acid. Indomethacin, naproxen, ibuprofen and piroxicam were used for comparisons.

PGE synthesis was concentration-relatedly inhibited by all the NSAIDs tested. The overall relative potencies, based on the approximate IC50 values, were indomethacin > naproxen > ibuprofen > piroxicam > pirazolac. The order based on recommended dose/IC50 (up to 600mg for a dose of pirazolac; the other doses are stated earlier) is: ibuprofen > naproxen > indomethacin > pirazolac > piroxicam. If our hypotheses stated above are correct, the findings suggest that pirazolac is less likely than some other NSAIDs drugs to cause gastric mucosal damage.

2. Acemetacin, BW755C and mepacrine

In another series of experiments with mucosal pieces, the NSAID acemetacin (E. Merck; [1-(p-chlorobenzoyl)-5-methoxy-2-methylindol-3-acetoxy] acetic acid), indomethacin or the dual cyclo-oxygenase/ lipoxygenase inhibitor BW755C (all 0.1 - 100μg/ml) concentration-relatedly reduced the amounts of PGE, 6-keto-PGF$_{1\alpha}$ and TXB$_2$, whereas mepacrine had little or no effect. The reductions by indomethacin 0.1-10μg/ml were: PGE 34-86%, 6-keto-PGF$_{1\alpha}$ 45-73%, TXB$_2$ 29-85%. With acemetacin 0.1-100μg/ml the mean reductions were PGE 19-74%, 6-keto-PGF$_{1\alpha}$, 11-79% and TXB$_2$ 0-80%. The order of potency was indomethacin > acemetacin = BW755C. The IC50 values for inhibition of PGE synthesis by indomethacin and acemetacin were 2 and 7 μM respectively. For inhibition of PGI$_2$ formation, as measured by the amounts of 6-keto-PGF$_{1\alpha}$, the respective EC50 values were 0.6 and 9. Evidence that acemetacin shows a better gastric tolerance than indomethacin is consistent with its weaker inhibition of gastric mucosal PG synthesis in vitro.

The amount of LTB$_4$ was reduced by BW755C, indomethacin and, to some extent, by acemetacin, whereas again mepacrine was ineffective. There was little or no change with any test drug on peptido-leukotriene (LTC$_4$/D$_4$) accumulation in the incubates. Roles played by leukotrienes in the gastric mucosa have not yet been fully defined, but they appear to be capable of damaging the tissue (BM Peskar, as described elsewhere in this book). BW755C concentration-relatedly inhibited LTB$_4$ accumulation but had no effect on LTC$_4$/D$_4$. Although indomethacin blocks cyclo-oxygenase, it can also inhibit leukotriene formation at higher concentrations, as shown by others and ourselves (Tavares et al., 1986). If LTB$_4$ is damaging to human gastric mucosa, inhibition of its synthesis by indomethacin and acemetacin might partly offset any damage that they cause through inhibition of PG formation or by other mechanisms.

REFERENCES

Caruso I and Bianchi Porro G. (1980). Gastroscopic evaluation of anti-inflammatory drugs. Br. Med. J. 1: 75-78.

CSM Update (1986). Non-steroidal anti-inflammatory drugs and serious gastrointestinal adverse reactions-2. Br. Med. J. 1, 292: 1140-1191.

Dearden JC and Nicholson RM. (1984). Correlation between gastric irritancy and anti-inflammatory activity of non-steroidal anti-inflammatory drugs. J. Pharm. Pharmacol 36: 713-715.

Ferreira SH. (1972). Prostaglandins, aspirin-like drugs and analgesia. Nature New Biol. 240: 200-203.

Ivey KJ, Silvoso GR and Krauss WJ. (1978). Effect of paracetamol on gastric mucosa. Br. Med. J. 1: 1586-1588.

Kauffmann GL and Whittle BJR. (1982). Gastric vascular actions of prostanoids and the dual effect of arachidonic acid. Am. J. Physiol. 242: G582-587.

Konturek SJ, Brzozowski T, Piastucki I, Rudecki T and Dembinska-Kiec A. (1983). Role of prostaglandin and thromboxane synthesis in gastric necrosis produced by taurocholate and ethanol. Dig. Dis. Sci. 28: 154.

Rainsford KD. (1984). Side effects of anti-inflammatory/analgesic drugs: epidemiology and gastrointestinal tract. Trends Pharmacol. Sci. 5: 156-159.

Tavares IA, Collins PO and Bennett A. (1987). Inhibition of prostanoid synthesis by human gastric mucosa. Alimentary Pharmacology and Therapeutics 1: 617-625.

Tavares IA, Sergis AN, Berry H and Bennett A. (1987). Synovial and blood polymorphonuclear leukocytes from arthritic patients metabolize arachidonic acid similarly. Progr. Lipid Res. 25: 577-578.

ASPECTS OF EICOSANOIDS IN INFLAMMATION

Per Hedqvist[1], Sven-Erik Dahlén[1], Johan Raud[1], Lennart Lindbom[1], Åsa Thuresson-Klein[2] and K.C. Nicolaou[3]

Department of Physiology and the Institute of Environmental Medicine, Karolinska Institutet, S-104 01 Stockholm Sweden[1]; Department of Pharmacology and Toxicology[2] University of Mississippi Medical Center, Jackson, MS 39216 and Department of Organic Chemistry, University of Pennsylvania[3], Philadelphia, PA 191 04

INTRODUCTION

The microvascular system has a key role in host defence and expression of the inflammatory process which is indispensible for the elimination of foreign and noxious agents. Regardless of the nature of the initiating stimulus, the sequence of microvascular events in early inflammation is with few exceptions characterized by the following partly overlapping reactions; (i) changes in arteriolar diameters and blood flow, (ii) increased venular permeability promoting macromolecular leakage and formation of tissue edema, and (iii) diapedesis and migration of leukocytes into the area of injury. It is also becoming increasingly clear that the waxing and waning of the inflammatory process, rather than being a static phenomenon, is the result of a continuous interplay between mediators, modulators, and feed back mechanisms.

The eicosanoids comprise a complex system of bioregulators, synthesized on demand in almost every tissue and demonstrating an impressing range of activities, in several cases with remarkable potency. They all derive from some polyunsaturated fatty acids, particularly arachidonic acid, which may be oxidized and further transformed in reactions initiated either by a cyclo-oxygenase yielding prostaglandins, prostacyclin and thromboxanes or, alternatively, by specific lipoxygenases giving rise to leukotrienes, lipoxins and a number of related hydroxy acids. Most of the eicosanoids thus formed either contract or relax vascular smooth muscle but some of them also have additional specific targets in the cardio-vascular system, such as the heart, blood cells, and the vascular endothelium.

The aim of this chapter is to briefly review recent observations pertaining to microvascular actions and interactions of some eicosanoids which are assumed to mediate or modulate significant events in early inflammation.

Specifically the following issues are addressed; the mechanisms for leukotriene-induced plasma leakage and diapedesis of leukocytes, microvascular potentials of the newly discovered lipoxins, and the capacity of prostaglandin E_2 to balance mast cell-dependent inflammation via inhibition of mediator release and enhancement of the target action of mediators. Studies of these aspects have been facilitated by the use of intravital microscopy (Lindbom and Arfors 1984, Björk et al 1984), which permits continuous observations of dynamic changes in blood flow, vascular permeability, and blood cell - endothelium interactions, and complementary electron microscopy (Thureson-Klein et al., 1986.) to unravel ultrastructural changes in connection with leukocyte activation and diapedesis .

MICROVASCULAR EFFECTS OF LEUKOTRIENES C_4, D_4 AND E_4

Studies of the metabolism of arachidonic acid by leukocytes and parallel structural work on slow reacting substance of anaphylaxis (SRS-A) in the late 1970-ies led to two major advances in the eicosanoid field; the discovery of the leukotriene (LT) family, with its principal members the dihydroxy acid LTB_4 and the cysteinyl-containing LTC_4, LTD_4 and LTE_4, and the identification of SRS-A as a mixture of the latter three leukotrienes. Since SRS-A had long been considered a mediator of anaphylaxis and inflammation (cf. Orange and Austen 1969) it is easy to understand that proinflammatory effects received special attention in the subsequent exploration of leukotriene activities.

When injected intradermally, the cysteinyl leukotrienes cause local edema in several species including man (Drazen et al. 1980; Hedqvist et al. 1980; Soter et al. 1983). In most cases they also cause vasoconstriction, and blunting of that response with vasodilative prostaglandins may potentiate the edema (Peck et al. 1981). The human skin is an exception, however, with LTC_4-E_4 causing a flare response (Bisgaard et al. 1982, Soter et al., 1983). Furthermore, when given systemically these leukotrienes apparently have the capacity to evoke generalized leakage of plasma, as noted in monkey and guinea pig (Smedegård et al. 1982; Hua et al. 1985). In the latter species the extent of plasma exudation was quite impressive, as indicated by 20% hemoconcentration 5 min after injection of 1 nmol x kg^{-1} of LTC_4.

The mechanisms for the edema-promoting effect of the cysteinyl leukotrienes have been characterized by means of intravital microscopy of the terminal vascular bed of the hamster cheek pouch (Dahlén et al. 1981; Björk et al. 1982a, 1983; Raud et al. 1988) (Fig. 1). In this *in vivo* model, LTC_4, LTD_4, and LTE_4, in the low nanomolar range, elicit constriction of the arterioles and intense leakage of plasma from the venules. In the latter respect, they are equiactive and approximately 1000 times as potent as histamine. The leakage of plasma is, however, not a consequence of the vasoconstriction, for example angiotensin II (Dahlén et al., 1981) or the novel peptide endothelin (Öhlén et al., 1989) cause similar intense arteriolar constriction as the cysteinyl leukotrienes without changing the microvascular permeability. In addition, blunting of the vasoconstrictor response makes these leukotrienes even more possessive edema-inducers. Furthermore, the leakage effect is selectively oriented towards postcapillary venules, and it is uninfluenced by depletion of circulating neutrophils or administration of antihistaminics and inhibitors of prostaglandin biosynthesis. Taken together, these observations indicate a direct action on the endothelial lining of the postcapillary venules. Recent ultrastructural work on the hamster cheek pouch, rabbit tennuissimus muscle, and guinea pig abdominal muscle has confirmed this (Hedqvist et al. 1987; Joris et al. 1987). In all three tissues, the leukotrienes elicit endothelial cell contraction and formation of junctional gaps, and extravasation appears to occur preferentially through these gaps.

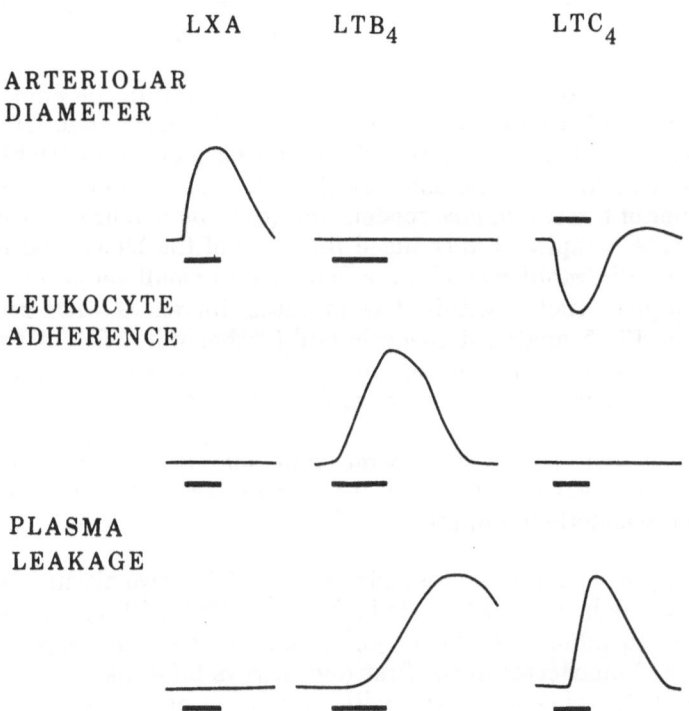

Fig. 1.   Comparison of the microvascular actions of LXA_4, LTB_4, and LTC_4 in the hamster cheek pouch (compiled from data in Dahlén et al., 1981; Björk et al., 1982; Dahlén et al 1987). LXA_4 causes arteriolar dilation, whereas LTB_4 has no effect on blood flow, and LTC_4 elicits vasoconstriction. Only LTB_4 is chemotactic for leukocytes. LXA_4 does not cause plasma leakage, whereas LTB_4 induces a delayed phase of leukocyte-dependent leakage from small and large venules. LTC_4 causes an immediate type of leakage which is leukocyte-independent, dissociated from vasoconstriction, and specifically located to postcapillary venules.

MICROVASCULAR EFFECTS OF LEUKOTRIENE B₄

There is considerable *in vitro* evidence indicating that LTB₄ is chemo-kinetic and chemotactic for leukocytes; i.e. it increases random and direction-al migration of the cells (Ford-Hutchinson et al., 1980; Goetzl and Picket, 1980; Malmsten et al., 1980). In addition, LTB₄ has been reported to stimu-late cAMP formation in leukocytes (Claesson, 1982), and to cause degranula-tion, superoxide generation, and mobilization of membrane-associated calcium in these cells (Serhan et al., 1983). Apparently LTB₄ is leukotactic also *in vivo*. Thus, intradermal injection of LTB₄ is associated with local accumulation of leukocytes in several species, including man (Bray et al., 1981; Soter et al., 1983), and neutrophils and macrophages may be harvested in large numbers after intraperitoneal injection of LTB₄ (Smith et al., 1980). When given systemically to rabbits and monkeys, LTB₄ causes a reversible drop in circulating leukocytes (Bray et al., 1981; Smedegård et al., 1982).

Intravital microscopy of the terminal vascular bed in the hamster cheek pouch and the rabbit tennuissimus muscle has disclosed that LTB₄ causes dramatic changes in the behaviour of circulating leukocytes (Dahlén et al., 1981; Björk et al. 1982a,b; Lindbom et al. 1982). Upon topical application of LTB₄ to either of the two *in vivo* models, marginating leukocytes begin to role at a slower rate, in spite of unchanged flow rate of the blood, and to stick to the endothelium in venules of all sizes and even in small veins. The adhesion of the leukocytes, visible within few minutes, increases with time and is followed after 10-15 min by diapedesis and further migration of the cells in the extravascular space. In addition to mobilizing leukocytes, LTB₄ promotes plasma leakage, but the mechanism differs from that of LTC₄-LTE₄. Thus, LTB₄ causes extravasation from both postcapillary and larger venules, and the reaction, which occurs with some time lag, is virtually abolished in neutropenic animals, suggesting that it is indirect and secondary to leukocyte adhesion to the endothelial lining.

According to electron microscopic studies of the two tissues (Thureson-Klein et al. 1984a,b, 1986, 1987; Hedqvist et al. 1987), LTB₄ causes all types of leukocytes to adhere to the endothelium. Subsequent diapedesis, with neutrophils and monocytes in the first row, always takes place between inter-digitating endothelial cells and virtually without formation of junctional gaps. It may also be deduced from the ultrastructural studies that LTB₄-induced extravasation of macromolecules is localized to the sites of adhering leuko-cytes and apparently occurs in the wake of migrating cells. With regard to effect of LTB₄ on the different types of leukocytes, the neutrophils are relatively resistant to degranulation, particularly in the tennuissimus muscle, whereas the basophils frequently release granular material. How-ever, the endothelium apparently remains intact even at sites where degranu-lated leukocytes attach. Only when LTB₄ is injected intraarterially and in high concentration may structural breakdown of endothelial cells become evident (Thureson-Klein unpublished), but in this case the chemotactic signal becomes misdirected and activated leukocytes fail to migrate into the extra-vascular space (Lundberg, et al. 1988). Therefore, it seems clear that LTB₄ applied extravascularly and in low concentrations better reflects the pre-sumed scenario in early inflammation, i.e. selective recruitment of leukocytes and extravasation of macromolecules along with migrating cells without signs of structural damage to the endothelial lining.

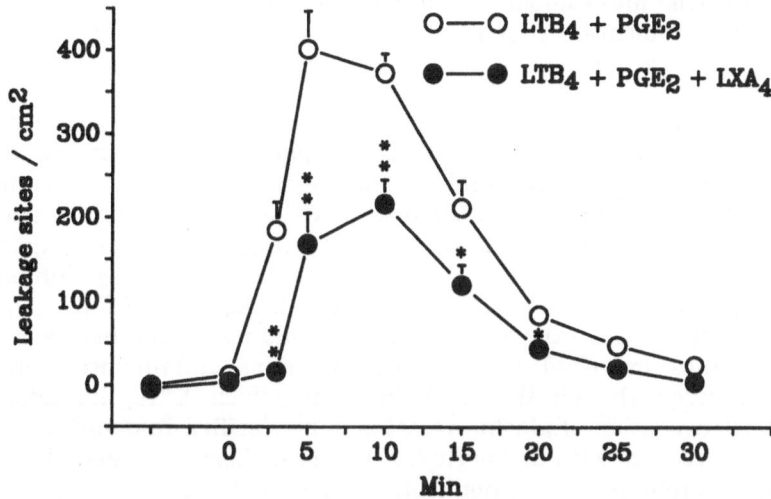

Fig. 2. Plasma extravasation provoked by topical application of LTB$_4$ (30 nM for 5 min)(open symbols) and LTB$_4$ in the presence of LXA$_4$ (300 nM)(filled symbols) to the microvasculature of hamster cheek pouches. PGE$_2$ (30 nM) added topically from -5 to +10 min in all experiments. Mean values ± SEM in 5+5 experiments. * : P < 0.05; **: P < 0.01.

MICROVASCULAR EFFECTS OF LIPOXIN A$_4$

Interaction between lipoxygenases acting at C-15 and C-5 of arachidonic acid has been shown to give rise to a new class of derivatives named lipoxins (LX), of which one major member is LXA$_4$ (5S,6R,15S-trihydroxy-7,9,13-trans-11-cis-eicosatetraenoic acid) (Serhan et al. 1984, 1986). The biological properties of LXA$_4$ have been explored using both biologically generated material and synthetic stereochemically defined compound (Nicolaou et al., 1985), in most cases with concordant results.

Several biological activities have been attributed to LXA$_4$, such as activation of protein kinase C (Hansson et al. 1986), inhibition of cytotoxicity of human NK cells (Ramstedt et al. 1985), constriction of guinea pig lung strips and human bronchi (Dahlén et al. 1987, 1988, 1989), and thromboxane release from guinea pig lung (Dahlén et al., 1987, Wikström et al., 1989). Lipoxin A$_4$ may also provoke superoxide generation and lysosomal enzyme release in human leukocytes (Serhan et al. 1984), but more recent investiga-

173

tions have mainly found a discrete chemokinetic action (Palmblad et al. 1988; Spur et al. 1988). With regard to the vascular system, LXA$_4$ causes arteriolar dilatation in rat kidney and hamster cheek pouch (Badr et al. 1987; Dahlén et al. 1987), relaxation of guinea pig aorta and human pulmonary artery but contraction of rat tail artery (Matsuda et al. 1989; Lam and Wong 1987). In the cheek pouch the vasodilatation response to LXA$_4$ was prompt and relatively short-lived and comparable to that of one of its precursors 15-HPETE. There was no indication that LXA$_4$ in concentrations up to 3 µM provoked increased vascular permeability or accumulation of leukocytes (see Fig. 1).

While LXA$_4$ per se seems to cause but vasodilatation in the hamster cheek pouch, other experiments with that particular preparation indicate that LXA$_4$ may be a potent inhibitor of the target action of inflammatory mediators (Hedqvist et al. 1989). Thus, LXA$_4$ both delayed and reduced the extravasation of plasma induced by LTB$_4$ (Fig. 2), however, apparently without affecting leukocyte adhesion to the endothelial lining. Inhibition of the leakage response was substantial with LXA$_4$ 300 nM and virtually complete after 3 µM. On the other hand, LXA$_4$ did not inhibit extravasation of macromolecules provoked by the directly acting inflammatory mediator histamine. Even though the mechanism by which LXA$_4$ inhibits LTB$_4$-induced extravasation of plasma remains to be clarified in detail, the results suggest interference with leukocyte function or leukocyte - endothelium interaction, rather than a direct action on the endothelial cells.

EFFECTS OF VASODILATIVE PROSTANOIDS IN INFLAMMATION

The antiphlogistic effect of non-steroidal anti-inflammatory drugs (NSAID:s) is well established and apparently correlates with inhibition of arachidonic acid metabolism. In particular the vasodilative PGE$_2$ and PGI$_2$ are generally accepted as proinflammatory agents, though they themselves provoke little or no edema or pain. The explanation for this apparent paradox is that they act in synergism with other inflammatory stimuli. Thus, they are believed to augment the response to pain producing agents by sensitizing the pain receptors (Ferreira 1972, 1978), and there is evidence that they potentiate evoked extravasation of plasma principally as a consequence of arteriolar dilation and increased blood flow (Williams 1983; Raud et al. 1988; Raud 1989). While this offers a straightforward explanation for the proinflammatory effects of vasodilative prostaglandins and consequently the pain relieving and edema suppressing therapeutic effects of NSAID:s, it should be observed that NSAID:s sometimes seem to enhance inflammatory reactions (Higgs et al. 1980; Hedqvist et al. 1984; Lundberg and Gerdin 1984), and several *in vitro* studies indicate that vasodilative prostaglandins may inhibit evoked release of mediators from granulocytes (Lichtenstein and Bourne 1971; Weissmann et al. 1980, Ham et al., 1983.), mast cells (Loeffler et al. 1971), and lung tissue (Walker 1973; Hitchcock 1978).

We have recently explored these seemingly discordant observations in experiments with the hamster cheek pouch (Raud et al. 1988, 1989a,b; Raud 1989). The results indicate that vasodilative prostaglandins may display both pro- and anti-inflammatory actions in one and the same tissue *in vivo*.

Thus, PGE_2 and PGI_2 strikingly enhanced the extravasation of plasma evoked by histamine, LTC_4, and LTB_4, as well as the LTB_4-induced accumulation of leukocytes (Fig. 3). Qualitatively and quantitatively the same potentiation was obtained with forskolin and nitroprusside in concentrations that matched the vasodilative effect of PGE_2 and PGI_2. Per se, the four enhancers had little or no capacity to cause plasma leakage or cell accumulation, indicating that their principal action was to make the terminal vascular bed more responsive to inflammatory mediators.

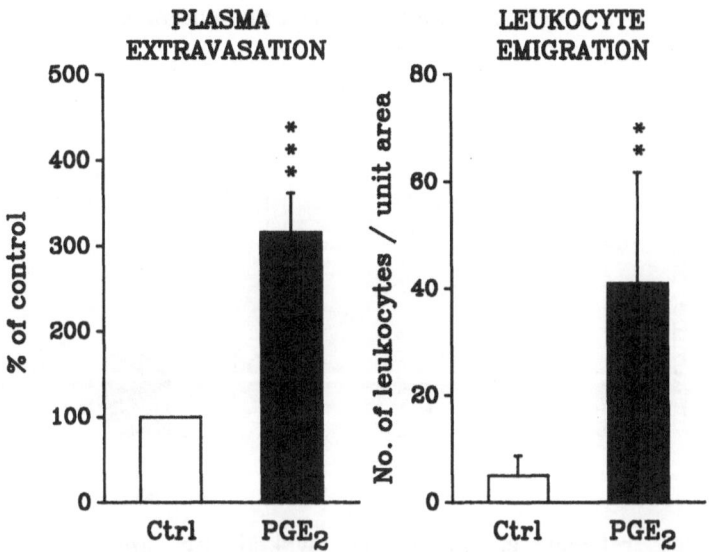

Fig. 3. Plasma extravasation and leukocyte diapedesis provoked by LTB_4 (20 nM) alone (Ctrl, open columns) and in the presence of PGE_2 (30 nM) (PGE_2, filled columns) in the hamster cheek pouch. Note that PGE_2 per se did not affect the two parameters. Mean values ± SD in 5+5 experiments. * : P < 0.05; **: P < 0.01.

A different pattern emerged in experiments where inflammation was induced by challenge with antigen or the mast cell secretagogue compound 48/80, both stimuli thus triggering release of endogenous mediators by activation of local mast cells. In this case, PGE_2 and PGI_2 inhibited the evoked leakage of plasma and accumulation of leukocytes. Forskolin also acted inhibitory, whereas nitroprusside enhanced the responses. The observed inhibition with PGE_2, PGI_2, and forskolin indicated an action on a plane distinct from the target level for inflammatory mediators and most likely on the process of mediator release from the mast cells. This interpretation gained support by the finding that PGE_2 substantially inhibited *in vivo* release of histamine evoked by antigen or compound 48/80 in the cheek pouch (Fig. 4). Furthermore, the NSAID:s indomethacin (Fig. 5) and diclofenac caused substantial enhancement of antigen-provoked inflammation, which could be referred to potentiation of mediator release (Fig. 4). Prostaglandin E_2 reversed the NSAID-induced potentiation both as regards mediator release and the ensuing inflammatory reactions (Figs. 4 and 5). The results summarized here indicate that vasodilative prostanoids may modulate the inflammatory process at two distinct levels and with opposite effects, as exemplified by inhibition of mediator release and enhancement of mediator

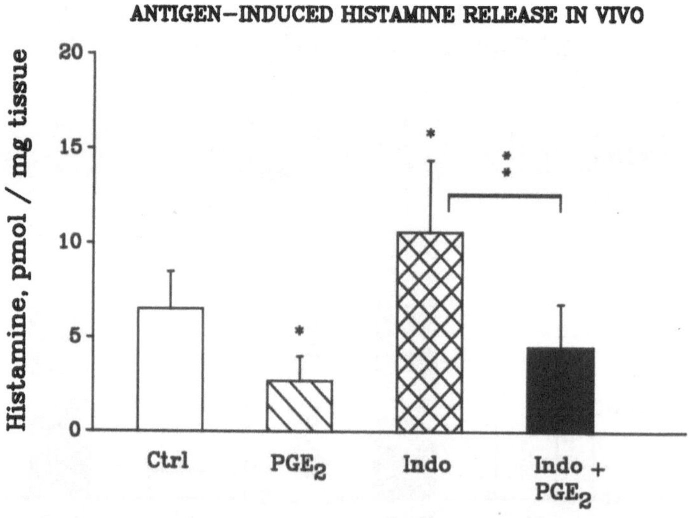

Fig. 4. Net release of histamine evoked by antigen challenge (ovalbumin 10 µg/ml topically for 5 min) in the hamster cheek pouch (Ctrl) is inhibited by PGE_2 (30 nM) and enhanced by indomethacin (6 µM, Indo). PGE_2 also reverses indomethacin-induced potentiation. Per se PGE_2 and indomethacind did not affect basal histamine release. Mean values ± SD, n=5-6. * : P < 0.05; **: P < 0.01; .

action. Furthermore, the differential effect of PGE_2, PGI_2 and forskolin versus that of nitroprusside on mediator release and on cAMP formation indicates that inhibition of mediator release is distinct from the process of vasodilatation, and might be linked to increased tissue levels of cAMP. Finally, the complete reversal by PGE_2 of the potentiating effect of NSAID:s on antigen-induced inflammation advocates a regulatory function on mediator release also by any of the endogenous entities.

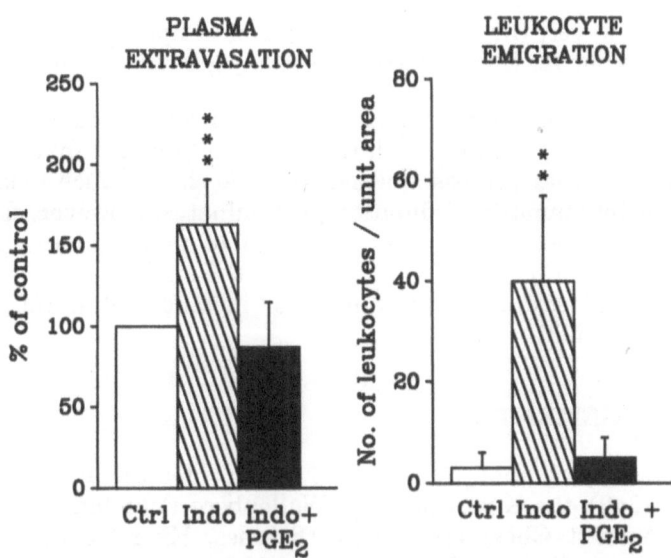

Fig. 5. Plasma extravasation and leukocyte diapedesis evoked by antigen challenge (ovalbumin 10 µg/ml topically for 5 min) alone (Ctrl) and in the presence of indomethacin (6 µM) or indomethacin + PGE$_2$ (30 nM) in hamster cheek pouches. Per se indomethacin or indomethacin + PGE$_2$ did not affect the two parameters. Mean values ± SD, n=5-6. **: P < 0.01; *** : P < 0.001 denote difference from Ctrl.

CONCLUSIONS

It is obvious that the eicosanoids display a number of biological actions with implication to the microvascular bed and the inflammatory process. The system is ubiquitous but also individual, as indicated by different cell populations usually manufacturing a single or a selected number of eicosanoids, which increases both the complexity and the versatility of the system. With regard to the leukotrienes they may be released from both blood borne and tissue residing white blood cells, and in minute concentrations they provoke local tissue edema and accumulation of phagocytizing cells. As a consequence they certainly have the potential to be important inflammatory mediators but several pieces of evidence remain to be collected before such a role can be established.

On the other hand, LXA$_4$ has microvascular actions (vasodilation, influence on leukocytes) that suggest mainly a modulatory role in inflammation. The inhibition by LXA$_4$ of leukocyte-dependent plasma extravasation may be an important mechanism for down-regulation of inflammation. Interestingly, LXA$_4$ may also inhibit actions of cysteinyl leukotrienes by specific antagonism at the level of the smooth muscle receptor (Dahlén et al.,

1987,1989). However, the relative contribution of lipoxins to the inflammatory process has not yet been investigated to any greater extent.

Finally, the vasodilative prostaglandins also seem to function primarily as modulators of inflammation, with the potential to both enhance and check dynamic events in that process. Judged from the cheek pouch model of mast cell-dependent inflammation inhibition predominates. However, factors such as the degree of local blood flow, the sites of prostaglandin production including the type preferentially formed, and the state of the tissue will all influence the final result and may in other instances alter the balance in favour of enhancement.

ACKNOWLEDGEMENTS

Supported by grants from the Swedish Medical Research Council (project 14X-4342), the Knut and Alice Wallenberg Foundation, the Swedish Association Against Chest and Heart Diseases, King Gustaf V Research Foundation, the Institute of Environmental Medicine, the Swedish Environment Protection Board (5324067-7), the National Institutet of Health (to KCN), the American Heart Association (to Å.T-K), Wenner-Gren Foundation and Karolinska Institutet.

REFERENCES

Badr, K.F., Serhan, C.N., and Nicolaou, K.C., 1987, The action of lipoxin A on glomerular microcirulatory dynamics in the rat. Biochem. Biophys. Res. Commun., 145:408-414.

Bisgaard, H., Kristensen, J. and Sondergaard, J, 1982, The effect of leukotriene C_4 and D_4 on cutaneous blood flow in humans. Prostaglandins, 23:797-801.

Björk, J., Hedqvist, P., and Arfors, K.-E., 1982a, Increase in vascular permeability induced by leukotriene B_4 and the role of polymorphonuclear leukocytes. Inflammation, 6:189-200.

Björk, J., Arfors, K.-E., Hedqvist, P., Dahlén, S.-E., and Lindgren, J.Å., 1982b, Leukotriene B_4 causes leukocyte migration in vivo. Microcirculation, 2:271-281.

Björk, J., Dahlén, S.-E., Hedqvist, P., and Arfors, K.-E., 1983, Leukotrienes B_4 and C_4 have distinct microcirculatory actions in vivo, in:"Advances in Prostaglandin, Thromboxane and Leukotriene Research", B. Samuelsson, R. Paoletti and P. Ramwell, eds, Vol. 12, pp.1-6, Raven Press, New York.

Björk, J., Smedegård, G., Svensjö, E., and Arfors, K.-E., 1984, The use of the hamster cheek pouch for intravital microscopy studies of microvascular events. Prog.Appl.Microcirc., 6:41-53.

Bray, M.A., Cunningham, F.M., Ford-Hutchinson, A.W., and Smith, M.J.H., 1981, Leukotriene B_4: a mediator of vascular permeability. Br.J.Pharmacol., 72:483-486.

Claesson, H.-E., 1982, Leukotrienes A_4 and B_4 stimulate the formation of cyclic AMP in human leukocytes. FEBS Lett., 139:305-308.

Dahlén, S.-E., Björk, J., Hedqvist, P., Arfors, K.-E., Hammarström, S., Lindgren, J.Å., and Samuelsson, B., 1981, Leukotrienes promote plasma leakage and leukocyte adhesion in postcapillary venules: In vivo effects with relevance to the acute inflammatory response. Proc.Natl.Acad.Sci.USA, 78:3887-3891.

Dahlén, S.-E., Raud, J., Serhan, C.N., Björk, J., and Samuelsson, B., 1987, Biological activities of lipoxin A include lung strip contraction and dilatation of arterioles in vivo. Acta Physiol.Scand., 130:643-648.

Dahlén, S.-E., Franzén, L., Raud, J., Serhan, C.N., Westlund, P., Wikström, E., Björck, T., Matsuda, H., Webber, S.E., Veale, C.A., Puustinen, T., Haeggström, J., Nicolaou, K.C. and Samuelsson, B., 1988, Actions of lipoxin A_4 and related compounds in smooth muscle preparations and on the microcirculation in vivo. In:"Lipoxins: Biosynthesis, Chemistry and Biological Activities", P.Y.-K. Wong, C.N. Serhan, eds, pp. 107-130, Plenum Press, New York.

Dahlén, S.-E., Veale, C.A., Webber, S.E., Marron, B.E., Nicolaou, K.C., and Serhan, C.N., 1989, Pharmacodynamics of Lipoxin A_4 in airway smooth muscle, Agents and Actions, 26:93-95.

Drazen, J.M., Austen, K.F., Lewis, R.A., Clark, D.A., Goto, G., Marfat, A., and Corey, E.J., 1980, Comparative airway and vascular activities of leukotrienes C-1 and D in vivo and in vitro. Proc.Natl.Acad.Sci.USA, 77:4354-4358.

Ferreira, S.H., 1972, Prostaglandins, aspirin-like drugs and analgesia. Nature New Biol. , 240:200-203.

Ferreira, S.H., Nakamura, M., and de Abreu Castro, M.S., 1978, The hyperalgesic effects of prostacyclin and prostaglandin E_2. Prostaglandins, 16:31-37.

Ford-Hutchinson, A.W., Bray, M.A., Doig, M.V., Shipley, M.E., and Smith, M.J.H., 1980, Leukotriene B, a potent chemokinetic and aggregating substance released from polymorphonuclear leukocytes. Nature, 286:264-265.

Goetzl, E.J., and Pickett, W.C., 1980, The human PMN leukocyte chemotactic activity of complex hydroxy-eicosatetraenoic acids (HETEs). J.Immunol., 125:1789-1791.

Ham, E.A., Soderman, D.D., Zanetti, M.E., Dougherty, H.W., McCauley, E., and Kuehl, F.A., 1983, Inhibition by prostaglandins of leukotriene B_4 release from activated neutrophils. Proc.Natl.Acad.Sci.USA, 80:4349-4353.

Hansson, A., Serhan, C.N. and Haeggström, J., 1986. Activation of protein kinase C by lipoxin A and other eicosanoids. Intracellular action of oxygenation products of arachidonic acid. Biochem. Biophys. Res. Commun., 134:1215-1222.

Hedqvist, P., Dahlén, S.-E., Gustafsson, L., Hammarström, S., and Samuelsson, B., 1980, Biological profile of leukotrienes C_4 and D_4. Acta Physiol.Scand., 110:331-333.

Hedqvist, P., Dahlén, S.-E., and Palmertz, U., 1984, Leukotriene-dependent airway anaphylaxis in guinea pigs. Prostaglandins, 28:605-608.

Hedqvist, P., Thureson-Klein, Å., Öhlén, A., Raud, J., Lindbom, L., and Dahlén S.-E., 1987, Neuropeptides and arachidonic acid derivatives as messengers in microvascular function, in:"Neuronal Messengers in Vascular Function", A. Nobin, C. Owman, B. Arneklo-Nobin, eds, pp.435-446, Elsevier, Amsterdam.

Hedqvist, P., Raud, J., Lindbom, L., Nicolaou, K.C., and Dahlén, S.-E., 1989, Lipoxin A_4 inhibits plasma leakage induced by leukotriene B_4 (submitted).

Higgs, G.A., Eakins, K.E., Mugridge, K.G., Moncada, S., and Vane, J.R., 1980, The effects of non-steroid anti-inflammatory drugs on leukocyte migration in carrageenin-induced inflammation. Eur.J.Pharmacol., 66:81-86.

Hitchcock, M., 1978, Effect of inhibitors of prostaglandin synthesis and prostaglandins E_2 and $F_{2\alpha}$ on the immunologic release of mediators of inflammation from actively sensitized guinea-pig lung. J.Pharmacol.Exp.Ther., 207:630-640.

Hua, X.-Y., Dahlén, S.-E., Hammarström, S., and Hedqvist, P., 1985, Leukotrienes C_4, D_4 and E_4 cause widespread and extensive plasma extravasation in the guinea pig. Naunyn-Schmiedebergs Arch.Pharmacol., 330:136-141.

Joris, I., Majno, G., Corey, E.J., and Lewis, R.A., 1987, The mechanism of vascular leakage induced by leukotriene E_4; Endothelial contraction. Am.J.Pathol., 126:19-24.

Lam, B.K., and Wong, P.Y.-K., 1988, Biosynthesis and biological activities of lipoxin A_5 and B_5 from eicosapentaenoic acid, in: "Lipoxins: Biosynthesis, Chemistry and Biological Activities", P.Y.-K. Wong, C.N. Serhan, eds, pp. 51-60, Plenum Press, New York.

Lichtenstein, L.M., and Bourne, H.R., 1971, Inhibition of allergic histamine release by histamine and other agents which stimulate adenyl cyclase, in:"Biochemistry of Acute Allergic Reactions:Second International Symposium", K.F. Austen, E.L. Becker, eds, pp. 161-174, Blackwell Scientific Publications, Oxford.

Lindbom, L., and Arfors, K.-E. 1984. The Tennuissimus Muscle Preparation as a Model for Intravital Microscopic Studies of Skeletal Muscle Circulatory Function. Prog.Appl.Microcirc., 6:32-40.

Lindbom, L., Hedqvist, P., Dahlén, S.-E., Lindgren, J.-Å., and Arfors, K.-E., 1982a, Leukotriene B_4 induces extravasation and migration of polymorphonuclear leukocytes in vivo. Acta Physiol.Scand., 116:105-108.

Loeffler, L.J., Lovenberg, W., and Sjoerdsma, A., 1971, Effects of dibutyryl-3',5'-cyclic adenosine monophosphate, phosphodiesterase inhibitors and prostaglandin E_1 on compound 48/80-induced histamine release from rat peritoneal mast cells in vitro. Biochem.Pharmacol., 20:2287-2297.

Lundberg, C., and Gerdin, B., 1984, The inflammatory reaction in an experimental model of open wounds in the rat. The effect of arachidonic acid metabolites. Eur.J.Pharmacol., 97:229-238.

Lundberg, C., Gardinali, M., Marceau, F., and Hugli, T.E., 1988, Effects of anaphylotoxins on vascular tissue *in vivo* and *in vitro*, in: "Endothelial Cells", U.S. Ryan, ed, Vol 2, pp. 243-257, CRC Press, Florida.

Malmsten, C.L., Palmblad, J., Udén, A.-M., Rådmark, O., Engstedt, L., and Samuelsson, B., 1980, Leukotriene B_4: A highly potent and stereospecific factor stimulating migration of polymorphonuclear leukocytes. Acta Physiol.Scand. , 110:449-451.

Matsuda, H., Dahlén, S.-E., Haeggström, J., Nicolaou, K.C., and Hedqvist, P., 1989, Lipoxins A_4 and B_4 relax isolated arteries from guinea pig and man. (submitted).

Nicolaou, K.C., Veale, C.A., Webber, S.E., Katerinopoulus, H., 1985, Stereo-controlled Total Synthesis of Lipoxins A, J. Am.Chem.Soc., 107:7515-7518.

Öhlén, A., Raud, J., Hedqvist, P., and Wiklund, P. 1988,· Microvascular effects of endothelin in the rabbit tennuissimus muscle and hamster cheek pouch, Microvasc. Res., in press.

Orange, R.P., and Austen, K.F., 1969, Slow reacting substance of anaphylaxis, Adv.Immunol. 10:105-144.

Palmblad, J., Gyllenhammar, H., and Ringertz, B., 1988, Effects of lipoxins A and B on functional responses of human granulocytes, in: "Lipoxins: Biosynthesis, Chemistry, and Biological Activities", P.Y-K. Wong, C.N. Serhan, eds, pp.137-145, Plenum Pressn, New York.

Peck, M.J., Piper, P.J., and Williams, T.J., 1981, The effect of leukotrienes C_4 and D_4 on the microvasculature of guinea pig skin. Prostaglandins, 21:315-321.

Ramstedt, U., Ng, J., and Wigzell, H., 1985, Action of novel eicosanoids lipoxin A and B on human natural killer cell cytotoxicity: Effects on intracellular cAMP and target cell binding. J.Immunol., 135:3434-3438.

Raud, J., 1989, Vasodilation and inhibition of mediator release as two distinct mechanisms for prostaglandin modulation of inflammation. (submitted).

Raud, J., Dahlén, S.-E., Sydbom, A., Lindbom, L., and Hedqvist, P., 1988, Enhancement of acute allergic inflammation by indomethacin is reversed by prostaglandin E_2:Apparent correlation with *in vivo* modulation of mediator release. Proc.Natl.Acad.Sci.USA, 85:2315-2319.

Raud, J., Sydbom, A., Dahlén, S.-E. and Hedqvist, P., 1989a, Prostaglandin E_2 prevents diclofenac-induced enhancement of histamine release and inflammation evoked by *in vivo* challenge with compound 48/80 in the hamster cheek pouch. Agents and Actions, in press.

Raud, J., Dahlén, S.-E., Sydbom, A., Lindbom, L. and Hedqvist, P., 1989b, Prostaglandin modulation of mast cell-dependent inflammation. Agents and Actions, 26:42-44.

Serhan, C.N., Radin, A., Smolen, J.E., Korchak, H., Samuelsson, B., and Weissmann, G., 1983, Leukotriene B_4 is a complete secretagogue in human neutrophils. Biochem.Biophys.Res.Commun., 107:1006-1012.

Serhan, C.N., Hamberg, M., and Samuelsson, B., 1984, Novel series of biologically active compounds formed from arachidonic acid in human leukocytes. Proc.Natl.Acad.Sci.USA, 81:5335-5339.

Serhan, C.N., Nicolaou, K.C., Webber, S.E., Veale, C.A., Dahlén, S.-E., Puustinen, T., and Samuelsson, B., 1986, Lipoxin A: Stereochemistry and biosynthesis. J.Biol.Chem., 261:16340-16345.

Smedegård, G., Hedqvist, P., Dahlén, S.-E., Revenäs, B., Hammarström, S., and Samuelsson, B., 1982, Leukotrienes C_4 affects pulmonary and cardiovascular dynamics in monkey. Nature, 295:327-329.

Smith, M.J.H., Ford-Hutchinson, A.W., and Bray, M.A., 1980, Leukotriene B: a potent mediator of inflammation. J.Pharm.Pharmacol., 32:517-518.

Soter, N.A., Lewis, R.A., Corey, E.J., and Austen, K.F., 1983, Local effects of synthetic leukotrienes (LTC_4, LTD_4,LTE_4 and LTB_4) in human skin. J.Invest.Dermatol., 80:115-119.

Spur, B.W., Jacques, C., Crea, A.E., and Lee, T.H., 1988, Lipoxins of the 5-series derived from eicosapentaenoic acid, in:"Lipoxins: Biosynthesis, Chemistry and Biological Actitivies", P.Y.-K. Wong, C.N. Serhan eds, pp. 147-154, Plenum Press, New York.

Thureson-Klein, Å., Hedqvist, P., and Lindbom, L., 1984a, Ultra-structure of polymorphonuclear leukocytes in postcapillary venules after exposure to leukotriene B_4 in vivo. Acta Physiol.Scand., 122:221-224.

Thureson-Klein, Å., Hedqvist, P., and Lindbom, L., 1984b, Ultra-structural effects of LTB_4 on leukocytes and blood vessels. Prostaglandins, 28:669-671.

Thureson-Klein, Å., Hedqvist, P., and Lindbom, L., 1986, Leukocyte diapedesis and plasma extravasation after leukotriene B_4: Lack of structural injury to the endothelium. Tissue Cell., 18:1-12.

Thureson-Klein, Å., Hedqvist, P., Öhlén, A., Raud, J., and Lindbom, L., 1987, Leukotriene B_4, platelet-activating factor and substance P as mediators of acute inflammation. Pathol.Immunopathol.Res. , 6:190-206.

Walker, J.L., 1973, The regulatory function of prostaglandins in the release of histamine and SRS-A from passively sensitized human lung tissue, in: "Advances in the Biosciences", S. Bergström, S. Bernhard, eds, Vol.9, pp. 235-240, Pergamon Press, New York.

Weissmann, G., Smolen, J.E., and Korchak, H., 1980, Prostaglandins and inflammation: Receptor/cyclase coupling as an explanation of why PGEs and PGI_2 inhibit functions of inflammatory cells, in:"Advances in Prostaglandin and Thromboxane Research", B. Samuelsson, P.W. Ramwell, R. Paoletti, eds., Vol. 8, pp. 1637-1646, Raven Press, New York.

Wikström, E., Westlund, P., Nicolaou, K.C., and Dahlén, S.-E., 1989. Lipoxin A_4 causes generation of thromboxane A_2 in the guinea-pig lung, Agents and Actions, 26:90-92.

Williams, T.J., 1983, Interactions between prostaglandins, leukotrienes and other mediators of inflammation. Br.Med.Bull., 39:239-242.

MODULATION OF THE INFLAMMATORY POTENTIAL OF THE 5-LIPOXYGENASE PATHWAY BY ALTERNATIVE FATTY ACIDS AND CYTOKINES

Robert A. Lewis

Syntex Research, Syntex Corporation
Palo Alto, CA 94304

INTRODUCTION

The inflammatory products of the 5-lipoxygenase pathway are considered to be locally-acting mediators, as compared to hormonal factors which can evoke their effects at great distances from the cell of origin. This is presumed to be correct because, despite the nanomolar potencies of several of these fatty acid metabolites for eliciting their effects, the quantities generated pathophysiologically are likely to be quite limited and the rate of metabolic inactivation in the circulation, significant. However, it is likewise clear that two classes of molecules that are more broadly bioavailable in the circulation, namely N-3 fatty acids provided in the diet by the oils of marine fish and certain cytokines, can have profound effects upon the generation of the 5-lipoxygenase products and certain of their elicited biological responses. Examples of such circulating regulators presetting the capacities for local mediator generation and response are the subject of this review.

ENZYMES OF THE 5-LIPOXYGENASE PATHWAY AND THEIR PRODUCTS

The 5-Lipoxygenase

In a variety of leukocyte types, the 5-lipoxygenase pathway metabolizes arachidonic acid to a hydroperoxy-fatty acid, which is reduced to a hydroxy-fatty acid, and to several leukotrienes. Subsequent to the action of 15-lipoxygenase on arachidonic acid, the 5-lipoxygenase also generates conjugated tetraene products, termed lipoxins.[1,2] The 5-lipoxygenase and subsequent enzymes in the cascade that it initiates exist in a limited number of cell types, including monocytes, macrophages, neutrophilic polymorphonuclear (PMN) leukocytes, eosinophils, basophils, and mast cells.[3,4] Although the 5-lipoxygenase recovered from supernatants of broken cell preparations after sedimentation at >100,000 xg[5-7] is not an intrinsic membrane protein, it is probably non-covalently membrane-associated for optimal function. The membrane association of enzyme and substrate is supported by the finding that the full catalytic activity of the 5-lipoxygenase purified from human PMN requires the back-addition of a membrane-rich fraction that was removed during the purification.[8] Purified 5-lipoxygenase enzymes derived from the rat basophilic leukemia cell (RBL-1), pig PMN, and human PMN[8-10] have apparent K_m values for arachidonic acid of 10 to 20 µM; these values are comparable to that of the cyclo-oxygenase[11] and lower than that of the 15-lipoxygenase[7,12] for the same substrate. Unlike the other polyunsaturated fatty acid lipoxy-genases, the 5-lipoxygenase has an obligatory functional requirement for ionic calcium.[8-10] Even when calcium ion is provided, the 5-lipoxy-genase, like the cyclooxygenase, responds to its hydroperoxide product with augmentation of its catalytic capacity.[13,14]

The action of the 5-lipoxygenase on arachidonic acid produces 5-hydroperoxyeicosatetraenoic acid (5-HPETE), which is short-lived in physiologic buffers and is degraded either non-enzymatically or cataly-tically via a peroxidase to the corresponding alcohol, 5-hydroxy-eicosa-tetraenoic acid (5-HETE). In a sequential catalytic step, the 5-lipoxygenase converts 5-HPETE to the epoxide leukotriene LTA_4. The less effective conversion of 5-HPETE to LTA_4 when the hydroperoxide is added directly to the purified enzyme[15] indicates that the second step is facilitated by the initial interaction of arachidonic acid with the 5-lipoxygenase. The oxygenation of arachidonic acid is carried out in conjunction with the extraction by the enzyme of a specific "pre-chiral" hydrogen from the seventh carbon (C-7); the conversion of the hydro-peroxide to the epoxide likewise involves the extraction of a specific "pre-chiral" hydrogen from C-10 in conjunction with closure of the epoxide ring.[8,16] 5-HETE can be adducted into lysophospholipids,[17] and some 5-HPETE could theoretically be covalently coupled into lysophospholipids before being reduced to the alcohol. 5-HETE can also be exported from leukocytes[18] and taken up by platelets, which, via action of their 12-lipoxygenase and subsequent reduction of the 12-hydroperoxide domain, produce 5S,12S-dihydroxy-6,10-_trans_-8,14-_cis_-eicosatetraenoic acid (12-_epi_-6-_trans_-8-_cis_-LTB_4).[1] 5-HETE can also enter leukocytes for conversion by 15-lipoxygenase to a 5,15-diol,[19] but 5-HETE is not believed to be a key substrate in the generation of the 5,6,15- or 5,14,15-triol conjugated tetraenes, lipoxins A and B.[2,20,21]

The 5-lipoxygenase can also accept certain polyunsaturated fatty acid substrates other than arachidonic acid. Eicosapentaenoic acid (EPA; 20:5, N-3) and docosahexaenoic acid (22:6, N-3) are provided in the diet of individuals consuming a significant quantity of marine fish oil, and via chain extension and desaturation, from the linolenic acid (18:3, N-3) derived from seaweed and related plant life. EPA is converted to its C-5 hydroperoxide with an apparent K_m of 13 µM,[6] which is comparable to that of the enzyme for arachidonic acid. Docosahexaenoic acid is a poor substrate, which is modestly converted to its C-7 or C-4 hydroperoxides.[22-24] Whereas 5-hydroperoxy-EPA (5-HPEPE) is readily converted to its epoxide leukotriene (LTA_5) by the 5-lipoxygenase,[22,24] the small quantities of 7- and 4-hydroperoxy-docosahexaenoic acids are not metabolized to leukotrienes.

LTB Synthetase/Epoxide Hydrolase and LTC Synthetase

Metabolism of LTA_4 to various 5,12-dihydroxy leukotrienes involves at least three routes: catalytic conversion by a specific epoxide hydrolase[25,26] to LTB_4 in the same cell that provided the LTA_4 via action of the 5-lipoxygenase; export from the cell of origin[27-31] and catalytic conversion by an epoxide hydrolase of another cell ["transcellular metabolism"][28,29] or of blood plasma;[32] or non-enzymatic hydrolysis to 5S,12S- and 5S,12R-dihydroxy-6,8,10-_trans_-14-cis-eicosatetraenoic acids (the 12-_epi_-6-_trans_-LTB_4 and 6-trans-LTB_4 diastereoisomers). The epoxide hydrolase has a favorable apparent K_m (20-30 μM) for LTA_4, which it converts to LTB_4[26] while simultaneously undergoing inactivation.[33] LTA_5 is an even more effective inactivator of the epoxide hydrolase and is less readily metabolized to LTB_5 than is LTA_4 to LTB_4.[24,33]

The microsomal enzyme that preferentially metabolizes LTA_4 to LTC_4, termed LTC synthetase, is a unique member of the family of glutathione-S-transferases. In contrast with the more classical cytosolic or microsomal glutathione-S-transferases, LTC synthetase does not utilize aromatic xenobiotics and aromatic chemical toxins as substrates.[34,35] The kinetics for solubilized, partially purified LTC synthetase from rat basophilic leukemia and guinea pig lung are similar.[35,36] The apparent K_m of LTC synthetase in a microsomal fraction from rat basophilic leukemia cells for LTA_4 is 5-10 μM and its apparent K_m for glutathione is 3-6 mM. Transcellular metabolism of LTA_4 to LTC_4 may also occur in endothelial cells[30] and platelets,[31] neither of which possesses 5-lipoxygenase activity. Since the LTC synthetase should be able to compete with the epoxide hydrolase for substrate LTA_4 on the basis of the relative K_m values, the relative presence of the terminal pathway enzymes should determine the ratios of generated LTB_4:LTC_4 in most cells containing the 5-lipoxygenase. As for LTA_4, LTA_5 is also a substrate for the LTC synthase, which yields LTC_5 as a product.

Eosinophils generate 25-50 ng of LTC_4 per 10^6 cells in response to activation with the calcium ionophore A23187,[37-39] but produce no LTB_4. Dispersed and purified human pulmonary mast cells, which have not been maintained in cell culture, yield LTC_4 without LTB_4, whether activated by A23187 or via IgE-dependent mechanisms.[40] Following a week of co-culture on murine 3T3 fibroblasts, partially purified human lung mast cells respond to IgE-Fc-dependent activation with augmented production of LTC_4 and of modest amounts of LTB_4.[41] In contrast, human pulmonary macrophages produce relatively little LTC_4, although they generate substantial quantities of LTB_4, in some cases >100 ng per 10^6 cells.[42-44] Human PMN produce about 40 ng LTB_4 per 10^6 cells in response to A23187; the variable and minimal quantity of LTC_4 produced by human PMN preparations is attributable to contamination with eosinophils.[45] Only the human monocyte can generate comparable quantities of LTB_4 and LTC_4 in response to calcium ionophore or transmembrane stimuli with the product ratio varying depending upon the agonist.[46-49]

Enzymes that Metabolize LTB_4 and LTC_4

During incubation periods of up to 30 minutes, metabolism of LTB_4 has been demonstrated only in PMN and not in eosinophils, monocytes, or pulmonary alveolar macrophages of the human. The enzymes responsible for processing of LTB_4 cause its ω-oxidation and thereby inactivate its biological activities. The LTB 20-hydroxylase, which oxidizes the C-20 methyl group to an alcohol,[50] is a unique enzyme, which differs from prostaglandin ω-oxidases and fatty acid ω-oxidase,[51-56] although each, as a member of the P450 oxidase family, uses the same coupled reductase.[55,56] The subsequent oxidation of the ω-hydroxy-LTB_4 can be effected by a cytosolic NAD+-dependent dehydrogenase or by the microsomal LTB 20-hydroxylase.[57] The K_m of the LTB_4 20-hydroxylase for its interaction with LTB_4 is 0.2-1.0 μM. Since LTB_4 is taken up into human PMN via a specific binding site or receptor,[58-61] LTB_4 from cell sources other than PMN would be readily metabolized. It is also possible that ω-OH-LTB_4 can also be taken up into the PMN, since it binds to the LTB_4 receptor.[62]

Further metabolism of LTC_4 occurs via two pathways, one of which is peptidolytic and the other, oxidative. Peptide cleavage of LTC_4 happens via the action of γ-glutamyl-transpeptidase, with removal of glutamic acid, to yield LTD_4. This process exists in cytochalasin B-treated mono-cytes,[59] but probably not in granulocytes.[63] However, since a variety of non-leukocyte cell types also show this activity as an exoenzyme,[64] peptidolytic cleavage of LTC_4 released by leukocytes would be significant in most tissues, including lung[65] and blood plasma.[66,67] A variety of peptidases, including an activity from human PMN-specific granules[63] and one in blood plasma,[66,67] can catalyze the subsequent cleavage of LTD_4 to LTE_4 with the release of glycine.

Oxidative metabolism of LTC_4, LTD_4, and LTE_4 leading to the generation of the S-diastereoisomeric sulfoxides of each and the 6-trans-(C-12)-diastereoisomers of LTB_4, occurs only in the extra-cellular environment of activated PMN and eosinophils[37,68,69] and of activated and highly concentrated monocytes.[70] The mechanism involves the cellular production of hydrogen peroxide via the respiratory burst, the secretion of the cell-specific peroxidase, and the interaction of enzyme, peroxide, and chloride ion to produce hypochlorous acid as the moiety which attacks the cysteinly-leukotriene. There are two major biologic differences between the peptidolytic pathway and the oxidative one. The former pathway does not require activated cells and does not eliminate the biological activities; the latter requires cell activation and results in functional catabolism.[37,68,69] It appears that in normal primates, the metabolic fate of LTE_4 is urinary excretion without additional modification; in rodents, LTE_4 is N-acetylated prior to excretion.[71-73] In vivo assessment for oxidative degradation of the cysteinyl-leukotrienes has not yet been reported.

EPA EFFECTS ON LEUKOCYTE BIOLOGY

The effects of eicosapentaenoic acid on the biology of human PMN in vivo could presumably include both those of EPA already incorporated into the leukocyte phospholipids and those of the cell-associated, but not covalently bound free fatty acid. However, it is not clear that the free fatty acid has any unique effects. The addition of exogenous EPA to human PMN in vitro, which almost surely allows some modest incorporation into phospholipids as well as presenting highly concentrated free fatty acid in the extracellular environment, has the same major effect on ionophore-activated PMN as the in vivo incorporation of EPA into cellular lipids during dietary manipulation of human subjects with subsequent ex vivo activation of the PMN: inhibition of the LTB synthetase/epoxide hydrolase.[22,24] The much greater membrane incorporation of EPA that occurs in in vivo studies additionally inhibits the hydrolytic release of arachidonic acid from its membrane phospholipid pools,[24] presumably by inhibiting the activation or activity of phospholipase A_2 (PLA_2) directly or indirectly.

In these experiments, PMN and monocytes of normal human subjects were purified before the subjects had begun ingesting a dietary supplement containing 3.2 grams/day of EPA-containing triglycerides and also at three and six weeks into the diet. The cells were activated ex vivo with the calcium ionophore A23187 on dose- and time-dependent bases, followed by lipid extraction, resolution on reverse phase high performance liquid chromatography, and quantitation by ultraviolet absorbance and/or radioimmunoassay of each 5-lipoxygenase product. A similar fish oil dietary protocol was subsequently carried out in subjects with active rheumatoid arthritis who were also taking non-steroidal anti-inflammatory drugs with or without addition of hydroxychloroquine. After six weeks on the dietary supplement, the PMN content of arachidonic acid and the stimulated biosynthesis of LTB_4 from PMN in each subject group were suppressed relative to the pre-dietary same-subject control measurements as were monocyte values in the study of normal subjects on the diet.[22,74] Monocytes from both normal subjects and rheumatoid arthritis patients that were harvested after six weeks on the diet were also inhibited for the production of the platelet activating factor (PAF; 1-O-alkyl-sn-2-acetyl-glyceryl-phosphorylcholine).[74,75] These results further support the suggestion that incorporated EPA suppresses PLA_2, since its substrate pool of alkyl-arachidonyl-glyceryl-phosphorylcholines yields both arachidonic acid and the precursor of PAF.

The studies involving the normal subjects on the fish oil supplement was also noteworthy because, whereas these regulatory effects were noted at six weeks into the dietary regimen, they could not be demonstrated at only three weeks of the diet. The most reasonable explanation, given that EPA was esterified into the leukocyte lipids at both times, is that the distribution of the EPA into PLA_2 substrate and/or PLA_2 regulatory phospholipid pools differed. This, in turn, would necessarily reflect a requirement that a leukocyte bone marrow precursor incorporated the EPA more than three weeks before the leukocytes were sampled and analyzed.

Differences in two biological functions of PMN could also be shown by comparing cells from the normal subjects at six weeks of the diet with those from the pre-diet period. By six weeks, the PMN had become one hundred-fold less sensitive to LTB_4 as a chemotactic factor and could respond maximally to only 30% of their highest level of chemotactic response in the pre-diet period. Additionally, whereas adherence of the PMN to bovine endothelial monolayers could be increased by preincubation of the endothelial cells with LTB_4 before dietary supplementation, six weeks of EPA-rich triglycerides abrogated the effect. Just as for the biochemical affects, the biological responses at three weeks on the diet were not different from the predietary control period.[22] After six weeks off the dietary supplement, all effects on the leukocytes had reverted to the pre-dietary state.

PMN chemotactic responses to N-formyl-met-leu-phe tripeptide and LTB_4 of cells from the rheumatoid arthritics were greatly decreased relative to those of normal subjects, when each subject group was on a normal diet. For the arthritic patients on the fish oil supplement for six weeks, an increase occurred in the chemotactic responsiveness of PMN to each stimulus.[74] We have hypothesized that the disease process chemotactically deactivated the PMN by in vivo presentation of chemotactic factors, so that an increased chemotactic responsiveness during the dietary manipulation represented the overriding influence of decreasing 5-lipoxygenase product generation in vivo. Likewise, the enhanced capacity of PMN to adhere to bovine aortic endothelium, pretreated with LTB_4, as noted for the leukocytes of normal subjects, was not demonstrable for PMN of rheumatoid arthritics, either before or after the fish oil supplementation, and could also represent in vivo deactivation.

CYTOKINES AND THE 5-LIPOXYGENASE PATHWAY

The biochemical and biological differences between the phagocytes of rheumatoid arthritis patients and those of normal subjects are also consistent with regulatory effects exerted by non-lipid products of cells in the inflammatory micrienvironment. The capacities of certain acidic monokines to enhance the leukotriene-generating responses of PMN and eosinophils to the calcium ionophore A23187 [76] may serve as an example. These monokines are produced by adherent human monocytes in culture with bacterial lipopolysaccharide. Although they do not directly elicit leukotriene production, they modestly enhance PMN biosynthesis of LTB_4 in response to A23187 and more than quadruple the generation of LTC_4 by A23187-activated eosinophyls.

Recombinant human granulocyte-macrophage colony-stimulating factor (GM-CSF) has also been shown to enhance A23187-evoked LTC_4 biosynthesis from human eosinophils in both time- and dose-dependent experiments; maximal augmentation occurs after 60 min preincubation with 40 pmolar GM-CSF.[77] Comparable augmentation of LTC_4 generation has been demonstrated for eosinophils that were cultured with recombinant human interleukin-3.[78] 5-lipoxygenase pathway production by mononuclear phagocytes can also be modulated by cytokines. Incubation of human alveolar macrophages for 24 hours with γ-interferon (IFN-γ) dose-dependently increases the cellular responsiveness to heat-aggregated IgG complexes for LTB_4 generation.[79] The same dose range (10-1000 U/ml) of γ-interferon has a parallel dose-response for increasing the number of IgG Fcγ receptors on the cultured alveolar macrophages. That IFN-γ does not affect LTB_4 synthesis by A23187, a receptor-independent stimulus, implies that the effect of IFN-γ is due to upregulation of receptors and proximal post-receptor portions of the activation cascade. That neither IFN-α nor IFN-ß had effects on IgG Fcγ receptor number or LTB_4 generation suggests receptor specificity for the IFN-γ. The parallel effects of IFN-γ on the number of cell activating receptors and the increased leukotriene-generating response to the augmented receptor number is reminiscent of the opposite effect of dexamethasone pretreatment of murine bone marrow-derived mast cells; this treatment was shown to decrease IgE receptor numbers and, in parallel, the antigen-dependent generation of LTC_4.[80]

REFERENCES

1. B. Samuelsson, S. Hammarström, M. Hamberg, and C. N. Serhan, Structural determination of leukotrienes and lipoxins, Adv. Prost. Thromb. Leuk. Res. 14:45 (1985).
2. B. J. Fitzsimmons, J. Adams, J. F. Evans, Y. Leblanc, and J. Rokach, The lipoxins: stereochemical identification and determination of their biosynthesis, J. Biol. Chem. 260:13008 (1985).
3. R. A. Lewis and K. F. Austen, The biologically active leukotrienes: biosynthesis, metabolism, receptors, functions, and pharmacology, J. Clin. Invest. 73:889 (1984).
4. D. W. MacGlashin, Jr., S. P. Peters, J. Warner, and L. M. Lichtenstein, Characteristics of human basophil sulfidopeptide leukotriene release: releasability defined as the ability of the basophil to respond to dimeric cross-links, J. Immunol. 136:2231 (1986).
5. B. A. Jakschik and C. H. Lee, Enzymatic assembly of slow reacting substance, Nature 287:51 (1980).
6. K. Ochi, T. Yoshimoto, S. Yamamoto, K. Taniguchi, and T. Miyamoto, Arachidonate 5-lipoxygenase of guinea pig peritoneal polymorphonuclear leukocytes: activation by adenosine-5' triphosphate, J. Biol. Chem. 258:5754 (1983).
7. R. J. Soberman, T. W. Harper, D. Betteridge, R. A. Lewis, and K. F. Austen, Characterization and separation of the arachidonic acid 5-lipoxygenase and linoleic acid ω-6 lipoxygenase (arachidonic acid 15-lipoxygenase) of human polymorphonuclear leukocytes, J. Biol. Chem. 260:4508 (1985).

8. C. A. Rouzer and B. Samuelsson, On the nature of the 5-lipoxygenase reaction in human leukocytes: enzyme purification and requirement for multiple stimulatory factors, Proc. Natl. Acad. Sci. USA 82:6040 (1985).

9. N. Ueda, S. Kaneko, T. Yoshimoto, and S. Yamamoto, Purification of arachidonate 5-lipoxygenase from porcine leukocytes and its reactivity with hydroperoxyeicosatetraenoic acids, J. Biol. Chem. 261:7982 (1986).

10. A. M. Goetze, L. Fayer, J. Bouska, D. Bornemeier, and G. W. Carter, Purification of a mammalian 5-lipoxygenase from rat basophilic leukemia cells, Prostaglandins 29:689 (1985).

11. S. Yamamoto, Purification and assay of PGH synthase from bovine seminal vesicles, in: "Methods in Enzymology, Vol 86," W. E. M. Lands and W. L. Smith, eds., Academic Press, New York (1982).

12. S. Narumiya, J. A. Salmon, L. H. Coltee, B. G. Weatherly, and R. J. Flower, Arachidonic acid 15-lipoxygenase from rabbit peritoneal polymorphonuclear leukocytes: partial purification and properties, J. Biol. Chem. 256:9583 (1981).

13. W. E. M. Lands, Interactions of lipid hydroperoxides with eicosanoid biosynthesis, J. Free Radic. Biol. Med. 1:97 (1985).

14. C. C. Reddy, M. K. Rao, A. M. Mastro, and R. W. Egan, Measurement of glutathione requiring enzymes involved in arachidonic acid cascade of rat basophil leukemia cells, Biochem. Int. 9:755 (1984).

15. C. A. Rouzer, T. Matsumoto, and B. Samuelsson, Single protein from human leukocytes possesses 5-lipoxygenase and leukotriene A_4 synthase activities, Proc. Natl. Acad. Sci. USA 83:857 (1986).

16. R. L. Maas, C. D. Ingram, D. F. Taber, J. A. Oates, and A. R. Brash, Stereospecific removal of the DR hydrogen atom at the 10-carbon of arachidonic acid in the biosynthesis of leukotriene A_4 by human leukocytes, J. Biol. Chem. 257:13515 (1982).

17. W. F. Stenson and C. W. Parker, Metabolism of arachidonic acid in ionophore-stimulated neutrophils: esterification of a hydroxylated metabolite into phospholipids, J. Clin. Invest. 64:1457 (1979).

18. J. D. Williams, T. H. Lee, R. A. Lewis, and K. F. Austen, Intracellular retention of the 5-lipoxygenase pathway product, leukotriene B_4, by human neutrophils activated with unopsonized zymosan, J. Immunol. 134:2624 (1985).

19. R. L. Maas, J. Turk, J. A. Oates, and A. Brash, Formation of a novel dihydroxy acid from arachidonic acid by lipoxygenase-catalyzed double oxygenation in rat mononuclear cells and human leukocytes, J. Biol. Chem. 257:7056 (1982).

20. C. N. Serhan, M. Hamberg, and B. Samuelsson, Trihydroxytetraenes: a novel series of compounds formed from arachidonic acid in human leukocytes. Biochem. Biophys. Res. Commun. 118:943 (1984).

21. C. N. Serhan, M. Hamberg, B. Samuelsson, J. Morris, and D. G. Wishka, On the stereochemistry and biosynthesis of lipoxin B, Proc. Natl. Acad. Sci. USA 83:1983 (1986).

22. T. H. Lee, R. L. Hoover, J. D. Williams, R. I. Sperling, J. R. Ravalese, III, B. W. Spur, D. R. Robinson, E. J. Corey, R. A. Lewis, and K. F. Austen, Effect of dietary enrichment with eicosapentaenoic and docosahexaenoic acids on in vitro neutrophil and monocyte leukotriene generation and neutrophil function, N. Engl. J. Med. 312:1217 (1985).

23. S. Fischer, C. von Schacky, W. Siess, T. Strasser, and P. C. Weber, Uptake, release and metabolism of docosahexaenoic acid (DHA C22:6 3) in human platelets and neutrophils, <u>Biochem. Biophys. Res. Commun.</u> 120:907 (1984).

24. T. H. Lee, J. M. Mencia-Huerta, C. Shih, E. J. Corey, R. A Lewis, and K. F. Austen, Effects of exogenous arachidonic, eicosapentaenoic, and docosahexaenoic acids on the generation of 5-lipoxygenase pathway products by ionophore-activated human neutrophils, <u>J. Clin. Invest.</u> 74:1922 (1984).

25. O. Rådmark, C. Malmsten, B. Samuelsson, D. A. Clark, G. Goto, A. Marfat, and E. J. Corey, Leukotriene A: stereochemistry and enzymatic conversion to leukotriene B, <u>Biochem. Biophys. Res. Commun.</u> 92:954 (1980).

26. O. Rådmark, T. Shimizu, M. Jörnvall, and B. Samuelsson, Leukotriene A_4 hydrolase in human leukocytes. Purification and properties, <u>J. Biol. Chem.</u> 259:12339 (1984).

27. C. A. Dahinden, R. M. Clancy, M. Gross, J. M. Chiller, and T. E. Hugli, Leukotriene C_4 production by murine mast cells: evidence for a role for extracellular leukotriene A_4, <u>Proc. Natl. Acad. Sci. USA</u> 82:6632 (1985).

28. J. E. McGee and F. A. Fitzpatrick, Erythrocyte-neutrophil interactions: formation of leukotriene B_4 by transcellular biosynthesis, <u>Proc. Natl. Acad. Sci. USA</u> 83:1349 (1986).

29. F. A. Fitzpatrick, W. Liggett, J. McGee, S. Bunting, D. Morton, and B. Samuelsson, Metabolism of leukotriene A_4 by human erythrocytes. A novel cellular source of leukotriene B_4, <u>J. Biol. Chem.</u> 259:11403 (1985).

30. S. J. Feinmark and P. J. Cannon, Endothelial cell leukotriene C_4 synthesis results from intercellular transfer of leukotriene A_4 synthesized by polymorphonuclear leukocytes, <u>J. Biol. Chem.</u> 261:16466 (1986).

31. C. R. Pace-Asciak, J. Klein, and S. P. Spielberg, Metabolism of leukotriene A_4 into C_4 by human platelets, <u>Biochim. Biophys. Acta</u> 877:68 (1986).

32. F. A. Fitzpatrick, J. Haeggström, E. Granström, and B. Samuelsson, Metabolism of leukotriene A_4 by an enzyme in blood plasma, <u>Proc. Natl. Acad. Sci. USA</u> 80:5425 (1983).

33. D. J. Nathaniel, J. F. Evans, Y. Leblanc, C. Leveille, B. J. Fitzsimmons, and A. W. Ford-Hutchinson, Leukotriene A_5 is a substrate and an inhibitor of rat and human neutrophil LTA_4 hydrolase, <u>Biochem. Biophys. Res. Commun.</u> 131:827 (1985).

34. M. K. Bach, J. R. Brashler, and D. R. Morton, Jr., Solubilization and characterization of the leukotriene C_4 synthetase of rat basophil leukemia cells: a novel, particulate glutathione-S-transferase. <u>Arch. Biochem. Biophys.</u> 230:455 (1984).

35. T. Yoshimoto, R. J. Soberman, R. A. Lewis, and K. F. Austen, Isolation and characterization of leukotriene C_4 synthetase of rat basophilic leukemia cells, <u>Proc. Natl. Acad. Sci. USA</u> 82:8399 (1985).

36. T. Yoshimoto, R. J. Soberman, B. Spur, and K. F. Austen, Properties of highly purified leukotriene C_4 synthase of guinea pig lung, <u>J. Clin. Invest.</u> 81:866 (1988).

37. P. F. Weller, C. W. Lee, D. W. Foster, E. J. Corey, K. F. Austen, and R. A. Lewis, Generation and metabolism of 5-lipoxygenase pathway leukotrienes by human eosinophils: predominant production of leukotriene C_4, <u>Proc. Natl. Acad. Sci. USA</u> 80:7626 (1983).

38. R. J. Shaw, O. Cromwell, and A. B. Kay, Preferential generation of leukotriene C_4 by human eosinophils, Clin. Exp. Immunol. 56:716 (1984).

39. W. R. Henderson, J. B. Harley, and A. S. Fauci, Arachidonic acid metabolism in normal and hypereosinophilic syndrome human eosinophils: generation of leukotriene B_4, C_4, D_4, and 15-lipoxygenase products, Immunology 51:679 (1984).

40. S. P. Peters, D. W. MacGlashan, Jr., E. S. Schulman, R. P. Schleimer, E. C. Hayes, J. Rokach, N. F. Adkinson, Jr., and L. M. Lichtenstein, Arachidonic acid metabolism in purified human lung mast cells, J. Immunol. 132:1972 (1984).

41. F. Levi-Schaffer, K. F. Austen, J. P. Caulfield, A. Hein, P. M. Gravallese, and R. L. Stevens, Co-culture of human lung-derived mast cells with mouse 3T3 fibroblasts: morphology and IgE-mediated release of histamine, prostaglandin D_2, and leukotrienes, J. Immunol. 129:494 (1987).

42. A. O. S. Fels, N. A. Pawlowski, E. B. Cramer, T. K. C. King, Z. A. Cohn, and W. A. Smith, Human alveolar macrophages produce leukotriene B_4, Proc. Natl. Acad. Sci. USA 79:7866 (1982).

43. J. MacDermott, C. R. Kelsey, K. A. Waddell, R. Richmond, R. K. Knight, P. J. Cole, C. T. Dollery, D. N. Landon, and I. A. Blair, Synthesis of leukotriene B_4 and prostanoids by human alveolar macrophages: analysis by gas chromatography/mass spectrometry, Prostaglandins 27:163 (1984).

44. T. R. Martin, L. C. Altman, R. K. Albert, and W. R. Henderson, Leukotriene B_4 production by the human alveolar macrophage: a potential mechanism for amplifying inflammation in the lung, Am. Rev. Respir. Dis. 129:106 (1984).

45. W. F. Owen, jr., R. J. Soberman, T. Yoshimoto, A. L. Sheffer, R. A. Lewis, and K. F. Austen, Synthesis and release of leukotriene C_4 by human eosinophils, J. Immunol. 138:532 (1987).

46. J. D. Williams, J. K. Czop, and K. F. Austen, Release of leukotrienes by human monocytes on stimulation of their phagocytic receptor for particulate activators, J. Immunol. 132:3034 (1984).

47. M. E. Goldyne, G. F. Burrish, P. Poubelle, and P. Borgeat, Arachidonic acid metabolism among human mononuclear leukocytes: lipoxygenase released pathways, J. Biol. Chem. 259:8815 (1984).

48. J. K. Czop and K. F. Austen, Generation of leukotrienes by human monocytes upon stimulation of their B-glucan receptor during phagocytosis, Proc. Natl. Acad. Sci. USA 82:2751 (1985).

49. J. D. Williams, J. L. Robin, R. A. Lewis, T. H. Lee, and K. F. Austen, Generation of leukotrienes by human monocytes pretreated with cytochalasin B and stimulated with formyl-methionyl-leucyl- phenylalanine, J. Immunol. 136:642 (1986).

50. W. Jubiz, O. Rådmark, C. Malmsten, G. Hansson, J. A. Lindgren, J. Palmblad, A. M. Udén, and B. Samuelsson, A novel leukotriene produced by stimulation of leukocytes with formylmethionylleucyl- phenylalanine, J. Biol. Chem. 257:6106 (1982).

51. W. S. Powell, Properties of leukotriene B_4 20-hydroxylase from polymorphonuclear leukocytes, J. Biol. Chem 259:3082 (1984).
52. S. Shak and I. M. Goldstein, Omega-oxidation is the major pathway for the catabolism of leukotriene B_4 in human polymorphonuclear leukocytes, J. Biol. Chem. 259:10181 (1984).
53. R. J. Soberman, R. W. Harper, R. C. Murphy, and K. F. Austen, Identification and functional characterization of leukotriene B_4 20-hydroxylase of human polymorphonuclear leukocytes, Proc. Natl. Acad Sci. USA 82:2292 (1985).
54. S. Shak and I. Goldstein, Leukotriene B_4 w-hydroxylase in human polymorphonuclear leukocytes, J. Clin. Invest. 76:1218 (1985).
55. D. E. Williams, S. E. Hale, R. T. Okita, and B. S. Masters, A prostaglandin omega-hydroxylase cytochrome P-450 (P-450PG-omega) purified from lungs of pregnant rabbits, J. Biol. Chem. 259:14600 (1984).
56. R. J. Soberman, R. T. Okita, B. Fitzsimmons, J. Rokach, B. Spur, and K. F. Austen, Stereochemical requirements for substrate specificity of LTB_4 20-hydroxylase, J. Biol. Chem. 262:12421 (1986).
57. H. Sumimoto, K. Takeshige, and S. Minakami, NAD+-dependent conversion of 20-OH-LTB_4 to 20-COOH-B by a cell-free system of human polymorphonuclear leukocytes, Biochem. Biophys. Res. Commun. 132:864 (1985).
58. D. W. Goldman and E. J. Goetzl, Specific binding of leukotriene B_4 to receptors on human polymorphonuclear leukocytes, J. Immunol. 129:1600 (1982).
59. R. A. Kreisle and C. W. Parker, Specific binding of leukotriene B_4 to a receptor on human polymorphonuclear leukocytes, J. Exp. Med. 157:628 (1983).
60. D. W. Goldman and E. J. Goetzl, Heterogeneity of human polymorphonuclear leukocyte receptors for leukotriene B_4: identification of a subset of high affinity receptors that transduce the chemotactic response, J. Exp. Med. 159:1027 (1984).
61. A. H. Lin, P. L. Ruppel, and R. R. Gorman, Leukotriene B_4 binding to human neutrophils, Prostaglandins 28:837 (1984).
62. R. M. Clancy, C. A. Dahinden, and T. E. Hugli, Oxidation of leukotrienes at the omega end: demonstration of a receptor for the 20-hydroxy derivative of leukotriene B_4 on human neutrophils and implications for the analysis of leukotriene receptors, Proc. Natl. Acad. Sci. USA 81:5729 (1984).
63. C. W. Lee, R. A. Lewis, E. J. Corey, and K. F. Austen, Conversion of leukotriene D_4 to leukotriene E_4 by a dipeptidase released from the specific granule of human polymorphonuclear leukocytes, Immunology 48:27 (1983).
64. S. S. Tate and A. Meister, Gamma-glutamyl transpeptidase: catalytic, structural and functional aspects, Monogr. Cell Biochem. 39:357 (1981).
65. T. W. Harper, J. Y. Westcott, N. Voelkel, and R. C. Murphy, Metabolism of leukotrienes B_4 and C_4 in the isolated perfused rat lung, J. Biol. Chem. 259:14437 (1984).
66. R. A. Lewis, J. M. Drazen, J. C. Figueiredo, E. J. Corey, and K. F. Austen, A review of recent contributions on biologically active products of arachidonate conversion, Int. J. Immunopharm. 4:85 (1982).

67. C. W. Parker, D. Koch, M. M. Huber, and S. F. Falkenhein, Formation of the cysteinyl form of slow reacting substance (leukotriene E_4) in human plasma, Biochem. Biophys. Res. Commun. 97:1038 (1980).

68. C. W. Lee, R. A. Lewis, E. J. Corey, A. Barton, H. Oh, A. I. Tauber, and K. F. Austen, Oxidative inactivation of leukotriene C_4 by stimulated human polymorphonuclear leukocytes, Proc. Natl Acad. Sci. USA 79:4166 (1982)

69. C. W. Lee, R. A. Lewis, A. I. Tauber, M. M. Mehrotra, E. J. Corey, and K. F. Austen, The myeloperoxidase-dependent metabolism of leukotrienes C_4, D_4, and E_4 to 6-trans-leukotriene B_4 diastereoisomers and the subclass-specific S-diastereoisomeric sulfoxides, J. Biol. Chem. 258:15004 (1983).

70. M. A. Neill, W. R. Henderson, and S. J. Klebanoff, Oxidative degradation of leukotriene C_4 by human monocytes and monocyte-derived macrophages, J. Exp. Med. 162:1634 (1985).

71. L. Örning, E. Norin, B. Gustafsson, and S. Hammarström, In vivo metabolism of leukotriene C_4 in germ-free and conventional rats: fecal excretion of N-acetyl leukotriene E_4, J. Biol. Chem. 261:766 (1986).

72. L. Örning, L. Kaijser, and S. Hammarström, In vivo metabolism of leukotriene C_4 in man: urinary excretion of leukotriene E_4, Biochem. Biophys. Res. Commun. 130:214 (1985).

73. S. Hammarström, L. Örning, N. Bernström, B. Gustafsson, E. Norin, and L. Kaijser, Metabolism of leukotriene C_4 in rats and humans. Adv. Prost. Thromb. Leuk. Res. 15:185 (1985).

74. R. I. Sperling, M. Weinblatt, J. L. Robin, J. Ravalese III, R. L. Hoover, F. House, J. S. Coblyn, P. A. Fraser, B. W. Spur, D. R. Robinson, R. A. Lewis, and K. F. Austen, Effects of dietary supplementation with marine fish oil on leukocyte lipid mediator generation and function in rheumatoid arthritis, Arth. Rheum. 30:988 (1987).

75. R. I. Sperling, J. L. Robin, K. A. Kylander, T. H. Lee, R. A. Lewis, and K. F. Austen, The effects of N-3 polyunsaturated fatty acids on the generation of platelet-activating factor-acether by human monocytes, J. Immunol. 139:4186 (1987).

76. A. J. Dessein, T. H. Lee, P. Elsas, J. R. Ravalese III, D. Silberstein, J. R. David, K. F. Austen, and R. A. Lewis, Enhancement by monokines of leukotriene generation by human eosinophils and neutrophils stimulated with calcium ionophore A23187, J. Immunol. 136:3829 (1986).

77. D. S. Silberstein, W. F. Owen, J. C. Gasson, J. F. DiPersio, D. W. Golde, J. C. Bina, R. J. Soberman, K. F. Austen, and J. R. David, Enhancement of human eosinophil cytotoxicity and leukotriene synthesis by biosynthetic (recombinant) granulocyte-macrophage colony-stimulating factor, J. Immunol. 137:3290 (1986).

78. M. E. Rothenberg, W. F. Owen Jr., D. S. Silberstein, J. Woods, R. J. Soberman, K. F. Austen, and R. L. Stevens, Human eosinophils have prolonged survival, enhanced functional properties, and become hypodense when exposed to human interleukin-3, J. Clin. Invest. 81:1986 (1988).

79. J. A. Rankin, C. E. Schrader, S. M. Smith, and R. A. Lewis, Recombinant gamma-interferon primes alveolar macrophages cultured in vitro for the release of leukotriene B_4 in response to IgG stimulation, J. Clin. Invest. (in press).

80. J. L. Robin, D. C. Seldin, K. F. Austen, and R. A. Lewis, Regulation of mediator release from mouse bone marrow-derived mast cells by glucocorticoids, J. Immunol. 135:2719 (1985).

INHIBITORS OF LEUKOTRIENE ACTION: POTENTIAL USE IN ASTHMA,

INFLAMMATORY BOWEL DISEASE, AND CUTANEOUS INFLAMMATION

A.F. Welton, P.C. Will, D.W. Morgan, H. Crowley,
M. O'Donnell, J. Hurley, and S. Shapiro

Hoffmann-La Roche, Inc.
340 Kingsland Street
Nutley, NJ 07110

INTRODUCTION

Research carried out in numerous laboratories has led to the hypothesis that metabolites of the Δ^5-lipoxygenase ($^5\Delta$-LO) pathway (e.g., leukotrienes and 5-HETE) may play an important role in mediating a number of inflammatory diseases including asthma, inflammatory bowel disease, and diseases associated with cutaneous inflammation. The purpose of this chapter is to briefly review the rationale supporting this hypothesis and to present the results of some experimental studies with promising Δ^5-LO inhibitors and leukotriene antagonists which would support the clinical evaluation of these types of drugs in the three disease states.

Asthma

The scientific rationale in support of a role for the peptidoleukotrienes ($LTC_4/D_4/E_4$) in mediating asthma is composed of a variety of observations such as:

a) Peptidoleukotrienes are very potent constrictors of isolated, in vitro preparations of guinea pig and ferret tracheal and parenchymal smooth muscle, and human bronchial smooth muscle (1-4).

b) The prolonged contraction induced by antigen in passively-sensitized human bronchi in vitro is antihistamine resistant (3) suggesting that other mediators, such as the leukotrienes, are primarily responsible for inducing the smooth muscle contraction. In additon, antihistamines have not proven useful yet in treating asthma.

c) Peptidoleukotrienes produce bronchoconstrictions when administered in vivo to guinea pigs and primates (5-8).

d) The peptidoleukotrienes induce bronchoconstriction, coughing, wheezing, chest tightness, and a reduction in maximum expiratory air flow when administered by inhalation in man (9-16). LTC_4 and LTD_4 are approximately 1000-times and LTE_4 approximately 100-times more potent than histamine and their onset of action is slower and their duration of action is more prolonged than histamine (15-16).

e) Peptidoleukotrienes are formed when sensitized human lung is challenged with antigen in vitro in quantities sufficient to elicit a bronchoconstrictive response (17, 18). Leukotrienes are also synthesized in vitro by human mast cells and eosinophils upon antigen challenge (19, 20).

f) Leukotrienes have been detected in sputum (21) and plasma (22) collected from patients with acute asthma and in the nasal washings (23) taken from atopic individuals following antigen challenge; and

g) Leukotrienes have a wide spectrum of biological activities which may contribute to asthmatic symptomatology in addition to contracting airway smooth muscle. These include the ability to contract pulmonary vascular smooth muscle (24), increase vascular permeability (4, 5) and increase mucus secretion in lung tissue (25).

Based on the circumstantial but convincing evidence detailed above, a number of pharmaceutical companies launched programs several years ago to identify peptidoleukotriene antagonists or Δ^5-LO inhibitors for evaluation in asthma reasoning that such compounds could prove to be new therapeutic agents for the treatment of this disease. Tables 1 and 2 describe the in vitro activity in our assay systems of a few of the most promising drug candidates to evolve from these efforts. Studies to evaluate the effects of known Δ^5-LO or dual Δ^5-LO/CO inhibitors on arachidonic acid metabolism in ionophore (A23187)-stimulated rat peritoneal macrophages were performed according to techniques described previously (26-28). The ^{3}H-LTD_4 binding studies on recently described LTD_4 antagonists were performed as indicated in Table 2.

TABLE 1

EFFECT OF Δ^5-LO INHIBITORS AND DUAL Δ^5-LO/CO INHIBITORS

ON ARACHIDONIC ACID METABOLISM IN IONOPHORE A23187-STIMULATED

MACROPHAGES

Compound	Structure	Peritoneal Macrophage[a]	
		LTB_4 IC_{50} (μM)	PGE_2
BW 755C		29	15
Phenidone		5	38
Quercetin		2	10
Nordihydroguaiaretic Acid (NDGA)		0.6	10
RS-43,179		0.3	66
AA861		0.2	5
Rev 5901		0.02	>100

[a]Rat peritoneal macrophages (4 x 10^6 cells/ml) were stimulated with ionophore A23187 (0.5 μM) for 20 minutes. LTB_4 and PGE_2 release was measured by RIA. Control release of LTB_4 and PGE_2 was approximately 15 pmole/10^6 cells and 5 pmole/10^6 cells, respectively.

TABLE 2

ACTIVITY OF LTD$_4$ ANTAGONISTS IN ^{3}H-LTD$_4$ BINDING

ASSAY UTILIZING GUINEA PIG LUNG HOMOGENATE MEMBRANES

Drug	Structure	^{3}H-LTD$_4$ Binding[a] IC$_{50}$ (µM)
FPL 55712		3
Ro 23-3544		5
SC-39070		2
LY 171,883		>10
ICI 198,615		0.001
ICI 204,219		0.0001
MCI-826		0.007

[a]Assay was performed at 20°C for 30 minutes in 10 mM Tris HCl (pH 7.4) containing 0.1% BSA, 5 mM Ca^{+2}, 5 mM Mg^{+2}, 3.5 nM ^{3}H-LTD$_4$ and 100 µg/ml of guinea pig lung homogenate membranes.

To date, the greatest successes in the development of drugs to treat asthma have been in the identification of LTD$_4$ antagonists with _in vivo_ activity which would support clinical evaluation. Progress in this area has been described in more detail in another chapter in this book

(29) and also in other recent reviews (30-31). Some experimental evidence to further support this statement is presented in Table 3 which compares the relative activities of several promising LTD_4 antagonists and Δ^5-LO inhibitors in a guinea pig model of antigen-induced, leukotriene synthesis-mediated bronchoconstriction (87). It can be seen that antagonists such as ICI 198,615 and MCI-826 are very potent in this model by the intravenous route and also are orally active whereas the Δ^5-LO inhibitors which were evaluated are much less active. These two LTD_4 antagonists thus are examples of compounds which show great promise as clinical candidates for evaluation as antiasthmatics.

Inflammatory Bowel Disease (IBD)

IBD is actually a family of chronic diseases of unknown etiology which are associated with an inflammation of the gastrointestinal tract, chronic diarrhea, and abdominal pain. These diseases include Crohn's ileitis or regional enteritis which localize in the distal small intestine and Crohn's colitis and ulcerative colitis which localize in the colon or rectum. The intestinal pathology associated with these diseases includes the accumulation of inflammatory cells, such as granulocytes and lymphocytes, in the intestinal mucosa and submucosa as well as edema, mucosal erosions and/or intestinal ulcerations.

Although the etiology of these diseases is unknown, most hypotheses include an important role for inflammatory mediators released during the initiation of the disease process, in the accumulation of inflammatory cells, and in the propagation of disease symptoms such as diarrhea and pain. Metabolites of Δ^5-LO are among the inflammatory mediators thought to have a role in IBD. This hypothesis is based, in part, on the known biological activities of LTB_4 and 5-HETE to induce neutrophil chemotaxis (32), increase neutrophil adherence (32), and activate neutrophils to release proteases, lipases, and oxygen radicals (33). The proinflammatory role of Δ^5-LO metabolites is also supported by the ability of the peptidoleukotrienes to alter capillary permeability within tissues (4,5,32). In this way the peptidoleukotrienes, LTB_4 and 5-HETE could synergize to promote an inflammatory reaction. Other evidence supporting the hypothesized role of Δ^5-LO inhibitors and other arachidonic acid metabolites in IBD includes the observations that:

a) Intestinal fluids from IBD patients have elevated levels of LTB_4 and E-type prostaglandins (34-36).

TABLE 3

ACTIVITY OF Δ^5-LO OR DUAL Δ^5-LO/CO INHIBITORS AND LTD$_4$

ANTAGONISTS IN AN IN VIVO ANTIGEN-INDUCED LEUKOTRIENE-MEDIATED

BRONCHOCONSTRICTION MODEL

Drug	% Inhibition of Bronchoconstriction	
	Intravenous 10 mg/kg[a]	Oral 100 mg/kg[b]
Δ^5-LO or Dual Δ^5-LO/CO Inhibitors		
Phenidone	92 ± 5 (6)[c]	46 ± 12
BW 755C	35 ± 5	14 ± 0
NDGA	29 ± 7	N.D.[d]
Rev 5901	60 ± 11 (9)[c]	N.D.[d]
AA861	94 ± 3 (3)[c]	12 ± 12
RS-43,179	27 ± 9	N.D.[d]
LTD$_4$ Antagonists		
FPL 55712	92 ± 1 (2)	N.D.[d]
Ro 23-3544	79 ± 9 (6)	N.D.[d]
ICI 198,615	97 ± 2 (0.06)	97 ± 1 (0.033)
MCI-826	97 ± 2 (0.03)	98 ± 1 (0.32)

[a]Actively sensitized guinea pigs pretreated with indomethacin, propranolol, and pyrilamine maleate as described previously (87) were exposed to test drug for 1 minute prior to antigen challenge.

[b]Guinea pigs prepared as described above were pretreated with test drug for 60 minutes prior to antigen challenge.

[c]Values presented are means ± S.E.M. (n=5 drug treated animals vs 5 control animals); Number in parenthesis is ID$_{50}$.

[d]Not Determined.

b) The intestinal mucosa from IBD patients synthesize increased amounts of the peptidoleukotrienes (37), LTB$_4$ (38), and various other prostaglandins and lipoxygenase products (39,40).

c) Δ^5-LO metabolites induce electrolyte secretion in intestinal tissues (41) suggesting a role in mediating the diarrhea associated with IBD.

d) The activity of phospholipase A_2, a key enzyme required for the release of arachidonic acid, is elevated in ileal mucosa from patients with Crohn's disease (42).

e) The use of cyclooxygenase inhibitors has been reported to exacerbate IBD (43,44) perhaps by shunting increased amounts of arachidonic acid through the Δ^5-LO pathway.

As was described above in our discussion on asthma, the type of information outlined above has provided the rationale within the pharmaceutical industry to develop modulators of leukotriene action in the treatment of IBD. Indeed Zipser et al. (45) have previously described the activity of a Δ^5-LO inhibitor, L-651,392, in a rabbit immune-complex model of intestinal inflammation. We, too, have been interested in IBD as a therapeutic target. Much of our interest has concentrated on evaluating leukotriene antagonists as well as Δ^5-LO inhibitors in animal models of intestinal inflammation.

A primary animal model of colonic inflammation, we and others have utilized in these studies involves treating the colon of Spague-Dawley rats with a dilute solution of acetic acid. This treatment has been shown to lead to distinct morphological changes in the treated colon over the next 24 hours consisting of ulceration of the mucosa, a decrease in goblet cell mucin, edema, hemorrhage and an increase in the number of neutrophils in the mucosa and submucosa (46,47). Alterations in arachidonic acid (AA) metabolism which are similar to those seen in human inflammatory bowel disease (e.g., increased metabolism of AA to 5-LO products leading to increased levels of LTB_4 and peptidoleukotrienes in the intestinal mucosa after acetic acid administration) have also been observed in this animal model (48,49). It has been suggested that Δ^5-LO metabolites might be associated with part of the pathology seen in the acetic acid-colitis model (especially neutrophil infiltration into the colon because of the ability of LTB_4 to induce neutrophil adherence and chemokinesis and the ability of peptidoleukotrienes to alter capillary permeability). This suggestion is supported by the data presented below demonstrating that Δ^5-LO inhibitors, dual Δ^5-LO/CO inhibitors, and LTD_4 antagonists inhibit neutrophil infiltration into the acetic acid challenged rat colon (50-52).

In Table 4 are presented the results of assaying Δ^5-LO or dual Δ^5-LO/CO inhibitors in this in vivo model. These compounds were as

TABLE 4

EFFECT OF Δ^5-LO INHIBITORS, DUAL Δ^5-LO/CO INHIBITORS, AND

SULFASALAZINE ON ACETIC ACID-INDUCED COLITIS

Compound	Dose (mg/kg)	Rat Acetic Acid Colitis Model[a] % Inhibition of Myeloperoxidase Accumulation[b]
Phenidone	10	50 ± 17
	100	58 ± 11[c]
	200	61 ± 15[c]
NDGA	30	12 ± 35
	100	70 ± 20[c]
	300	105 ± 14[c]
Quercetin	100	54 ± 24[c]
RS-43,179	25	65 ± 1[c]
Sulfasalazine	30	5 ± 34
	100	52 ± 14[c]
	300	64 ± 24[c]

[a]Male rats were pretreated orally, twice daily for two days with the test drug. On the third day, they were again treated with a single dose and then challenged two hours later with two ml of 2.5% acetic acid which was injected into the proximal colon as described previously (47,52). The animals were treated again with drug 3 hours later, and 24 hours after acetic acid treatment the animals were sacrificed and scrappings of the colon were assayed for myeloperoxidase, a marker for neutrophil infiltration.

[b]% inhibition = [(acetic acid group)-(drug group)]/[acetic acid group)-(control group)] x 100. All are myeloperoxidase specific activities. The data presented are the mean ± S.E.M. (n=4 to 10 drug treated animals vs 8 control).

[c]$p < 0.05$ vs acetic acid/vehicle group by ANOVA and Student's t test.

effective as sulfasalazine, a standard therapeutic used in treating IBD, in preventing neutrophil accumulation (as assayed by myeloperoxidase levels) into the colonic mucosa of acetic acid challenged animals (53). It is has been suggested that the efficacy of sulfasalazine in treating IBD may be due to inhibition of Δ^5-LO (54) or LTB_4 antagonism (55). In fact, these properties might explain the efficacy of sulfasalazine in this acetic acid-colitis model. Regardless, the results presented in Table 4 support a role for Δ^5-LO metabolites in mediating neutrophil accumulation in colonic tissue in this rat model. Furthermore, the activity of Δ^5-LO inhibitors in this rat model and the rabbit immune-complex model (52) described above, support the clinical testing of such drugs in patients with IBD.

A major interest at Roche has also been the potential use of leukotriene antagonists in IBD. For this reason we have tested the activity of this type of compound in the rat acetic acid colitis model (52,56). Initial studies were performed with FPL 55712 and Ro 23-3544, a Roche leukotriene antagonist described previously (57). The results of these studies are presented in Table 5. When rats were orally treated with FPL 55712 at doses between 10 to 100 mg/kg, there was no significant effect on acetic acid-induced neutrophil accumulation. This contrasts with the results obtained when FPL 55712 was given intraperitoneally which indicate a significant reduction of inflammation. Ro 23-3544, on the other hand, was orally active at doses above 10 mg/kg. These results demonstrate that both FPL 55712 and Ro 23-3544 can reduce the accumulation of neutrophils in the colon of rats and that Ro 23-3544 is orally active in this model.

TABLE 5

EFFECT OF RO 23-3544, FPL 55712 AND SULFASALAZINE ON ACETIC

ACID-INDUCED COLITIS

Treatment	Route	Dose (mg/kg)	% Inhibition of Myeloperoxidase Accumulation[a,b]
Ro 23-3544	p.o.	3	22 ± 49
	p.o.	10	28 ± 32
	p.o.	30	55 ± 31^{c}
	p.o.	60	72 ± 10^{c}
	p.o.	90	84 ± 22^{c}
FPL 55712	p.o.	10	32 ± 22
	p.o.	30	37 ± 23
	p.o.	100	34 ± 36
	i.p.	10	$81 \pm\ 8^{c}$
	i.p.	100	94 ± 11^{c}
Sulfasalazine	p.o.	30	5 ± 34
	p.o.	100	52 ± 14^{c}
	p.o.	300	64 ± 24^{c}

[a]Studies were performed as described in Table 4.

[b]% Inhibition = [(Acetic acid group)-(Drug group)]/[Acetic acid group)-(Control group)] x 100. All are myeloperoxidase specific activities. The values presented are the means ± S.E.M. (n=6 to 10 drug treated animals vs 8 control animals).

[c]$p < 0.05$ vs. acetic acid/vehicle group by Student's t-test.

The effects of Ro 23-3544 on acetic acid-induced pathology in the rat colon were also evaluated. The effect of Ro 23-3544 (60 mg/kg) was compared to that of sulfasalazine (100 mg/kg). The only parameter of the histology which was significantly affected by sulfasalazine was the infiltration of polymorphonuclear leukocytes (PMNs) into the submucosa. Treatment with Ro 23-3544, however, reduced the PMN infiltration into the mucosa, the submucosa and the muscularis. There was also a significant reduction of the submucosal hemorrhage and the submucosal congestion. The histological observation of a reduction of PMN infiltration substantiates the results described previously in Table 5 which inferred a decrease in neutrophil accumulation from a decrease in the level of assayable myeloperoxidase.

Although Ro 23-3544 is a structural analog of FPL 55712 (see structures in Table 2) and was originally characterized as a LTD_4 antagonist (57), we have continued to expand its pharmacological profile in a number of other test systems. Table 6 summarizes what we now know about the profile of Ro 23-3544. This compound is a relatively selective peptidoleukotriene antagonist in guinea pig bronchoconstriction tests since it demonstrated no activity as an antagonist of histamine, PAF, or arachidonic acid-induced bronchoconstrictions (57). We have observed in this model, however, that it inhibited LTB_4-induced bronchoconstriction in guinea pigs. In vitro, Ro 23-3544 was also observed to be weak antagonist of LTB_4-induced chemotaxis and of ^{3}H-LTB_4 binding to HL-60 cells. Other studies have also demonstrated this compound was a weak inhibitor of Δ^5-LO from RBL-1 cells. Thus, at this time, we are not absolutely sure of the mechanism of action of this compound in the acetic acid-induced colitis model. Recent studies with a structurally unique and very potent LTD_4 antagonist, ICI 204,219 (58), however, have indicated that at 30 mg/kg orally this compound also was active in the acetic acid model (84 ± 13% inhibition of myeloperoxidase levels induced by acetic acid challenge). This confirms that LTD_4 antagonists from different structural series are active in the model. Furthermore, the data presented in Table 7 demonstrate that when Ro 23-3544 (10 µM) was administered with LTB_4 (1 µM) in vivo into the lumen of the distal large bowel, it was ineffective at antagonizing neutrophil accumulation stimulated by LTB_4. However, when Ro 23-3544 (10 µM) was given concomitantly with LTD_4 (1 µM), there was a significant reduction in the LTD_4-mediated neutrophil accumulation. These results suggest that Ro 23-3544 can block LTD_4 actions in the rat colon in vivo and lend

TABLE 6

CHARACTERIZATION OF RO 23-3544 IN STANDARD TEST SYSTEMS

FOR LEUKOTRIENE INHIBITORS

Test Systems	Activity	
	Ro 23-3544	FPL 55712
In vitro peptidoleukotriene (SRS-A)-induced guinea pig ileum contraction, IC_{50}	50 nM	50 nM
In vitro, LTD_4-induced guinea pig tracheal contraction, K_b	0.25 µM	1.3 µM
In vitro, ^3H-LTD_4 binding to lung homogenate, IC_{50}	5 µM	3 µM
In vitro, LTB_4-induced chemotaxis, IC_{50}	20 µM[a]	N.D.[b]
In vitro, ^3H-LTB_4 binding to HL-60 cells, IC_{50}	1-10 µM	10 µM
In vitro, Δ^5-lipoxygenase inhibition (RBL-1 enzyme), IC_{50}	2 µM	>10 µM
In vivo, LTD_4-induced bronchoconstriction in guinea pigs, ID_{50} or IC_{50}	4.6 mg/kg, i.v.; 0.01 % aerosol	2.0 mg/kg, i.v.; 0.5% aerosol
In vivo, LTB_4-induced bronchoconstriction in guinea pigs, IC_{50}	0.002% aerosol	3.0% aerosol

[a]This effect may not be specific for LTB_4 since more recent studies also suggest an effect on formyl-methionyl-leucylphenylalanine-induced chemotaxis.

[b]Not Determined.

support to LTD_4 antagonism as a mechanism of action for Ro 23-3544 in acetic acid-colitis. Currently, studies to investigate the in vivo effect of Ro 23-3544 on arachidonic acid metabolism in the colon are being conducted.

In summary, data from patients with IBD has suggested that Δ^5-LO metabolites may play a significant role in mediating a portion of the symptomatology associated with this disease. Studies conducted in our laboratories in an animal model of intestinal inflammation also support

TABLE 7

THE EFFECT OF RO 23-3544 ON LEUKOTRIENE-STIMULATED
INCREASES IN MYELOPEROXIDASE IN THE RAT COLON

Treatment In Vivo	Myeloperoxidase Specific Activity[a] (Units/gram)
Saline Control	0.25 ± 0.07
10 μM Ro 23-3544	0.38 ± 0.07
1 μM LTB$_4$	0.55 ± 0.17
1 μM LTB$_4$ + 10 μM Ro 23-3544	0.75 ± 0.18^b
1 μM LTD$_4$	0.86 ± 0.13^b
1 μM LTD$_4$ + 10 μM Ro 23-3544	0.41 ± 0.07^c

[a]Data presented is the mean ± S.E.M. (n=8 animals).

[b]$p < 0.05$ vs Saline Control by Student's t-test.

[c]$p < 0.05$ vs 1 μM LTD$_4$ by Student's t-test.

this hypothesis because of the observed efficacy of both Δ^5-LO inhibitors and leukotriene antagonists in this model. This information encourages the clinical evaluation of these modulators of leukotriene action in patients with IBD.

Diseases Associated With Cutaneous Inflammation

Certain skin disorders are associated with a cutaneous inflammatory reaction which may be mediated, in part, by Δ^5-LO products. One such disease is psoriasis, a disease of unknown etiology characterized by increased epidermal cell turnover (associated with scaling of the lesional skin), emigration of neutrophils into the lesional dermis and epidermis (observed to be an early event in the evolution of psoriatic plaques), and dilation of the vasculature in the affected area often leading to erythema and edema. As indicated below, several lines of evidence suggest that $^5\Delta$-LO metabolites are important mediators of the pathophysiology of psoriasis; since:

a) Increased levels of free arachidonic acid (59), LTB$_4$ (60-62), 5-HETE (60), and LTC$_4$/LTD$_4$ (63) have been found in the epidermis of patients with psoriatic lesions.

b) $^5\Delta$-LO activity is higher in involved than in uninvolved psoriatic skin (64).

c) Topical administration of the cyclooxygenase (65,66) inhibitor, indomethacin, exacerbates pre-existing psoriatic lesions (possibly by redirecting arachidonic acid metabolism through the Δ^5-LO pathway).

d) Cultured mouse and human keratinocytes synthesize LTB_4 and LTD_4 when stimulated with ionophore (67,68) and cultured epidermal cells synthesize LTB_4 (83,84,85).

e) LTB_4 has been shown to stimulate epidermal proliferation in vivo in guinea pigs (69).

f) The intracutaneous application of LTB_4 to human skin has been shown to result in the production of a transient wheal and flare reaction followed by infiltration of neutrophils into the site of application (70-72). As stated above, the influx of neutrophils is one of the earliest pathological events seen in psoriatic lesions.

g) Topical application of LTB_4 results in the production of intra-epidermal abscesses histologically similar to lesions observed in pustular psoriasis (73); and

h) Peptidoleukotrienes express potent biological actions when injected intradermally into human skin leading to a wheal and flare reaction caused by alteration of capillary permeability and vasodilation (71,72,74).

On the basis of the above information, it has been hypothesized that the peptidoleukotrienes, which have profound effects on the dermal vasculature, could act synergistically with LTB_4, a chemotactic agent, in mediating psoriatic pathophysiology.

In addition to psoriasis, the biological activities seen with leukotrienes are also consistent with their playing a role in allergic skin diseases such as atopic dermatitis. This possibility is supported by studies which have identified LTB_4-like immunoreactivity (75,86) and LTC_4-like immunoreactivity (76) in affected skin areas in patients with atopic dermatitis.

Not surprisingly, the above information has also lead to an interest within the pharmaceutical industry in the utility of inhibitors of leukotriene action in the treatment of psoriasis. Indeed, this is one of the first therapeutic targets for most Δ^5-LO inhibitors which are being developed within the industry. As in the case of asthma and IBD, we, at Roche, have also been interested in cutaneous inflammation as a therapeutic target for leukotriene antagonists.

The mouse arachidonic acid (AA) - induced ear edema model has become a widely utilized model for identifying drugs to evaluate clinically as topical antiinflammatory agents acting through inhibiting leukotriene action (77). In this model, it has been shown that AA applied topically to the ear results in the synthesis of LTB_4, peptidoleukotrienes, 5-HETE, 12-HETE, 15-HETE and PGE_2 (78). These biochemical changes are accompanied by edema and neutrophil infiltration into the site of AA application and are maximal within 60 minutes of AA application to the ear. Selective Δ^5-LO inhibitors have been shown to inhibit formation of Δ^5-LO metabolites and dual inhibitors have been shown to inhibit formation of both Δ^5-LO metabolites and PGE_2. Both types of inhibitors have also been shown to prevent edema formation (78,79).

The results we obtained in this model with standard Δ^5-LO or dual Δ^5-LO/CO inhibitors are presented in Table 8. Included in this evaluation was RS-43,179 (Lonapalene), a Syntex compound which also is being evaluated clinically. Published reports on a topical gel formulation of this compound used in patients with psoriasis suggest, in one study, efficacy equivalent to that of fluocinolone acetonide gel, a topical steroid (80). In a recent study in patients with plaque psoriasis, RS-43179 was also found to be therapeutically effective in reducing erythema, induration, and desquamation while selectively reducing LTB_4 levels in the lesional skin (81). These studies certainly support the likelihood that modulators of leukotriene action will find a use in treating skin inflammatory disorders.

As indicated in Table 9, several types of LTD_4 antagonists are also as active in the AA-induced mouse ear edema test as are Δ^5-LO or dual Δ^5-LO/CO inhibitors. This suggests an important role for these peptidoleukotrienes in inducing the edema response in this animal model. One of the compounds which we are quite interested in, in this regard, is Ro 23-3544. As discussed in the previous section on IBD, the pharma-

TABLE 8

EFFECT OF 5-LO OR DUAL 5-LO/CO INHIBITORS ON

AA-INDUCED EAR EDEMA IN MICE

Compound	Dose (mg)	AA-Induced Ear Edema[a] % Inhibition
Phenidone	0.1	39[b]
	0.2	43[c]
	0.5	56[d]
	1.0	65[d]
	2.0	72[d]
AA 861	0.5	71[d]
	1.0	73[d]
NDGA	0.5	42[d]
	1.0	59[d]
RS-43,179	1.0	61[d]
Rev 5901	0.1	32[a]
	0.25	41[b]
	0.5	50[c]

[a]Test substance was applied to the ear of CD-1 mice in a constant volume of 25 µl of acetone. Arachidonic acid, at a dose of 0.5 mg/25 µl, was then applied topically to the same ear 30 minutes later. The mice were sacrificed one hour later and ear edema was measured by weighing 6 mm biopsy punch (52,79). Data was obtained in experiments in which 8 drug treated animals were compared with 8 control animals.

[b]$p \leq 0.05$ vs AA control by Student's t-test.

[c]$p \leq 0.01$ vs AA control by Student's t-test.

[d]$p \leq 0.001$ vs AA control by Student's t-test.

cological profile of Ro 23-3544 has been expanded to cover biological activities, in addition to LTD_4 antagonism, which might contribute to its activities in vivo (See Table 6). Thus, we are currently trying to assess the possible mechanisms of action of Ro 23-3544 in the skin by the topical route.

We have established that Ro 23-3544, when applied topically, will antagonize LTD_4-induced increases in vascular permeability in the skin of Sprague-Dawley rats or Hartley guinea pigs. In the model systems developed to assess this property, it has been determined that LTD_4 (0.01 to 10 µg/site) injected intradermally into anesthetized animals

TABLE 9

EFFECT OF PEPTIDOLEUKOTRIENE ANTAGONISTS

ON AA-INDUCED EAR EDEMA IN THE MOUSE

Treatment	Dose (mg)	AA-Induced Ear Edema[a] % Inhibition
FPL 55712	0.5	6
	1.0	48[b]
	2.0	73[b]
Ro 23-3544	0.2	21[b]
	0.5	42[b]
	1.0	63[b]
	2.0	65[b]
ICI 198,615	1.0 mg	50[b]
MCI-826	1.0 mg	46[b]

[a]Test performed as described in Table 8.

[b]$p \leq .05$ vs AA control by Student's t-test.

will induce dose-related changes in capillary permeability which can be observed by the migration of intravenously administered Evans blue dye into the skin injection site (6). Intravenously administered LTD_4 antagonists will block this response (5,6); whereas Δ^5-LO and CO inhibitors will not (unpublished observations). Topically administered Ro 23-3544 and FPL 55712 were also studied for their ability to antagonize the skin response elicited by 0.4 µg LTD_4/injection-site (82). In these studies, it was observed that optimum activity was obtained by pretreating the animals with these drugs 2 hours (guinea pig) or 4 hours (rat) before LTD_4 challenge. The results of dose response evaluations with Ro 23-3544 and FPL 55712 at these time points are described in Table 10. When topically applied, both Ro 23-3544 and FPL 55712 were able to antagonize LTD_4-induced responses. In the guinea pig, FPL 55712 appeared to be slightly more potent than Ro 23-3544 whereas in the rat the potencies were reversed. In general, the two compounds demonstrated activity across the same dose ranges. A comparison of Tables 9 and 10 demonstrate that Ro 23-3544 and FPL 55712 were more potent in the

TABLE 10

TOPICAL ACTIVITY OF RO 23-3544 AND FPL 55712 AS

ANTAGONISTS OF LTD_4-INDUCED SKIN CAPILLARY PERMEABILITY

RESPONSES IN GUINEA PIGS AND RATS

Drug	mg Applied	% Inhibition (Mean ± S.E.M.)[a] Guinea Pig[b]	Rat[c]
Ro 23-3544	1.0	N.D.[d]	28 ± 4
	2.5	11 ± 3	50 ± 6
	5.0	33 ± 3	59 ± 6[d]
	7.5	43 ± 4	N.D.[d]
	12.5	49 ± 4	67 ± 5
FPL 55712	0.5	25 ± 1	N.D.[d]
	2.5	N.D.[d]	30 ± 14
	5.0	41 ± 3	43 ± 5
	7.5	N.D.	55 ± 2
	12.5	47 ± 4	65 ± 2

[a]Experiments were performed with 3 drug treated and 3 control animals (4 spots per animal).

[b]Measured 2 hours after topical administration.

[c]Measured 4 hours after topical administration.

[d]N.D. = not determined.

AA-induced mouse ear edema test than in the LTD_4-induced rat and guinea pig cutaneous capillary permeability models. This may be due to differences in the skin permeability of the drugs in the rat, guinea pig, and mouse. It also may be due to the method of administration of the challenge agent in the models. AA is applied directly onto the top of the skin whereas LTD_4 was injected under the skin.

The results of the studies in the LTD_4-induced skin capillary permeability tests demonstrate that, by the topical route, Ro 23-3544 is able to act as a LTD_4 antagonist and imply that this is a likely mechanism by which Ro 23-3544 could be acting in the AA-induced mouse ear edema model. Other mechanisms will also be studied, however. In any case, the interesting profile of activity seen with Ro 23-3544 in vitro and in these animal models would support a conceptual clinical study of this compound in various dermatological disorders in which leukotrienes may have a pathological role, and, indeed, such studies are ongoing.

Summary

In this chapter we have presented the rationale for hypothesizing that modulators of leukotriene action, including Δ^5-LO inhibitors , dual Δ^5-LO/CO inhibitors, and LTD_4 antagonists, may be useful agents to treat at least three types of inflammatory diseases. It is likely that as our knowledge of the role of Δ^5-LO metabolites in other diseases increases, new diseases may also be targets for these types of drugs. The results of clinical studies, which are currently ongoing, are anxiously awaited to see which of the currently hypothesized clinical targets will be the benefactor of the extensive research which has gone into the development of the various types of drugs which inhibit leukotriene action.

REFERENCES

1. R.A. Lewis, K.F. Austen, J.M. Drazen, D.A. Clark, A. Marfat and E.J. Corey, Slow reacting substance of anaphylaxis: Identification of leukotrienes C-1 and D from human and rat sources, Proc. Natl. Acad. Sci. USA 77:3710 (1980).

2. P.J. Piper and M.N. Samhoun, The mechanism of action of leukotrienes C_4 and D_4 in guinea pig isolated perfused lung and parenchymal strips of guinea pig, rabbit and rat, Prostaglandins 21:793 (1981).

3. G.K. Adams, and L.M. Lichtenstein, Antagonism of antigen-induced contraction of guinea pig and human airways, Nature 270:255 (1977).

4. R.D. Krell, D.W. Snyder, D. Aharony, B.-S. Tsai, and R.E. Giles, Pharmacologic description of peptide leukotriene receptors in conducting airways of guinea pig and ferret, Prostaglandins 28:614 (1984).

5. A.F. Welton, H.J. Crowley, D.A. Miller, and B. Yaremko, Biological activities of a chemically synthesized form of leukotriene E_4, Prostaglandins 21:287 (1981).

6. A.F. Welton, M. O'Donnell, W. Anderson, H. Crowley, A. Medford, B. Simko and B. Yaremko, Role of cyclooxygenase products in some of the biological effects of chemically synthesized leukotrienes (B_4, C_4, D_4, and E_4), Advances in Prostaglandin, Thromboxane and Leukotriene Research, 12:145 (1983).

7. J.M. Drazen, K.F. Austen, R.A. Lewis, D.A. Clark, G. Goto, A. Marfat, and E.J. Corey, Comparative airway and vascular activities of leukotrienes C-1 and D in vivo and in vitro, Proc. Natl. Acad. Sci. USA 77:4354 (1980).

8.   R. Patterson, K.E. Harris, L.J. Smith, P.A. Greenberger, M.A. Shaughnessy, P.R. Bernstein, and R.D. Krell, Airway response to leukotriene D_4 in Rhesus monkeys, Int. Archs. Allergy Appl. Immunol. 71:156 (1983).

9.   M.C. Holroyde, R.E.C. Altounyan, M. Cole, M. Dixon, and E.V. Elliott, Bronchoconstriction produced in man by leukotrienes C and D, Lancet 2:17 (1981).

10. M. Griffin, J.W. Weiss, A.G. Leitch, E.R. McFadden Jr., E.J. Corey, K.F. Austen, and J.M. Drazen, Effects of leukotriene D on the airways in asthma, N. Engl. J. Med. 308:436 (1983).

11. E. Adelroth, M. Morris, F.E. Hargreave, and P.M. O'Byrne, Airway responsiveness to leukotrienes C_4 and D_4: Relationship to airway responsiveness to methacholine, Am. Rev. Respir. Dis. 131:A4 (1985).

12. J.W. Weiss, J.M. Drazen, N. Coles, E.R. McFadden, Jr., P.F. Weller, E.J. Corey, R.A. Lewis, and K.F. Austen, Bronchoconstriction effects of leukotriene C in humans, Science 216:196 (1982).

13. L.J. Smith, P.A. Greenverger, R. Patterson, R.D. Krell, and P.R. Bernstein, The Effect of inhaled leukotriene D_4 in humans, Am. Rev. Respir. Dis. 131:368 (1985).

14. J.W. Weiss, J.M. Drazen, E.R. McFadden, Jr., P. Weller, E.J. Corey, R.A Lewis, and K.F. Drazen, Airway constriction in normal humans produced by inhalation of leukotriene D: potency, time course, and effect of aspirin therapy, J. Am. Med. Assoc. 249:2814 (1983).

15. H. Bisgaard, S. Groth, and F. Madsen, Bronchial hyperreactivity to leukotriene D_4 and histamine in exogenous asthma, Br. Med. J. 290:1468 (1985).

16. N.C. Barnes, P.J. Piper, and J.F. Costello, Comparative effects of inhaled leukotriene C_4, leukotriene D_4, and histamine in normal human subjects, Thorax 39:500 (1984).

17. S.E. Dahlen, G. Hansson, P. Hedqvist, T. Bjorck, E. Granstrom, and B. Dahlen, Allergen challenge of lung tissue from asthmatics elicits bronchial contraction that correlates with the release of leukotrienes C_4, D_4, and E_4, Proc. Nat'l. Acad. Sci. USA 80:1712 (1983).

18. T. Vigano, A. Toia, G. Galli, F. Berti, M.T. Crivellari, M. Mezzetti, and G.C. Folco, Adenosine and eicosanoid release from immunologically challenged human lung fragments, Advances in Prostaglandins, Thromboxanes, and Leukotriene Research. 17B:992 (1987).

19. D.W. MacGlashan, R.P. Schieimer, S.P. Peters, E.S. Schulman, G.K.

Adams, H.H. Newball, and L.M. Lichtenstein, Generation of leuko-trienes by purified human lung mast cells, J. Clin. Invest. 70:747 (1982).

20. R.J. Shaw, G.M. Walsh, O. Cromwell, R. Mogbel, C.J.F. Spry, and A.B. Kay, Activated human eosinophils generate SRS-A leukotrienes following IgG-dependent stimulation, Nature 316:150 (1985).

21. A.B. Kay, The sputum in bronchial asthma. in: "Asthma", Clark and Dogfrey, ed., Chapman and Hall, London (1983).

22. J.T. Zakrzewski, N.C. Barnes, P.J. Piper, and J.F. Costello, Measurement of leukotrienes in arterial and venous blood from normal and asthmatic subjects by radioimmunoassay, Br. J. Clin. Pharmacol. 19:574 P. (1985).

23. P.S. Creticos, S.P. Peters, N.F. Adkinson, Jr. R.M. Naclerio, E.C. Hayes, P.S. Norman, and L.M. Lichtenstein, Peptide-leukotriene release after antigen challenge in patients sensitive to ragweed, N. Engl. J. Med. 310:1626 (1984).

24. C.J. Hanna, M.K. Bach, P.D. Pare, and R.R. Schellenberg, Slow-reacting substances (leukotrienes) contract human airway and pulmonary vascular smooth muscle in vitro, Nature 290:343 (1981).

25. Z. Marom, J.H. Shelhamer, M.K. Bach, D.R. Morton, and M. Kaliner, Slow-reacting substances, leukotrienes C_4 and D_4 increase the release of mucus from human airways in vitro, Am. Rev. Respir. Dis. 126:449 (1982).

26. A.F. Welton, L.D. Tobias, C. Fiedler-Nagy, W. Anderson, W. Hope, K. Meyers, and J.W. Coffey, The effect of flavonoids on arachidonic acid metabolism, in: "Plant Flavonoids in Biology and Medicine", Cody, V., Middleton, Jr., E., Harborne, J.B., (eds): Alan R. Liss, New York (1987).

27. A.F. Welton, J. Hurley, and P. Will, Flavonoids and arachidonic acid metabolism, in: "Plant Flavonoids in Biology and Medicine II: Biochemical, Cellular, and Medicinal Properties", Cody, V., Middleton Jr., E., Jr., Harborne, J.B., and Beretz, A. (eds)., Alan R. Liss, New York (1988).

28. C. Fiedler-Nagy, , B.H. Wittreich, A. Georgiadis, W.C. Hope, A.F. Welton and J.W. Coffey, Comparative study of natural and synthetic retinoids as inhibitors of arachidonic acid release and metabolism in rat peritoneal macrophages, Dermatologica 175:81 (1987).

29. A.F. Welton and M. O'Donnell, New Pharmacologic Agents Which Antagonize Leukotriene D_4 and PAF, in "Prostanoids and Drugs," G. Floco and G. Velo (eds)., Plenum Press, New York (1989).

30. J.H. Fleisch, L.E. Rinkema, C.A. Whitesitt, and W.S. Marshall,

Development of cysteinyl leukotriene receptor antagonists, Advances in Inflammation Research 12:173 (1988).

31. R.D. Krell, Federation Proceedings (in press).

32. A.W. Ford-Hutchinson, Leukotrienes: Their formation and role as inflammatory mediators, Fed. Proc. 44:25 (1985).

33. J.T. O'Flaherty, Neutrophil degranulation: Evidence pertaining to its mediation by the combined effects of leukotriene B_4, platelet activating factor, and 5-HETE, J. Cell. Physiol. 122:229 (1985).

34. S.R. Gould, Assay of prostaglandin-like substances in feces and their measurement in ulcerative colitis, Prostaglandins 11:489 (1976).

35. K. Lauritsen, L.S. Laursen, K. Bukhave, and J. Rask-Madsen, Effects of topical 5-aminosalicylic acid and prednisolone on prostaglandin E_2 and leukotriene B_4 levels determined by equilibrium in vivo dialysis of rectum in relapsing ulcerative colitis, Gastroenterology 91:837 (1986).

36. D.S. Rampton, G.E. Sladen, and L.J.F. Youlten, Rectal mucosal prostaglandin E_2 release and its relation to disease activity, electrical potential difference, and treatment in ulcerative colitis, Gut 21:591 (1980).

37. B.M. Peskar, K.W. Dreyling, B.A. Peskar, B. May, and H. Goebell, Enhanced formation of sulfidopeptide-leukotrienes in ulcerative colitis and Crohn's disease: inhibition by sulfasalazine and 5-aminosalicyclic acid, Agents Actions 18:381 (1986).

38. P. Sharon, and W.F. Stenson, Enhanced synthesis of leukotriene B_4 by colonic mucosa in inflammatory bowel disease, Gastroenterology 86:453 (1984).

39. N.K. Boughton-Smith, C.J. Hawkey, and B.J.R. Whittle, Biosynthesis of lipoxygenase and cyclooxygenase products from [^{14}C]-arachidonic acid by human colonic mucosa, Gut 24:1176 (1983).

40. M. Ligumsky, F. Karmeli, P. Sharon, U. Zor, F. Cohen, and D. Rachmilewitz, Enhanced thromboxane A_2 and prostacyclin production by cultured rectal mucosa in ulcerative colitis and its inhibition by steroids and sulfasalazine, Gastroenterology 81:444 (1981).

41. M.W. Musch, R.J. Miller, M. Field, and M.I. Siegel, Stimulation of colonic secretion by lipoxygenase metabolites of arachidonic acid, Science 217:1255 (1982).

42. T. Bolin, R. Heuman, R. Sjodahl, and C. Tagessan, Decreased lysophospholipase and increased phospholipase A_2 activity in ileal mucosa from patients with Crohn's disease, Digestion 29:55 (1984).

43. D.S. Rampton, and G.E. Sladen, Prostaglandin synthesis inhibitors

in ulcerative colitis: Flurbiprofen compared with conventional treatment, <u>Prostaglandins</u> 21:417 (1981).

44. H.J. Kaufmann, and H.L. Taubin, Nonsteroidal antiinflammatory drugs activate quiescent inflammatory bowel disease, <u>Annals Int. Med.</u> 107:513 (1987).

45. R.D. Zipser, M. Pinzani, and C.C. Nast, Effect of sulfasalazine and the leukotriene inhibitor L-651,392 in rabbit colitis: Evidence that LTB_4 production contributes to inflammation, <u>Gastroenterology</u> 92:1711 (1987).

46. B.R. MacPherson, and C.J. Pfeiffer, Experimental production of diffuse colitis in rats, <u>Digestion</u> 17:135 (1978).

47. N.S. Mann, H.C. Kwaan, and S.K. Mann, E.C. Cheung, Effect of epsilon amino caproic acid on experimental acetic acid colitis, <u>Am. J. Proct. Gastro. Colon Rectal Surg.</u> 31:11 (1980).

48. P. Sharon, and W.F. Stenson, Enhanced synthesis of leukotriene B_4 by colonic mucosa in inflammatory bowel disease, <u>Gastroenterology</u> 86:543 (1984).

49. P. Sharon, and W.F. Stenson, Metabolism of arachidonic acid in acetic acid colitis in rats: similarity to human inflammatory bowel disease, <u>Gastroenterology</u> 88:55 (1985).

50. P. Conzentino, P.C. Will, A. Lin, and T.S. Gaginella, Effect of Δ^5lipoxygenase (LO) inhibitors on acetic acid induced colitis in the rat, <u>Pharmacologist</u> 28:163 (1986).

51. P.C. Will, P. Conzentino, W. Allbee, G. Roberts, A. Lin, L. Iverson, W. Weiss, F. Cochran, D. Morgan, and T.S. Gaginella, Effect of inhibitors of Δ^5lipoxygenase on acetic acid-induced colitis in the rat. In Preparation.

52. P.C.Will, G. Roberts, W. Allbee, P. Conzentino, T.S. Gaginella and A. Welton, Efficacy of leukotriene antagonists in animal models of intestinal inflammation. In Preparation.

53. J.E. Krawisz, P. Sharon, and W.F. Stentson, Quantitative assay for acute intestinal inflammation based on myeloperoxidase activity: assessment of inflammation in rat and hamster models, <u>Gastro-enterology</u> 87:1344 (1984).

54. B.M. Peskar, K.W. Dreyling, B.A. Peskar, B. May, and H. Goebell, Enhanced formation of sulfidopeptide-leukotrienes in ulcerative colitis and Crohn's disease: Inhibition by sulfasalazine and 5-amino salicylic acid, <u>Agents Actions</u> 18:381 (1986).

55. M.A. Peppercorn, Sulfasalazine and related new drugs, <u>J. Clin. Pharmacol.</u> 27:260 (1987).

56. P.C. Will, W. Allbee, T.S. Gaginella, A.F. Welton, L. Iverson, W.

Weis, G. Roberts, P. Conzentino, and J. Edgcomb, Colonic anti-inflammatory activity of ablucast, an orally active leukotriene antagonist, <u>4th International Conference of the Inflammation Research Association Abstracts</u>, October, 1988.

57. M. O'Donnell, A.F. Welton, H. Crowley, D. Brown, R. Garippa, N. Cohen, G. Weber, B. Banner, and R.J. Lopresti, Pharmacological profile of Ro 23-3544, a new aerosol active leukotriene receptor antagonist, <u>Adv. Prostaglandin Thromboxane, and Leukotriene Res.</u> 17:512 (1987).

58. C. Buckner, J. Fedyna, R. Krell, J. Robertson, R. Keith, V. Matassa, F. Brown, P. Bernstein, Y. Yee, J. Will, R. Fishleder, R. Saban, B. Hesp, and R. Giles, Antagonist by ICI 204,219 of leuko-triene receptors in guinea pig and human airways, <u>Fed. Proc.</u> 2(5):A1264 (1988).

59. S. Hammarström, M. Hamberg, B. Samuelsson, E. Duell, M. Stawiski, and J.J. Voorhees, Increased concentrations of non-esterified arachidonic acid, prostaglandin E_2 and prostaglandin $F_{2\alpha}$ in epidermis of psoriasis, <u>Proc. Natl. Acad. Sci. USA</u> 72:5130 (1975).

60. J. Grabbe, B.M. Czarnetzki, T. Rosenbach, and M. Mardin, Identifi-cation of chemotactic lipoxygenase products of arachidonate metabo-lism in psoriatic skin, <u>J. Invest. Dermatol.</u> 82:477 (1984).

61. S.D. Brain, R.D.R. Camp, P.M. Dowd, A. Kobza-Black, P.M. Wollard, A.I. Mallet, and M.W. Greaves, Psoriasis and leukotriene B_4, <u>Lancet</u> 2:763 (1982).

62. S. Brain, R. Camp, P. Dowd, A.K. Black, and M.J. Greaves, The release of leutotriene B_4-like material in biologically active amounts from the lesional skin of patients with psoriasis, <u>Invest. Dermatol.</u> 83:70 (1984).

63. S.D. Brain, R.D.R. Camp, A. Kobza-Black, P.M. Dowd, M.W. Greaves, A.W. Ford-Hutchinson, and S. Charleson, Leukotrienes C_4 and D_4 in psoriatic skin lesions, <u>Prostaglandins</u> 29(4):611 (1985).

64. V.A. Ziboh, T. Casebolt, C.L. Marcelo, and J.J. Voorhees, Enhance-ment of 5-lipoxygenase activity in soluble preparations of human psoriatic plaque, <u>J. Invest. Dermatol.</u> 80:359 (1983).

65. H. Kayayama, and A. Kawada, Exacerbation of psoriasis induced by indomethacin, <u>J. Dermatol.</u> 8:323 (1981).

66. J.J. Voorhees, Leukotrienes and other lipoxygenase products in the pathogenesis and therapy of psoriasis and other dermatoses, <u>Arch. Dermatol.</u> 119:541 (1983).

67. V.A. Ziboh, C.L. Marcelo, and J.J. Voorhees, Induced lipoxygenation

of arachidonic acid in mouse epidermal keratinocytes by calcium ionophore A23187, J. Invest. Dermatol. 76:307 (1981).

68. S.D. Brain, R.D.R. Camp, I.M. Leigh, and A.W. Ford-Hutchinson, The synthesis of leukotriene B_4-like material by cultured human keratinocytes, J. Invest. Dermatol. 78:328 (1982).

69. C.C. Chan, L. Duhamel, and A.W. Ford-hutchinson, Leukotriene B_4 and 12-hydroxyeicosatetraenoic acid stimulate epidermal proliferation in vivo in the guinea pig, J. Invest. Dermatol. 85:333 (1985).

70. N.A. Sorter, R.A. Lewis, E.J. Corey, and K.F. Austen, Local effects of synthetic leukotrienes (LTC_4, LTD_4, LTE_4, and LTB_4) in human skin, J. Invest. Dermatol. 80:115 (1983).

71. W.A. Bray, A.W. Ford-Hutchinson, and M.J.H. Smith, Leukotriene B_4: An inflammatory mediator in vivo, Prostaglandins 22:213 (1981).

72. R.D.R. Camp, A.A. Coutts, M.W. Greaves, A.B. Kay, and M.J. Walport, Responses of human skin to intradermal injections of leukotrienes C_4, D_4, and B_4, Br. J. Pharmacol. 80:497 (1983).

73. R. Camp, R.R. Jones, S. Brain, P. Wollard, and M. Greaves, Production of intraepidermal microabscesses by topical application of leukotriene B_4, J. Invest. Dermatol. 82:202 (1984).

74. H. Bisgaard, J. Kristensen, and J. Sondergaard, The effect of leukotrienes C_4 and D_4 on microcirculatory flow in humans, Br. J. Dermatol. 109:124 (1983).

75. T. Ruzicka, T. Simmet, B.A. Peskar, and O. Braun-Falco, Leukotrienes in skin of atopic dermatitis, Lancet 1:222 (1984).

76. S.F. Talbot, P. Atkins, E. Goetzl, and B. Zweiman, Patterns of LTC_4 release in human allergic skin reactions, J. Allergy and Clin. Immunol. 75:183 (1985).

77. A.F. Welton, and W.A. Scott, Therapeutic approaches to arthritis through modulation of lipid mediators, Adv. in Inflamm. Res. 11: 313 (1986).

78. J.L. Humes, E.E. Opas, and R.J. Bonney, Arachidonic acid metabolites in mouse ear edema, Adv. in Inflammation Res. 11:57 (1986).

79. J.M. Young, B.M. Wagner, and D.A. Spires, Tachyphylaxis in 12-0-tetracecanoylphorbol acetate- and arachidonic acid-induced ear edema, J. Invest. Dermatol. 80:48 (1983).

80. A. Lassus, and S. Forsstrom, A dimethoxynaphthalene derivative (RS-43179 gel) compared with 0.025% fluocinolone acetonide gel in the treatment of psoriasis, Br. J. Dermatol. 113:103 (1985).

81. R. Camp, A. Kobza-Black, F. Cunningham, A. Mallet, and M. Greaves, Pharmacological effects of topical lonapalene in psoriasis, J. Invest. Dermatol. 90:550 (1988).

82. H. Crowley, B. Yaremko, and A.F. Welton, Topical activity of FPL 55712, a leukotriene receptor antagonist in rats and guinea pigs, XII International Congress of Allergology and Clinical Immunology Abstracts (1985).

83. J. Grabbe, T. Rosenbach, and B.M. Czarnetzki, Production of LTB_4-like chemotactic arachidonate metabolites from human keratinocytes, J. Invest. Dermatol. 85:527 (1985).

84. V.A. Ziboh, T.L. Casebolt, C.L. Marcelo, and J.J. Voorhees, Biosynthesis of lipoxygenase products by enzyme preparations from normal and psoriatic skin, J. Invest. Dermatol. 83:426 (1984).

85. N. Fincham, R. Camp, and I. Leigh, Synthesis of arachidonate lipoxygenase products by epidermal cells, J. Invest. Dermatol. 84:447 (1985).

86. T. Ruzicka, T. Simmet, B.A. Peskar, and J. Ring, Skin levels of arachidonic acid-derived inflammatory mediators and histamine in atopic dermatitis and psoriasis, J. Invest. Dermatol. 86:105 (1986).

87. W.H. Anderson, M. O'Donnell, B.A. Simko, and A.F. Welton, An in vivo model for measuring antigen-induced SRS-A-mediated bronchoconstriction and plasma SRS-A levels in the guinea pig, Br. J. Pharmacol. 78:67 (1983).

NOVEL 5-LIPOXYGENASE INHIBITORS IN INFLAMMATION AND ASTHMA

G.A. Higgs

Wellcome Research Labs, Beckenham, Kent, BR3 3BS, UK
Present address: Celltech Ltd., 216 Bath Road
Slough, Berks, UK

INTRODUCTION

The discovery of mammalian lipoxygenases which convert arachidonic acid to oxygenated products with potent inflammatory and anaphylactic properties has led to growing speculation that these enzymes are central to certain disease processes (Samuelsson, 1983; Higgs, Moncada and Vane, 1984). This speculation has been supported by the demonstration of lipoxygenase activity in a number of different tissues following stimulation. For example, pulmonary tissues synthesize the peptido-leukotrienes (LTC_4, D_4 and E_4), which are products of 5-lipoxygenase, in response to immunological challenge. These leukotrienes comprise the activity originally referred to as 'slow reacting substance of anaphylaxis' (SRSA), they are powerful constrictors of airway smooth muscle and are thought to be mediators of anaphylactic bronchoconstriction. Phagocytic leukocytes also convert arachidonic acid to leukotrienes and the major product in polymorphonuclear leukocytes (PMNs) is the di-hydroxy acid LTB_4. Leukotriene B_4, along with some of the mono-hydroxy lipoxygenase products is chemotactic and it has been suggested that LTB_4 production by activated PMNs represents a local control mechanism for the accumulation of leukocytes at inflammatory sites.

In the same study in which lipoxygenase activity was first revealed in platelets, Hamberg and Samuelsson (1974) also showed that the enzyme was inhibited by the acetylenic analogue of arachidonic acid, ETYA. This compound, which has four triple bonds in place of the four double bonds in arachidonic acid, inhibited cyclo-oxygenase as well. In both reactions, ETYA competes with arachidonic acid for the enzymes; however, with ETYA, hydrogen abstraction cannot occur and so the peroxidation that is normally catalyzed by cyclo-oxygenase or lipoxygenase is blocked. Selective inhibition of 5-, 12- or 15-lipoxygenases has also been described but there are no reports that these compounds act as lipoxygenase inhibitors in vivo. In fact, there is no shortage of substances which inhibit lipoxygenase in vitro. These include radical scavengers, anti-oxidants and some anti-inflammatory drugs (for review see Bhattacherjee et al., 1988). In vivo, however, many of these substances have no activity at all and none act as selective inhibitors of 5-lipoxygenase. The absence of selective inhibitors which are active in vivo has, therefore, prevented a proper investigation of the role of leukotrienes in disease processes.

NOVEL INHIBITORS

The hypothesis that iron plays a key role in lipoxygenase catalysis led to the synthesis of some amide analogues of arachidonic acid in which strong coordination to iron is possible (Corey et al, 1984). Analogues containing a hydroxamic acid moiety are potent and selective inhibitors of leukotriene synthesis. A novel series of acetohydroxamic acids has now been synthesized for evaluation as potential enzyme inhibitors. Phenoxycinnamyl and tetrahydro-naphthylpropenyl acetohydroxamic acids (BW A4C and BW A797C) were prepared by reducing the appropriate oximes, followed by acetylation and selective O-deacetylation (Jackson et al, 1988).

INHIBITION OF LEUKOTRIENE SYNTHESIS IN VITRO AND IN VIVO

The acetohydroxamic acids caused a concentration-dependent inhibition of LTB_4 generation in homogenates of human PMNs while concentrations required to inhibit the production of TXB_2 (a cyclo-oxygenase product) were up to 24 times higher (Tateson et al, 1988). Similar activities were reported for nordihydroguaiaretic acid NDGA) and nafazatrom.

In vivo, however, only BW A4C and BW A797C caused a selective inhibition of LTB_4 production after oral administration to rats (Tateson et al, 1988). The effects of lipoxygenase inhibitors on the ex vivo synthesis of LTB_4 and TXB_2 in ionophore-stimulated whole blood taken up to six hours after oral administration of the drugs was measured. Nafazatrom produced only a slight and transitory reduction in LTB_4 synthesis and NDGA had no effect at all. Both BW A4C and BW A797C caused a dose-dependent and prolonged suppression of LTB_4 synthesis with no effects on TXB_2. Six hours after dosing, ED_{50} values for inhibition of 5-lipoxygenase in vivo were approximately 10mg/kg.

THE EFFECT OF LIPOXYGENASE INHIBITORS ON BRONCHIAL ANAPHYLAXIS

The effects of acetohydroxamic acids in a model of bronchial anaphylaxis in the guinea-pig have been investigated (Payne et al, 1988). Animals were sensitized to ovalbumin and challenged with aerosolized antigen. Bronchoconstriction was measured as the increase in pulmonary inflation pressure in pump-ventilated anaesthetized guinea-pigs. The animals were pre-treated with mepyramine (2mg/kg i.v.) and indomethacin (10mg/kg i.v.) in order to minimise the effects of endogenous histamine or thromboxane. The residual cyclo-oxygenase and histamine-independent bronchoconstriction was markedly reduced by additional pre-treatment with the leukotriene antagonist FPL 55712 (10mg/kg i.v.). This indicated that there is a significant 'leukotriene-dependent' component of anaphylactic bronchospasm in this model. BW A4C and BW A797C caused a dose-dependent reduction in the 'leukotriene-dependent' bronchospasm up to a maximal effect which was equivalent to that obtained with FPL 55712. The duration of action of these novel lipoxygenase inhibitors corresponded to the plasma concentration of unchanged drug. These results indicate that the novel acetohydroxamic acids prevent anaphylactic bronchospasm by the selective inhibition of leukotriene synthesis by arachidonate 5-lipoxygenase.

THE EFFECT OF LIPOXYGENASE INHIBITORS ON INFLAMMATION

To investigate the role of lipoxygenase products in inflammation and to determine the possible therapeutic value of lipoxygenase inhibitors, the acetohydroxamic acids have been tested in a series of animal models of acute inflammation (Higgs et al, 1988).

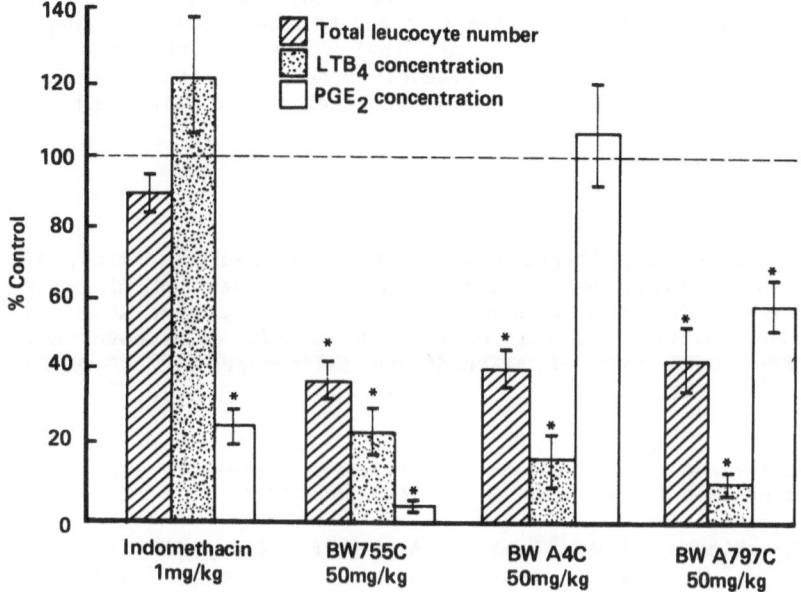

Fig. 1. The effects of oral administration of drugs on total leukocyte numbers and concentrations of LTB_4 and PGE_2 in inflammatory exudates. * indicates that $p < 0.05$ compared with control values (Bhattacherjee et al, 1988)

The concentration of LTB_4 found in 6 hour inflammatory exudates, induced in rats by the subcutaneous implantation of carrageenin-soaked polyester sponges were reduced dose-dependently by BW A4C (ED_{50} = 2.6mg/kg p.o.) and BW A797C (ED_{50} = 14.3 mg/kg p.o.). These compounds had relatively little effect on PGE_2 synthesis at the inflammatory site. The selective inhibition of lipoxygenase in inflamed tissue was accompanied by a reduction in the numbers of migrating leukocytes (Fig 1). It is possible that the reduction in leukocyte migration may be due to the inhibition of the synthesis of LTB_4 which is a potent chemotactic agent (Ford-Hutchinson et al, 1980).

The novel lipoxygenase inhibitors had no effect on irritant induced oedema or hyperalgesia in rate or mice. In contrast, yeast-induced pyrexia in rats was reduced by BW A4C and BW A797C but there was not a dose correlation between the anti-pyretic effects of these drugs and the inhibition of lipoxygenase. From these experiments, it would appear that cyclo-oxygenase products are the major mediators of vascular and pain responses in acute inflammation and that lipoxygenase products are relatively unimportant in these models.

SUMMARY

A new series of arachidonate 5-lipoxygenase inhibitors have been shown to have potent, selective and long lasting effects in vivo. These compounds also attenuate 'leukotriene-dependent' anaphylactic bronchospasm, accumulation of inflammatory leukocytes and the development of fever in experimental models. It only remains to be determined if these compounds have any therapeutic value in man.

REFERENCES

Bhattacherjee, P., Boughton-Smith, N.K., Follenfant, R.L., Garland, L.G., Higgs, G.A., Hodson, H.F., Islip, P.J., Jackson, W.P., Moncada, S., Payne, A.N., Randall, R.W., Reynolds, C.H., Salmon, J.A., Tateson, J.E. and Whittle, B.J.R., 1988. The effects of a novel series of selective inhibitors of arachidonate 5-lipoxygenase on anaphylactic and inflammatory responses. Ann. N.Y. Acad. Sci., 524: 307-320.

Corey, E.J., Cashman, J.R., Kantner, S.S. and Wright, S.W., 1984. Rationally designed, potent competitive inhibitors of leukotriene biosynthesis. J. Am. Chem. Soc., 106: 1503-1504.

Ford-Hutchinson, A.W., Bray, M.A., Doig, M.V., Shipley, M.W. and Smith, M.J.H., 1980. Leukotriene B, a potent chemokinetic and aggregating substance released from polymorphonuclear leukocytes. Nature, 286: 264-265.

Hamberg, M. and Samuelsson, B., 1974. Prostaglandin endoperoxides. Novel transformations of arachidonic acid in human platelets. Proc. Natl. Acad. Sci. USA, 71: 3400-3404.

Higgs, G.A., Follenfant, R.L. and Garland, L.G., 1988. Selective inhibition of arachidonate 5-lipoxygenase by novel acetohydroxamic acids : III. Effects on acute inflammatory responses. Br. J. Pharmacol., 94: 547-551.

Higgs, G.A., Moncada, S. and Vane, J.R., 1984. Eicosanoids in inflammation. Ann. Clin. Res. 16: 287-299.

Jackson, W.P., Islip, P.J., Kneen, G., Pugh, A. and Wates, P.J., 1988. Acetohydroxamic acids as potent, selective, orally active 5-lipoxygenase inhibitors. J. Med. Chem., 31 : 499-500.

Payne, A.N., Garland, L.G., Lees, I.W. and Salmon, J.A., 1988. Selective inhibition of arachidonate 5-lipoxygenase by novel acetohydroxamic acids: II. Effects on bronchial anaphylaxis in anaesthetised guinea-pigs. Br. J. Pharmacol., 94: 540-546.

Samuelsson, B., 1983. Leukotrienes: mediators of immediate hypersensitivity reactions and inflammation. Science, _220_: 568-575.

Tateson, J.E., Randall, R.W., Reynolds, C.H., Jackson, W.P., Bhattacherjee, P., Salmon, J.A. and Garland, L.G., 1988. Selective inhibition of arachidonate 5-lipoxygenase by novel acetohydroxamic acids: I. Biochemical assessment _in vitro_ and _ex vivo_. Br. J. Pharmacol., _94_: 528-539.

EICOSANOIDS AS REGULATORS OF EICOSANOID RELEASE IN MACROPHAGES: IMPACT

FOR EXACERBATION OF TISSUE DAMAGE BY NON-STEROIDAL ANTI-INFLAMMATORY DRUGS

Iván L. Bonta and Graham R. Elliott

Department of Pharmacology, Faculty of Medicine
Erasmus University Rotterdam, P.O.B. 1738
3000 DR Rotterdam, The Netherlands

BACKGROUND AND SCOPE

Macrophages are an important source of eicosanoids, releasing both cyclooxygenase and lipoxygenase metabolites of arachidonic acid (AA). Macrophages are also equipped with receptors for these essential fatty acid products. Hence eicosanoids released from macrophages not only influence the activity of surrounding cells but also modify the state of activation of the macrophage itself. Previous studies have shown that both, leukotrienes (LTs), which are metabolites of the lipoxygenase pathway, and cyclooxygenase inhibitors activate macrophages, whilst PGE_2, a cyclooxygenase metabolite, suppresses cell activation as indicated by the release of lysosomal enzymes. LTC_4 has been shown to stimulate PGE_2 synthesis, indicating that the action of this mediator is self-limiting and that eicosanoid formation is partially regulated by interactions between the different metabolites. These earlier findings prompted us to further investigate the possibility that PGE_2 suppresses, and cyclooxygenase inhibitors stimulate, macrophage functions via effects on LT synthesis. In this article, besides reviewing the most salient previous observations, account of recent experiments on the modulation of this synthesis by PGE_2 and non-steroidal anti-inflammatory drugs (NSAIDs) will be given. Most of the work is now in the process of publication in extenso (Elliott et al. 1988) and therefore, in the present article several technical details are omitted. While the regulatory role of PGE_2 on macrophage functions is an earlier proposal (Bonta & Parnham 1982), presently the focus of discussion will be on the balance between synthesis of lipoxygenase metabolites and PGE_2, which maintains the macrophage in a dynamic state.

LEUKOTRIENE C_4 AUGMENTATION OF LYSOSOMAL ENZYME SECRETION

It is becoming increasingly apparent that eicosanoids, products of arachidonic acid (AA) metabolism, are important modulators of macrophage cyclooxygenase and lipoxygenase pathways. For example, mouse resident peritoneal macrophage cyclooxygenase and 5'-lipoxygenase activities were inhibited by metabolites of the lipoxygenase pathway (Hume et al. 1986). Synthesis of cyclooxygenase metabolites by rat peritoneal macrophages was stimulated by the lipoxygenase products (Feuerstein et al. 1981,

Schenkelaars & Bonta 1986) while PGE_2 inhibited synthesis of the cyclooxygenase metabolites, TxB_2 and 6-keto-$PGF_{1\alpha}$ (Elliott et al. 1985). Such interactions between eicosanoids may be important for regulation of macrophage functions, as demonstrated by Schenkelaars and Bonta (1986) who reported that LTC_4 stimulated the secretion of the lysosomal enzyme beta-glucuronidase (GUR). This secretory response was enhanced by the non-steroidal anti-inflammatory drugs (NSAIDs) indomethacin and aspirin which possess cyclooxygenase inhibitory activity. Exogenously added PGE_2 prevented this stimulation of enzyme release. Of relevance to these interactions are reports showing that PGE_1 inhibited, and indomethacin stimulated, human neutrophil LTB_4 formation (Ham et al. 1983, Docherty & Wilson 1987). Therefore, in the light of published data, it appeared conceivable that indomethacin and aspirin stimulated macrophage GUR release by promoting synthesis of LTs, as a consequence of the inhibition of PGE_2 synthesis. In order to investigate this possibility we investigated the effect of PGE_2, indomethacin and aspirin on A23187-stimulated LTB_4 release by carrageenin-elicited rat peritoneal macrophages. In support of the findings in rat macrophages occasional experiments with mouse peritoneal macrophages will be also discussed.

CALCIUM FLUX-STIMULATED RELEASE OF EICOSANOIDS AND AUGMENTED LIPOXYGENASE ACTIVITY BY INHIBITORS OF CYCLOOXYGENASE

We used a non-physiological agent, A23187, to induce a physiological change, i.e. stimulate calcium flux. A23187 was used primarily as a LT stimulation (Docherty & Wilson 1987). Thus we could investigate regulatory events associated with LTB_4 formation. Specifically, the role played by PGE_2 in the mobilization and subsequent metabolism of AA to LTB_4, events thought to be associated with the increase in calcium flux was examined. A23187 (10^{-6}M) stimulated macrophage PGE_2, TxB_2 and LTB_4 synthesis and release as shown in Fig.1.

Indomethacin and aspirin enhanced A23187-stimulated LTB_4 synthesis and inhibited A23187-stimulated PGE_2 and TxB_2 formation (Figs. 2 and 3).

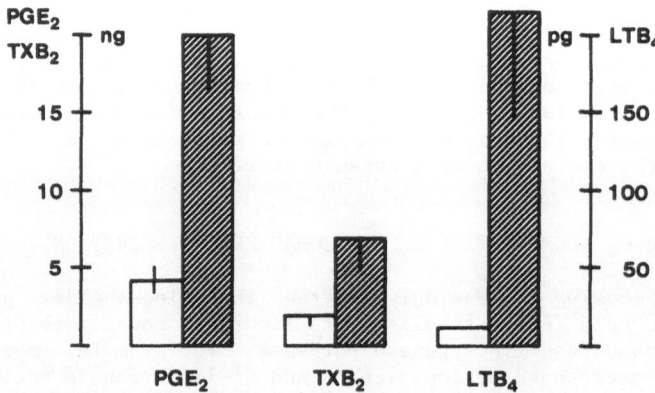

Fig. 1. A23187 (hatched bars) stimulation of eicosanoid release in rat elicited peritoneal macrophages.

These NSAIDs, also inhibited the basal formation of cyclooxygenase metabolites (data not shown), but had no detectable stimulatory effect on the basal synthesis of LTB$_4$. In similarity with these results on rat macrophages, indomethacin also promoted the A23187-stimulated LTB$_4$ release in peritoneal macrophages of mice (Elliott et al. 1988a).

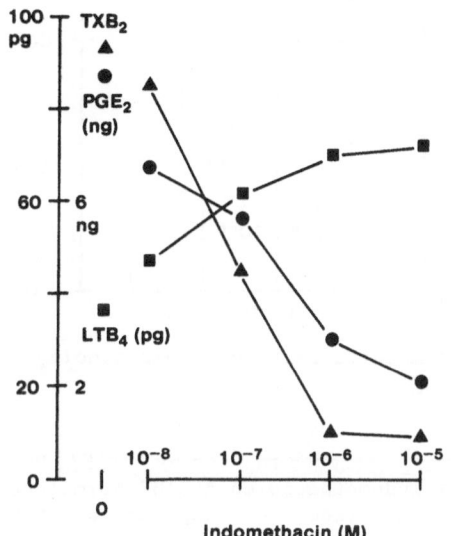

Fig. 2. Indomethacin effect on A23187 stimulated release of eicosanoids.

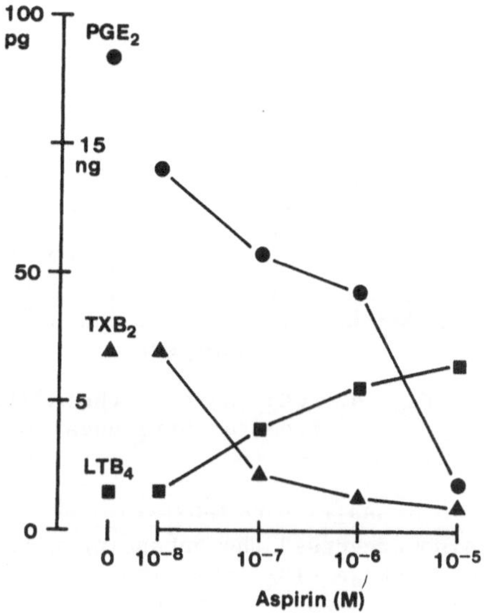

Fig. 3. Aspirin effect on A23187 stimulated release of eicosanoids.

The finding that the NSAIDs promoted A-23187-stimulated LTB$_4$ synthesis supports our contention that endogenously formed PGE$_2$ could have a regulatory function. However, we cannot say to what extent the stimulatory effect of the cyclooxygenase inhibitors on LTB$_4$ formation was due to removal of the inhibitory PGE$_2$. A switching of AA from the cyclooxygenase to the lipoxygenase path i.e. "substrate shunting", could also have contributed to the increase observed. Basal synthesis of LTB$_4$ was too low to assay, even in the presence of aspirin and indomethacin. It would appear therefore, that cyclooxygenase inhibitors can influence LT formation only if the lipoxygenase enzyme is stimulated by some other agent, i.e. they are not direct activators of the lipoxygenase.

PROSTAGLANDIN E$_2$ COUNTERACTS THE RELEASE OF EICOSANOIDS

We reported earlier that PGE$_2$ caused a decrease in release of TxB$_2$ and 6-keto-PGF$_{1\alpha}$ from carrageenin-stimulated macrophages (Elliott et al. 1985). This indicated that PGE$_2$ counteracts augmented production of cyclooxygenase metabolites. Now we observed that PGE$_2$ inhibited the calcium ionophore stimulated release of not only the cyclooxygenase-product TxB$_2$, but also the simultaneous release of the lipoxygenase-product LTB$_4$ as well (Fig.4).

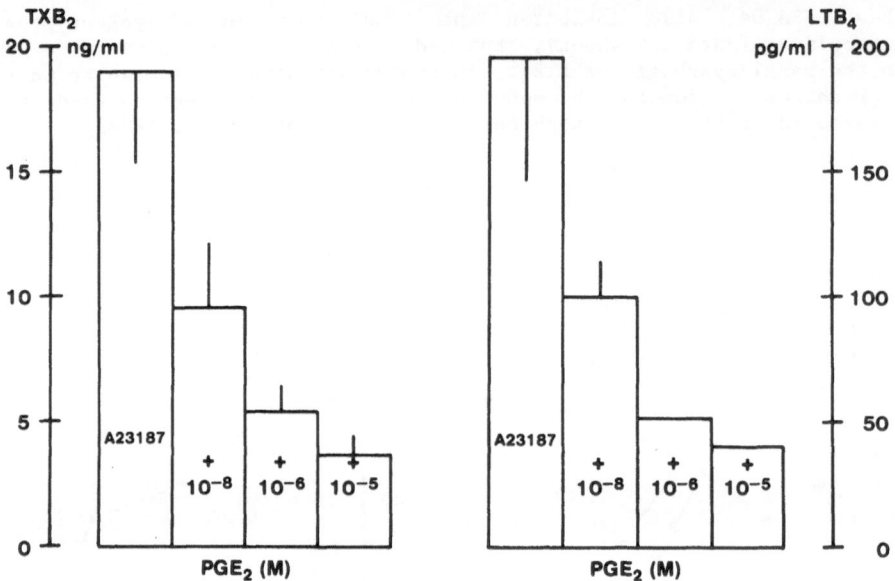

Fig. 4. PGE$_2$ inhibits the A23187-stimulated release of eicosanoids from rat peritoneal macrophages.

In addition to inhibiting the eicosanoid release induced by A23187, PGE$_2$ also reversed the enhancing effect of indomethacin on A23187-stimulated macrophage LTB$_4$ formation. The enhancing effect of aspirin on LTB$_4$ release was inhibited by PGE$_2$ to a similar extent as that of indomethacin. However, PGE$_2$ failed to decrease the enhanced release of LTB$_4$ and TxB$_2$ following the challenge of macrophages with 8×10^{-6}M of AA. The experiment with indomethacin is shown in Fig.5, while with respect to the results with aspirin and AA reference is made to the original paper (Elliott et al. 1988b).

In the here presented work we have shown that exogenously added PGE$_2$ inhibited A23187-stimulated LTB$_4$ synthesis. The lowest concentration of PGE$_2$ used (10^{-8}M) inhibited A23187-stimulated LTB$_4$ formation markedly (Fig.4). In the presence of the calcium ionophore rat peritoneal macrophages released about 0.5×10^{-9}M PGE$_2$ (calculated from the original data which served to derive Fig.1), indicating that endogenously formed PGE$_2$ could also play a role in regulating LT synthesis. This extends our previous finding that PGE$_2$ inhibits the synthesis and release of TxB$_2$ and 6-keto-PGF$_{1\alpha}$ induced by carrageenin (Elliott et al. 1985). It is reasonable to assume that PGE$_2$ would also modify the effect of other agents or factors which, in similarity with A23187 stimulate AA turnover.

PGE$_2$ inhibited both lipoxygenase (LTB$_4$) and cyclooxygenase (TxB$_2$) metabolite release. PGE$_2$ also inhibited the further increase in LTB$_4$ formation observed when cells were incubated with A23187 together with indomethacin or aspirin. Furthermore, PGE$_2$ had no effect on AA stimulated LTB$_4$ or TxB$_2$ synthesis. It is unlikely therefore, that PGE$_2$ acted on specific enzymes within the AA cascade. A more likely explanation is that PGE$_2$ limited the availability of AA. PGE$_2$ is thought to exert its immunomodulatory effects by stimulating cAMP synthesis (Bonta & Parnham 1982). Not shown in the present paper is our observation that db-cAMP partially inhibited A23187-stimulated LTB$_4$ and

230

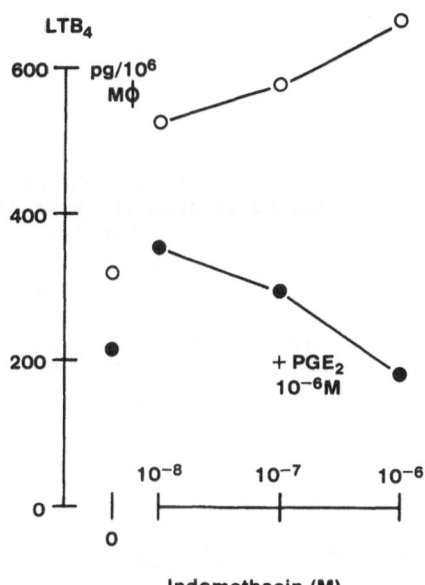

Fig. 5. PGE$_2$ (closed circles) counteracts indomethacin-augmentation (open circles) of A23187-stimulated release of LTB$_4$.

TxB$_2$ formation (Elliott et al. 1988b). In support of this interpretation carrageenin-stimulated eicosanoid synthesis has also been demonstrated to be inhibited by db-cAMP (Elliott et al. 1985). Furthermore, we observed that both PGE$_2$ and cAMP synthesis were decreased when macrophages were incubated with indomethacin (Elliott et al. 1988b). This finding is consistent with the proposal that endogenously formed PGE$_2$ is important for the maintenance of macrophage cAMP concentrations (Lim et al. 183). There are several possible mechanisms by which cAMP and db-cAMP, could reduce the concentration of AA available to the different enzymes, for example, stimulation of AA reacylation and inhibition of phospholipase (PL) activity. Indeed, Lapetina et al. (1981) reported that cAMP stimulated the reincorporation of AA into platelet phosphatidylinositol and Hirata et al. (1984) demonstrated that cAMP blocked deactivation of the PLA$_2$ inhibitory polypeptide, lipocortin, by agents such as A23187 and phorbol esters. Our results suggest that PGE$_2$ inhibits macrophage LTB$_4$ synthesis by limiting the availability of AA.

CYCLOOXYGENASE INHIBITORS AND EXACERBATION OF TISSUE DAMAGE

NSAIDs, such as aspirin and indomethacin, which are used to treat chronic inflammatory conditions are recognized to act, at least foremostly, by inhibiting the cyclooxygenase pathway. Schenkelaars and Bonta (1986) demonstrated that both aspirin and indomethacin enhanced LT-stimulated macrophage lysosomal enzyme release. This finding, while having been published in detail earlier, is in context of results discussed in this article, shown here again (Fig.6).

It is clear that NSAID augmentation of lysosomal enzyme secretion was concomitant with inhibition of PGE_2 release. It is almost certain that the two events are in causal relation with each other (Schenkelaars & Bonta 1986). We have now shown that the two NSAIDs, aspirin and indomethacin, also enhance A23187-stimulated LTB_4 synthesis and that this effect is reversed by added PGE_2. Indomethacin has also been shown to promote neutrophil superoxide production although the authors suggested that this was due to an inhibition of diacylglycerol lipase activity (Dale & Penfield 1987). Our results, together with other findings (Docherty & Wilson 1987, Schenkelaars & Bonta 1986) provide experimental evidence for the theoretical proposal of Rang and Dale (1987) namely that the use of NSAIDs in chronic conditions, such as e.g. rheumatoid arthritis could, by inhibiting PGE_2 synthesis and stimulating LT production, exacerbate tissue damage in the long term.

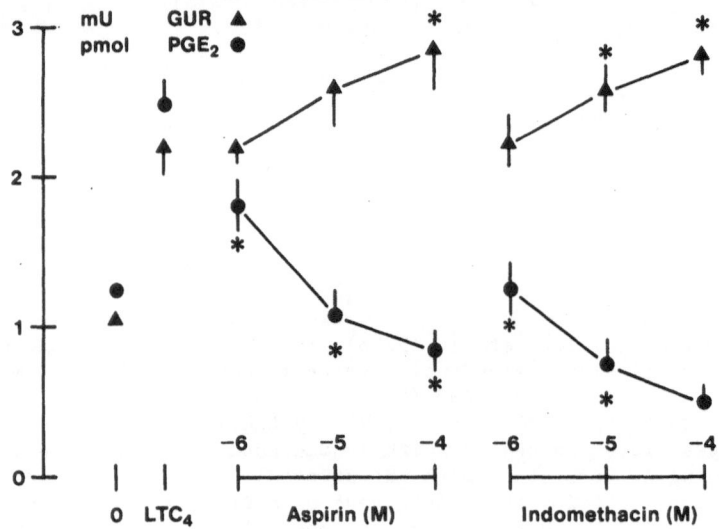

Fig. 6. NSAIDs augment LTC_4-stimulated secretion of β-glucuronidase (GUR).

CONCLUDING REMARKS

The studies discussed in this article show that the eicosanoid producing functions and the lysosomal enzyme secreting capacity of macrophages are positively related to the release of lipoxygenase metabolites and negatively to the production of the cyclooxygenase metabolite PGE_2. The results as summarized in Fig.7 indicate that LTC_4 and/or inhibitors of cyclooxygenase enhance the function of macrophages, whereas PGE_2 suppresses these cells.

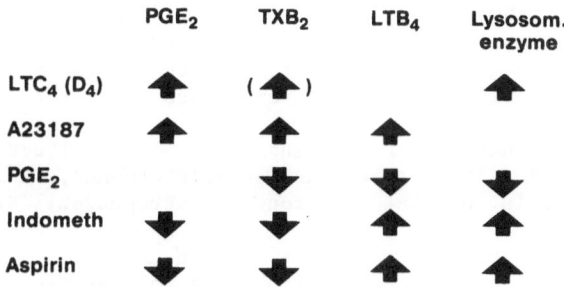

Fig. 7. Releasing activity of macrophages as influenced by
eicosanoids and NSAIDs.

Also we presented evidence that calcium flux-induced release of LTB_4 is
augmented by inhibitors of cyclooxygenase, but counteracted by PGE_2.
These results are in favour of the concept that the dynamic state of
activation of macrophages is maintained by balanced interactions between
endogenous PGE_2 and leukotrienes. PGE_2 stimulation of cAMP formation and
reduced production of PGE_2, as a consequence of decreased availability
of AA by increase of cAMP, are further complicating factors in the
balanced state of macrophage activity. Finally, we provided evidence for
the speculative possibility that NSAIDs, probably by removing the
regulatory function of endogenous PGE_2, promote the synthesis of the
pro-inflammatory LTB_4 and augment the secretion of tissue-damaging
lysosomal enzyme.

ACKNOWLEDGEMENTS

The original experiments, which are discussed in this article, have
been financially sponsored by Sigma-Tau Pharmaceutical Co., Rome.

REFERENCES

Bonta, I. L., and Parnham, M. J., 1982, Immunomodulatory-antiinflammatory
    functions of E-type prostaglandins. Minireview with emphasis on
    macrophages mediated effects, Int. J. Immunopharmacol., 4:103.
Dale, M. M., and Penfield, A., 1987, Comparison of the effects of indome-
    thacin, RHC80267 and R59022 on superoxide production by 1,oleoyl-2,
    acetyl glycerol and A23187 in human neutrophils, Br. J. Pharmacol.,
    92:63.
Docherty, J. C., and Wilson, T. W., 1987, Indomethacin increases the
    formation of lipoxygenase products in calcium ionophore stimulated
    human neutrophils, Biochem. Biophys. Res. Commun., 2:534.
Elliott, G. R., Van Batenburg, M. J., and Bonta, I. L., 1985, Differen-
    tial regulation of the cyclooxygenase pathway in starch elicited rat
    peritoneal macrophages by prostaglandin E_2, U-44069, a stable
    endoperoxide analogue and dibutyryl-cyclic AMP, Eur. J. Pharmacol.,
    114:71.

Elliott, G. R., Tak, C., Pellens, C., Ben-Efraim, S., and Bonta, I. L., 1988a, Indomethacin stimulation of macrophage cytostasis against MOPC-315 tumor cells is inhibited by both prostaglandin E_2 and nor-dihydroguaiaretic acid, a lipoxygenase inhibitor, Cancer Immunol. immunother., 17:133

Elliott, G. R., Lauwen, A. P. M., and Bonta, I. L., 1988b, Prostaglandin E_2 inhibits and indomethacin and aspirin enhance, A23187-stimulated LTB_4 synthesis by rat peritoneal macrophages, Br. J. Pharmac., Submitted.

Feuerstein, N., Foegh, M., and Ramwell, P. W., 1981, Leukotriene C_4 and D_4 induce prostaglandin and thromboxane release from rat peritoneal macrophages, Br. J. Pharmac., 72:389.

Ham, E. A., Soderman, D. D., Zanetti, M. A., Dougherty, H. W., McCauley, E., and Keuhl, F. A., 1983, Inhibition by prostaglandins of leuko-triene B_4 release from activated neutrophils, Proc. Natl. Acad. Sci. USA, 80:4349.

Hirata, F., Matsuda, L., Notsu, Y., Hattori, T., and Del Carmine, R., 1984, Phosphorylation at a tyrosine residue of lipomodulin in mito-gen-stimulated murine thymocytes, Proc. Natl. Acad. Sci. USA, 81: 4717.

Humes, J. L., Opas, E. E., Galavage, M., Soderman, D., and Bonney, R. J., 1986, Regulation of macrophage eicosanoid production by hydroperoxy and hydro-eicosatetraenoic acids, Biochem. J., 233:199.

Lapetina, E. G., Billah, M. M., and Cuatrecasas, P., 1981, The phospha-tidylinositol cycle and regulation of arachidonic acid production. Nature, 292:367.

Lim, L. K., Hunt, N. H., and Weidermann, M. J., 1983, Reactive oxygen production, arachidonate metabolism and cyclic AMP in macrophages, Biochim. Biophys. Res. Comm., 114:549.

Rang, H. P., and Dale, M. M., 1987, Drugs used to suppress inflammatory and immune reactions. In: Pharmacology, H. P. Rang, and M. M. Dale, eds., Churchill Livingstone, pp.206-207.

Schenkelaars, E. J., and Bonta, I. L., 1986, Cyclooxygenase inhibitors promote the leukotriene C_4 induced release of beta-glucuronidase from rat peritoneal macrophages: prostaglandin E_2 suppresses, Int. J. Immunopharmacol., 8:305.

EICOSANOID REGULATION OF MACROPHAGE-MEDIATED ANTI-TUMOR FUNCTION

Iván L. Bonta[1], Graham R. Elliott[1] and Shlomo Ben-Efraim[2]

[1]Dept. of Pharmacology, Faculty of Medicine, Erasmus Univ.
Rotterdam, P.O.B. 1738, 3000 DR Rotterdam, The Netherlands
[2]Dept. of Human Microbiology, Sackler School of Medicine
Tel Aviv University, Tel Aviv, Israel

EICOSANOIDS MODULATE MACROPHAGE ACTIVATION STATE

When phospholipids deliver free arachidonic acid (AA), it can be in macrophages metabolized either into the cyclooxygenase pathway or into lipoxygenase products. The release of eicosanoids is intimately related to the activation state of macrophages. The production of the cyclooxygenase metabolite PGE_2 is inversely correlated with the activation state. Furthermore PGE_2, via receptor-mediated activation of adenylate cyclase, is involved in elevated levels of intracellular cyclic AMP in macrophages. Increased levels of cyclic AMP are associated with inhibition of macrophage functions and PGE_2 which activates the adenylate cyclase, is recognized as deactivator of macrophages. In this context, inhibitors of cyclooxygenase promote the activation of macrophages, as i.a. shown by enhanced release of lysosomal enzymes (Schenkelaars & Bonta 1986). In contrast to the above, the lipoxygenase pathway favours the activation of macrophages. Several immunological events are associated with increased biosynthesis of leukotrienes (LTs) (Rola-Pleszczynski & LeMaire 1986). Macrophages were shown to be responsive to exposure of either LTC_4 or LTD_4, both of them inducing the release of several products of the cyclooxygenase pathway. Using the secretion of a lysosomal enzyme as a marker of cell activity, LTC_4 was also shown to trigger the activation of macrophages. Thus LTC_4 proved to enhance the enzyme secretion of macrophages, whereas PGE_2 inhibited this event. Because lysosomal enzyme release was observed with a lower concentration of LTC_4 than necessary to induce the biosynthesis of PGE_2 it was proposed that the enzyme secretion is the primary event and that the subsequent release of PGE_2 serves to limit the activating function of the peptidoleukotriene. In that case full expression of LT induced activation would only be observed in the absence of endogenous PGE_2. Indeed, it was shown that inhibitors of cyclooxygenase promote the LTC_4-induced release of a lysosomal enzyme (Schenkelaars & Bonta 1986). The finding that LTs promote the production of PGE_2, – the cyclooxygenase metabolite which suppresses macrophages – indicates that the action of LTs is self-limiting and that eicosanoid formation is, at least partially, regulated by interactions between the different metabolites of AA. The more recent observation, showing that the calcium flux-induced release of LTB_4 is counteracted by PGE_2 and augmented by inhibitors of cyclooxygenase (Elliott et al. 1988b), gives further support to the concept that the

235

dynamic state of activation of macrophages is maintained by balanced interactions between endogenous PGE_2 and leukotrienes. Macrophage cytotoxicity or cytostasis towards tumor cells is a characteristic expression of macrophage activation. Studies, which were aimed to investigate the role of eicosanoids in the anti-tumor function of macrophages, represented a logical move.

FACTORS MEDIATING ANTI-TUMOR FUNCTION OF MACROPHAGES

Tumor tissues transplanted between rodents possessing identical histocompatibility antigens can lead to immunologic rejection of the tumor. This has led investigators to propose that tumors, including those which spontaneously occur in man, may result, at least in part, from failure of the immune response of the host to recognize and subsequently destroy cells bearing tumor antigens. This concept of immune surveillance directed the attention to the antitumor potential of macrophages, which are increasingly recognized as surveillance cells of the immune system. Whereas the antitumor potential of quiescent macrophages is negligible, macrophages, when appropriately activated, inhibit tumor cell growth during cocultures in vitro and destroy susceptible tumor targets by a non-phagocytic process (Adams & Hamilton 1984). This process may include a variety of different mechanisms. Even when their activity is not cytotoxic, or cytocidal, macrophages can inhibit tumor cell growth through cytostatic activity. The two activities can be readily distinguished and measured separately: cytocidal effect as release of ^{51}Cr from prelabelled tumor cells, whereas inhibition of ^3H-thymidine incorporation in the tumor cell is a readily measurable parameter of cytostasis. Nevertheless, the two events may be interrelated and several mechanisms, - non of which excluding the others - have been proposed to be valid for both events. Some of these suggestions comprised that direct cell-to-cell contact is important (Leibovici et al. 1986). Others have indicated that a soluble mediator, released by macrophages upon activation, is necessary. While not pretending completeness, such mediators could include neutral proteases (Adams & Hamilton 1984), cell damaging protein factors i.e., a group of products referred to commonly as Tumor Necrosing Factor (Matthews 1981) and more recently the involvement of interleukin 1 has been proposed (Onozaki et al. 1985). O_2 metabolites, - which are also products of stimulated macrophages - have also deleterious effects on tumor cells (Nathan et al. 1980).

In the original experiments to be discussed in this article, we exclusively used peritoneal resident macrophages from BALB/c mice. The target tumor cells were also of mouse origin and included two cell lines which are unsensitive to interleukine-1 (IL-1): MOPC-315 plasmacytoma cells and P-815 mastocytoma cells. The third tumor cell line used was the WEHI-3B myeloma, which is sensitive to the cytostatic action of IL-1.

MACROPHAGE CYTOSTASIS IS INTERRELATED WITH EICOSANOID RELEASE

Evidence is accumulating in favour of the view that cyclooxygenase and lipoxygenase metabolites of arachidonic acid (AA) can exert opposing effects on macrophage functions. For example, the lipoxygenase product LTC_4 stimulated the secretion of macrophage beta-glucuronidase, a lysosomal enzyme. This effect was inhibited by PGE_2, a cyclooxygenase metabolite, and enhanced by indomethacin, a cyclooxygenase inhibitor (Schenkelaars & Bonta 1986). Indomethacin has also been shown to enhance, and PGE_2 to inhibit LTB_4 synthesis in macrophages (Elliott et al. 1986). It appears therefore that indomethacin could stimulate macrophage functions by removing the inhibitory action of PGE_2 on LT formation, so increasing the effective concentration of these lipoxygenase metabolites. We have also reported that mouse resident peritoneal macrophages could be activated by indomethacin, in vitro, to inhibit growth of MOPC-315 tumor cells. Further, macrophage cytostasis was enhanced by LTD_4 (Ophir et al. 1987, Bonta & Ben-Efraim 1987). Thus in similarity with their effect on enzyme secretion and eicosanoid release, cyclooxygenase and lipoxygenase metabolites appeared to have opposing effects on expression of macrophage cytostatic function. Subsequently we have further explored this phenomenon by examining the actions of PGE_2 and nordihydroguaiaretic acid (NDGA), a lipoxygenase inhibitor, on indomethacin stimulated macrophage cytostasis. The results are now being published in extenso (Elliott et al. 1988a). A brief account of this study is given as follows.

Assessment of cytostasis of resident peritoneal macrophages from BALB/c mice towards MOPC-315 cells was carried out by a method published in detail elsewhere(Ophir et al. 1987). Briefly, a coculture of macrophages and tumor cells in a ratio 100:1 was incubated with the test substances or the respective vehicles for 24h. Thereafter ^{3}H-thymidine (^{3}HTdR) was added for another 16h incubation, that was terminated by harvesting the cells onto glass fibre filtermats which were punched out to feed into a beta counter to measure the cellular incorporation of radioactivity. In parallel experiments macrophages were cultured alone. Values for tumor cell ^{3}HTdR incorporation in the coculture experiments were obtained by the formula:

$$cpm (MOPC-315 + macrophages) - cpm\ macrophages$$

The effect of indomethacin and NDGA on macrophage LTB_4 release has been measured by radioimmunoassay in the supernatant following 15 min incubation with the calcium ionophore A23187 (10^{-6}M), a stimulator of the lipoxygenase pathway. Indomethacin and NDGA were added at the beginning of the incubation.

Thymidine incorporation of MOPC-315 was decreased in the presence of macrophages. This cytostatic activity was further stimulated by indomethacin 10^{-5}M, the effect of which was reversed by PGE_2 (Fig. 1A). The stimulatory effect of indomethacin on macrophage cytostasis was also reversed by NDGA (Fig. 1B). LTB_4 synthesis in macrophages (576 ± 85 pg/ml) was also stimulated by indomethacin 10^{-7}M (1022 ± 288) and inhibited by NDGA 10^{-5}M (72 ± 42).

The observations that the stimulatory effect of indomethacin on macrophage cytostasis required the concentration of 10^{-5}M, whereas LTB_4 synthesis was stimulated by 10^{-7}M reinforce the earlier proposal (Ophir et al. 1987) that the full effects of LTs are only observed in the absence of cyclooxygenase metabolites, in particular PGE_2. Thus, two interrelated processes could be important for indomethacin stimulated macrophage cytostasis. First, inhibition of cyclooxygenase activity; second, stimulation of LT formation. The stimulation by indomethacin of LT synthesis could have been due to substrate shunting or to removal of the inhibitory PGE_2. It is reasonable to postulate that NDGA reversed

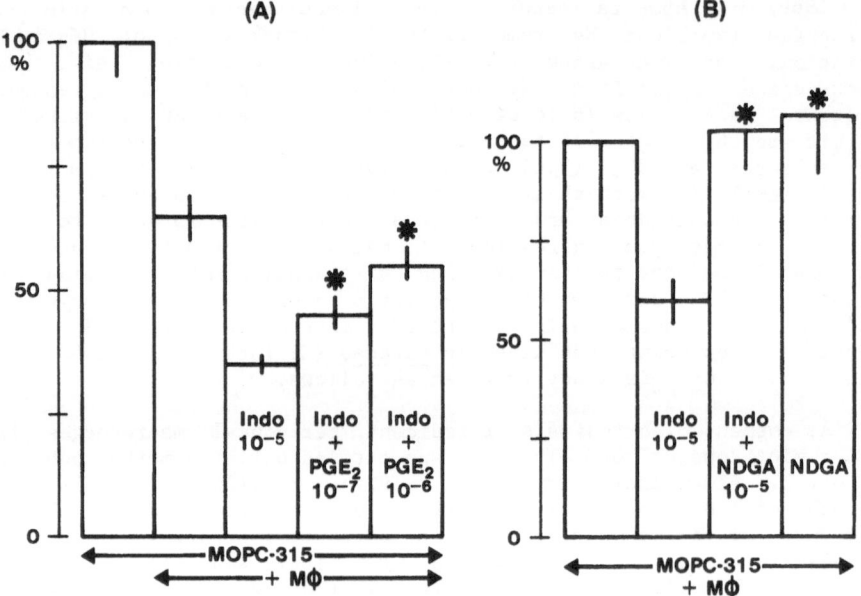

Fig. 1. Indomethacin-stimulation of macrophage cytostasis. ^{3}H-thimidine uptake of MOPC-315 cells (A) or MOPC-315 plus macrophages (B) is arbitrarily set as 100 percent. Doses of substances are shown as molar concentrations. Significance (Mann-Whitney U-test) was calculated from the absolute values that are published elsewhere. * = P < 0.005 vs indomethacin.

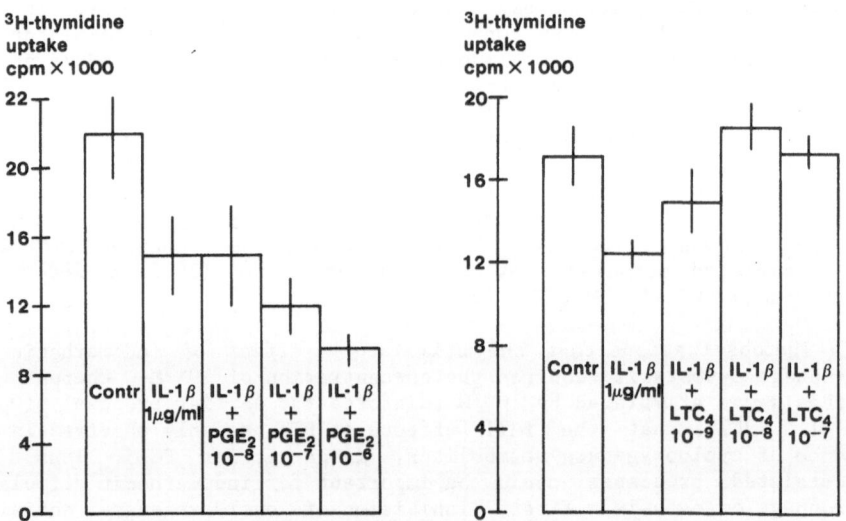

Fig. 2. PGE_2 enhances and LTC_4 counteracts the effect of IL-1 on WEHI-3B cells.

the indomethacin-stimulated cytostasis by inhibiting lipoxygenase activity. It would appear that impairment of the lipoxygenase pathway leads to suppression of the cytostatic function of macrophages that have been activated by removal of endogenous PGE_2. This is complementary to the earlier finding which showed that LTD_4 additively enhanced the indomethacin stimulated macrophage cytostasis towards MOPC-315. It is reasonable to postulate that the NDGA-induced suppression of macrophage cytostasis towards MOPC-315 cells is subsequent to impairment of lipoxygenase in the macrophages. Congruent results have been obtained with A23187 activated macrophage cytostasis against P-815 cells using AA-861, which is more specific than NDGA in causing inhibition of lipoxygenase (van Hilten et al. 1988).

Macrophages release a host of products on activation, including interleukin-1 (IL-1), tumor necrosing factor (TNF), active oxygen species and lysosomal enzymes, all of which could be involved in cytostasis. The release of some of these products was shown to be promoted by LTs and inhibited by PGE_2 (Rola-Pleszczynski & LeMaire 1985, Schenkelaars & Bonta 1986). The MOPC-315 cell line is resistent to the effects of IL-1 and TNF (data not shown). However, we cannot exclude any of the other possible mechanisms. Activated macrophages can exert cytostasis also by cell-to-cell contact (Leibovici 1986). Provided this was involved in our experiments, it could also explain why we need so large a macrophage/tumor cell ratio.

EICOSANOID INTERACTION WITH INTERLEUKIN-1

The interleukines-1 (IL-1) are a family of polypeptides, produced by monocytes and/or macrophages and have been implicated in the antitumor function of these cells. Indeed recombinant human Hr Il-1 has recently been reported to directly inhibit the growth of some tumor cell lines in vitro indicating that IL-1 could posses antitumor functions in vivo (Onozaki et al. 1985). Some actions of IL-1 are thought to be mediated via the stimulation of PGE_2 (Dinarello et al. 1986). Further, the synthesis of IL-1 is inhibited by PGE_2 and stimulated by LTs. Thus AA metabolites (eicosanoids) are both mediators through which IL-1 can work and modulators of IL-1 synthesis (Farrar & Humes 1985, Kunkel et al. 1986, Rola-Pleszczynski & LeMaire 1985). It is conceivable, therefore, that the cytostatic effect of IL-1 on tumor cell growth could be modified by eicosanoids. We found that WEHI-3B cells, a murine myeloid monocytic leukemia cell line, were sensitive to the cytostatic action of HrIL-1 (α and β). Using this model we investigated the interactions between IL-1, PGE_2 and LTC_4 and the possible mechanisms involved. This work is now being published in extenso elsewhere (Elliott et al. 1988c). A brief account is given here, but concerning technical details, reference is made to the original paper.

HrIL-1 inhibited WEHI-3B cell growth in a dose related manner (10-10,000 u/ml). PGE_2, at high concentrations (1000ng/ml) also inhibited cell growth. When added together, HrIL-1 and PGE_2 inhibited WEHI-3B growth in a synergistic manner. In contrast to the effects of the cyclooxygenase product, the lipoxygenase metabolite LTC_4 reversed the cytostatic action of HrIL-1 (Fig.2).

Thus the cytostatic effect of HrIL-1 was enhanced synergistically by PGE_2 and reversed by LTC_4. To our knowledge, this is the first time that eicosanoids have been shown to modify the effect of IL-1 itself. The mechanism by which HrIL-1 is not clear. We could not detect the release of eicosanoids from WEHI-3B cells stimulated with the calcium ionophore A23187, indicating that HrIL-l acts did not act by modifying the bioconversion of AA. Our results indicate that PGE_2 and LTC_4 are important modifiers of the effects of IL-l and are more than just mediators through which IL-l sometimes works. There is, in fact, a complex network of interactions between IL-1 and eicosanoids through which the synthesis and functions of IL-1 are regulated. Our results further emphasize the importance of interactions between macrophage derived mediators, which not only affect macrophage functions but also regulate associated systems.

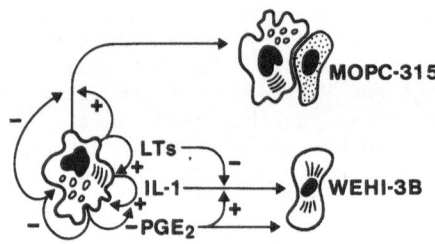

Fig. 3. Schematic representation of eicosanoid modulation of cell-to-cell contact-mediated and IL-1 mediated macrophage cytostasis.

CONCLUSIONS

As presented above, in studies derived from our laboratory and from others, the balance between lipoxygenase and cyclooxygenase metabolites is important in controlling macrophage-mediated cytostasis of tumor cell growth in vitro. The effects are dependent on whether the target tumor cell line required cell-to-cell contact with the activated macrophage or not (Fig.3).

With the MOPC-315 cell line, representing tumor cells which, to be inhibited in their growth, require cell-to-cell contact, we have shown that indomethacin stimulation of macrophage cytostasis can be counteracted by PGE_2 and by the lipoxygenase inhibitor NDGA. The results are congruent with the earlier finding, which showed that LTD_4 reinforces the effect of indomethacin on macrophage cytostasis. It is not unconceivable that macrophage-derived O_2-metabolites are involved in this kind of cytostasis. Using WEHI-3B cells which do not require contact with macrophages to be inhibitited by macrophage-secreted cytostatic factor(s), we observed that the inhibition by IL-1 was synergistically enhanced by PGE_2 and counteracted by LTC_4. In conclusion thus, it appears that inhibitors and/or products of the lipoxygenase and cyclooxygenase enzymes are capable of modulating macrophage cytostasis both, by influencing the macrophage itself and by interferring with the direct effect of a macrophage-derived cytokine, IL-1, on the tumor cell.

ACKNOWLEDGEMENTS

The original experiments discussed in this article have been financially sponsored by the Dutch Cancer Foundation (Koningin Wilhelmina Fonds). Some of the work quoted was carried out during a sabbatical stay of Ivan L. Bonta as Elected Fellow of the Mortimer and Raymond Sackler Institute of Advanced Studies, Tel Aviv University, Israel. Shlomo Ben-Efraim is presently spending his sabbatical as Visiting Professor at the Faculty of Medicine, Erasmus University Rotterdam. Figure 3 has been originally drafted by Graham R. Elliott.

REFERENCES

Adams, D. O., and Hamilton, T. A., 1984, The cell biology of macrophage activation. Am. Rev. Immunol., 2:283.

Bonta, I. L., and Ben-Efraim, S., 1987, Leukotrienes and prostaglandins mutually govern the antitumor potential of macrophages. In: "Prostaglandins in Cancer Research", M. G. Santoro, ed., Springer Verlag pp. 193-201.

Dinarello, C. A., Cannon, J. G., Mier, J. W., Bernheim, H.A., LoPreste, G., Lynn, D. L., Love, R. N. Well, A. C., Auron, P. E. Ruben, R. C., Rich, A., Wolff, S. M., and Putney, S. D., 1986, Multiple biological activities of human recombinant interleukin-1. J. Clin. Invest., 77:1734.

Elliott, G. R., Tak, C., Pellens, C., Ben-Efraim, S., and Bonta, I. L., 1988a, Indomethacin stimulation of macrophage cytostasis against MOPC-315 tumor cells is inhibited by both prostaglandin E_2 and nordihydroguaiaretic acid, a lipoxygenase inhibitor. Cancer Immunol. Immunother., 27:133.

Elliott, G. R., Lauwen, A. P. M., and Bonta, I. L., 1988b, Prostaglandin E_2 inhibits and indomethacin and aspirin enhance, A23187-stimulated leukotriene B_4 synthesis by rat peritoneal macrophages. Br. J Pharmac., 96:265.

Elliott, G. R. Tak, C., and Bonta, I. L., 1988c, Prostaglandin E_2 enhances, and leukotriene C_4 inhibits, interleukin-1 inhibition of WEHI-3B cell growth. Cancer Immunol. Immunother., 28:74.

Farrar, W. L., and Humes, J. L., 1985, The role of arachidonic acid metabolism in the activities of interleukin-1. J. Immunol., 135: 1153.

Hilten, J. A. van, Elliott, G. R., and Bonta, I. L., 1988, Specific lipoxygenase inhibition reverses macrophage cytostasis towards P815 tumor cells in vitro induced by the calcium ionophore A23187. Prostaglandins, Leukotrienes and Fatty Acids, 34:187.

Kunkel, S. L., Chensue, S. W., and Phan, S. H., 1986, Prostaglandins as endogenous modulators of interleukin-1 production. J. Immunol. 136:186.

Leibovici, J., Hoenig, S., and Pinchassov, A., 1986, In vitro effect of levan-activated macrophages on Lewis lung carcinoma cells. Int. J. Immunopharmac., 8:471.

Matthews, N., 1981, Production of an anti-tumor cytotoxin by human monocytes. Immunol., 44:135.

Nathan, C. F., Arrick, B. A., Murray, H. W., Desantis, N. M., and Cohn, Z. A., 1980, Tumor cell anti-oxidant defenses. Inhibition of the glutathione redox cycle enhances macrophage-mediated cytolysis. J. Exp. Med., 153:766.

Onozaki, K., Matsushima, K., Aggarwai, B. B., and Oppenheim, J. J., 1985, Human interleukin-1 is a cytocidal factor for several tumor cell lines. J. Immunol., 135:3962.

Ophir, R., Ben-Efraim, S., and Bonta, I. L., 1987, Leukotriene D_4 and indomethacin enhance additively the macrophage cytostatic activity in vitro towards MOPC-315 tumor cells. Int. J. Tiss. Reac., 9:189.

Rola-Pleszczynski, M., and LeMaire, I., 1985, Leukotrienes augment interleukin-1 production by human monocytes. J. Immunol., 135:3958.

Schenkelaars, E. J., and Bonta, I. L., 1986, Cyclooxygenase inhibitors promote the leukotriene C_4 induced release of beta-glucuronidase from rat peritoneal macrophages: Prostaglandin E_2 suppresses Int. J. Immunopharmac., 8:305.

INTERACTIONS BETWEEN ANTI-INFLAMMATORY DRUGS AND CANCER CHEMOTHERAPY

A. Bennett and J.D.Gaffen

Department of Surgery
King's College School of Medicine and Dentistry
The Rayne Institute
123 Coldharbour Lane
London, SE5 9NU, England

As a result of experiments indicating relationships of prostaglandins (PGs) to human mammary cancer (Bennett et al, 1977), we studied the effects of PG synthesis inhibitors on murine NC transplanted carcinomas in vivo and in vitro. Flurbiprofen or indomethacin (INDO) prolonged the survival of the host mice (Bennett et al, 1979, 1982), and potentiated the effect of the combined cytotoxic drug regimen of methotrexate (MTX) plus melphalan (MEL) (Berstock et al, 1979; Bennett et al, 1982; Berstock et al, 1982). This drug combination was used in the same ratio as in a human breast cancer study then being carried out by another group in our Department. However, we later found that the beneficial interaction with INDO on the NC tumour in vivo also occurs with just MTX alone (Bennett et al, 1987). Other experiments described below using cell culture support this finding.

Our in vitro studies have helped to determine the interactions between INDO, MTX and other cytotoxic drugs using cultures of NC mouse cancer cells, human cancer cells, and normal epithelium-like cells from human embryonic intestine. The aims were to see if the INDO interaction is confined to MTX, to determine the mechanism of action, and to examine the effect on normal cells. This chapter deals first with a brief account of our published in vitro studies on these aspects, and then proceeds to a description of some latest unpublished work.

As with the mouse in vivo experiments, INDO increased the killing by MTX of NC cells in culture (Gaffen et al, 1985), probably by enhancing the cellular uptake or retention of MTX (Gaffen et al, 1986; Bennett et al, 1987). However, INDO did not increase the cytotoxicity of MEL to the mouse NC cells in vitro (Bennett et al, 1988).

The potential therapeutic importance of this finding is that INDO also increased the killing of 2 human breast cancer cell lines (DU4475 and T47D), but not the normal epithelium-like cells from human embryonic intestine (Bennett et al, 1988). This sparing of the gut epithelial cells is also reflected by the inability of INDO to potentiate the killing of 2 human colon cancer cell lines by MTX (Bennett et al, 1988). Thus INDO may be useful for increasing the cytotoxicity of MTX for human breast cancer, without increasing the damage to the gut. An evaluation of this possibility must await the outcome of a clinical investigation, which remains to be attempted. The drug combination seems unlikely to enhance the treatment of colon cancers, and in any case malignancies of the human large bowel are known to be rather resistant to MTX.

With regard to the mechanism of this MTX/INDO interaction on the mouse NC cells, inhibition of PG formation by INDO is probably not important in the potentiation of MTX, since the effect in vitro was not counteracted by adding PGE_2 (Bennett et al, 1988) or mimicked by the other cyclo-oxygenase inhibitors flurbiprofen or piroxicam (Bennett et al, 1987, 1988). However, this conclusion is only tentative since we do not know whether PGE_2 alone is the best choice to see if the effect of indomethacin can be overcome, or whether flurbiprofen and piroxicam have other actions that counteract the response to a reduction of PG synthesis.

INDO can inhibit cAMP phosphodiesterase and calcium binding, but the interaction with MTX seems unlikely to be due to either of these mechanisms since it was not mimicked by theophylline (Bennett et al, 1987) or by the calcium antagonists verapamil or nifedipine (Gaffen, Stamford, Melhuish, Chambers and Bennett, unpublished).

Other recent studies which have not yet been published form the basis of the rest of this chapter. The aims were to determine whether (a) the potentiation of MTX cytotoxicity to human breast cancer cells is due to increased MTX uptake or retention (as appears to be the case with the mouse NC cancer cells), (b) whether the dual lipoxygenase/ cyclo-oxygenase inhibitor BW755C affects NC cancer cells and/or their response to MTX, (c) whether the anti-inflammatory steroid prednisolone (used clinically in cytotoxic drug regimens) affects NC cells or their response to MTX, and (d) whether prednisolone affects DU4475 human breast cancer cells and/or their response to MTX.

MATERIALS AND METHODS

Cells and cell culture. DU4475 cells originated from a metastatic cutaneous nodule from a 70-year-old female caucasian patient with advanced

244

breast cancer (Langlois et al, 1979). They were maintained as a suspension in RPMI 1640 culture medium containing 5% newborn bovine serum (NBS), 300mg/L of L-glutamine and 50 units/ml of both penicillin and streptomycin. The NC carcinoma arose spontaneously in the mammary region of a WHT/Ht mouse and has been passaged serially in this strain (Hewitt et al, 1976). NC carcinoma cells, obtained from a mouse with peritoneal metastases following i.p. injection of tumour (Bennett et al, 1987), were maintained as a suspension in MEM containing 10% NBS, 292 mg/L L-glutamine, antibiotics as above, and 1% nonessential amino acids prepared as directed by Flow Laboratories.

Drugs and solvents. INDO was dissolved in water containing sodium bicarbonate (final pH 7.8). MTX (Lederle) and BW755C (Wellcome Research Laboratories) were dissolved in 154 mM saline; the MTX solution was adjusted to pH 8.4 with 0.1M NaOH. Prednisolone was made up in ethanol/water (70:30). All the water was double-distilled in glass, and the solutions were sterilised by filtration.

Determination of cell growth. For both the DU4475 and NC cells, growth in suspension was determined by microturbidimetry (Gaffen et al, 1985). Cells were pelleted by centrifugation, resuspended in 1 ml trypsin/EDTA solution (0.05:0.02% w/v) and incubated for 30 s at 37°C. After rapidly adding 9 ml medium, the cells were gently disaggregated by repeated passage into and out of a pipette. The cell numbers were determined in a Coulter counter and adjusted so that 100µl contained 25,000 for the NC cells or 100,000 for the DU4475 cells. Aliquots of 100 or 200µl of medium containing drugs at x2 or x1.5 the desired final concentration (NC cells and DU 4475 cells respectively), or vehicle only were added to each of the 96 wells of a microtest plate, followed by 100µl of the cell suspension or medium alone. After incubation for 4 days (5% CO_2 humidified air, 37°C), the absorbance of 600nM light in each well was determined with a Dynatech microplate reader.

Concentration-growth curves for the DU4475 cells were obtained with MTX 2.5-10ng/ml alone or with prednisolone 1µg/ml.

Methotrexate uptake studies. 'MTX uptake' into the DU4475 cells was studied using a method modified from Henderson et al (1978). Bulk cultures of DU4475 cells were generated by inoculating 10-12 x 10^6 disaggregated cells into 120cm^2 glass culture flasks containing 100-120ml of RPMI 1640 medium + 5% NBS, and fed with fresh medium every second day. After 4-5 days at 37°C they were harvested by centrifugation (10min at 225 x g in 200ml aliquots), disaggregated, as described earlier, counted, and resuspended in glass centrifuge tubes (2x10^6 cells in 1.8ml medium). The tubes were then pre-incubated for 15 min at 37°C under the conditions described previously, in the presence of drugs or vehicle only. Radio-labelled MTX (0.2ml of 20µM [3',5',7' ^{3}H]-methotrexate sodium salt, 250mCi/mmol, Amersham UK) in phosphate buffered saline pH 7.4. was then added to each tube and the cells incubated at 37°C for 3hr in the presence

of either INDO 1μg/ml or vehicle.   Control samples were treated
identically except that the tubes were placed in an ice/water bath 5 min
before and during incubation with the isotope. The cell suspensions were
washed twice with ice-cold PBS (8 ml and then 10ml), and were centrifuged
at 700 x g for 5 min at $4^{O}C$ after each wash. Each cell pellet was
suspended in 1ml distilled water, and transferred to a glass counting vial
using 2 aliquots of scintillation fluid (final volume 10ml). Active
accumulation of label was taken as the difference in the radioactivity
between the experimental and control samples.

Mechanism by which indomethacin increases the cytotoxicity of
methotrexate to DU4475 human breast cancer cells. When the human breast
cancer cells were incubated with [^{3}H]-MTX for 3hr the median amount of
radioactivity retained by cells incubated with INDO 1μg/ml was 41% higher
than controls (P<0.01, Wilcoxon matched pairs signed-ranks test; n = 6).

Effect of BW755C on NC cancer cells and methotrexate cytotoxicity.
With the dual cyclo-oxygenase/ lipoxygenase inhibitor BW755C 1 or 10μg/ml,
the growth of the NC cells was respectively 15 ± 9 and 29 ± 4% (mean ±
sem) less as judged by microturbidimetry (P <0.2 and <0.001; n = 6).
However, BW755C did not affect the reduction by MTX 8ng/ml.

Prednisolone effect on NC cancer cells and methotrexate cytotoxicity.
Prednisolone 0.1 or 1μg/ml reduced the growth of NC cancer cells by 28 ± 7
and 33 ± 4% respectively as judged by microturbidimetry (P <0.01 and
<0.001; n = 7-9). The reduction of growth by MTX 8 ng/ml plus
prednisolone 0.1 or 1μg/ml was respectively 12 ± 6 and 22 ± 9% greater
than with MTX alone (P<0.05).

Prednisolone effect on methotrexate toxicity to DU4475 human breast
cancer cells. Prednisolone 1μg/ml slightly reduced the growth of the
DU4475 cells (5 ± 2%, P<0.05, n = 6). The effect of prednisolone combined
with MTX 2.5-10ng/ml was greater (18±3-32±5% respectively) than with MTX
alone (P<0.001, Student's t-test for paired data on overall difference).

DISCUSSION

Since INDO 1 μg/ml increased the amount of tritium in the human breast
cancer cells incubated with [^{3}H]-MTX, the mechanism of the INDO/MTX interaction might be the same as in the mouse NC carcinoma cells. Increased
MTX cytotoxicity with INDO in both these cell lines may be due to greater
MTX uptake or retention. The biochemical process involved is not yet
known, but we are investigating the effect of INDO on the formation of MTX
polyglutamate metabolites.

An inhibitory effect of BW755C or prednisolone on PG formation was
not expected to affect the cytotoxicity of MTX to the NC cells, since

flurbiprofen or piroxicam did not mimic the effect of INDO, and PGE_2 did not counteract the potentiation by INDO (Bennett et al, 1987, 1988). An important question is therefore whether a reduced formation of 5-lipoxygenase products by these drugs affects the NC cells or their response to MTX. However, we have not measured lipoxygenase product formation by NC cells, and we have not eliminated the possibility that other actions such as a simultaneous reduction of both lipoxygenase and cyclo-oxygenase products is needed for the anticancer effects of BW755C and prednisolone. Although both these drugs inhibited the growth of the NC cells, only prednisolone in combination with MTX produced an effect greater than MTX alone. Perhaps this reflects different mechanisms by which these drugs inhibit lipoxygenase; prednisolone can inhibit phospholipase A_2, and it may also decrease the amount of intracellular calcium which is essential for 5-lipoxygenase activity (Zor et al, 1987),

It is of particular clinical interest that prednisolone 1μg/ml increased the killing of DU4475 human breast cancer cells, and appears to potentiate the cytotoxicity of MTX. These findings may help explain the value of including prednisolone in cytotoxic drug regimens.

Acknowledgements. We thank the King's Joint Research Committee, the CRC and MRC for their support.

REFERENCES

Bennett, A., Charlier, E.M., McDonald, A.M., Simpson, J.S., Stamford, I.F. and Zebro, T. (1977). Prostaglandins and breast cancer. Lancet ii, 624-626.

Bennett, A., Houghton, J., Leaper, D.S. and Stamford, I.F. (1979). Cancer growth, response to treatment and survival time in mice: Beneficial effect of the prostaglandin synthesis inhibitor flurbiprofen. Prostaglandins, 17, 179-   191.

Bennett, A., Berstock, D.A. and Carroll, M.A. (1982). Increased survival of cancer-bearing mice treated with inhibitors of prostaglandin synthesis alone or with chemotherapy. Br. J. Cancer, 45, 762-768.

Bennett, A., Gaffen, J.D., Melhuish, P.B. and Stamford, I.F. (1987). Studies on the mechanism by which indomethacin increases the anticancer effect of methotrexate. Br. J. Pharmacol, 91: 229-235.

Bennett A., Gaffen J.D. and Chambers, E. (1988). Cyclo-oxygenase inhibitors and cell killing by cytotoxic drugs. In: Proceedings of the Taipei Conference on Prostaglandin and Leukotriene Research, in press.

Berstock, D.A., Houghton, J. and Bennett, A. (1979). Improved anticancer effect by combining cytotoxic drugs with an inhibitor of prostaglandin synthesis.   Cancer Treat. Rev.6 (Suppl), 69-71.

Berstock, D.A., Carroll, M.A. and Bennett, A. (1982). Murine cancer: the interaction of flurbiprofen with high-dose chemotherapy. 5th International Conference on Prostaglandins, abstract 149.

Gaffen, J.D., Bennett, A, Barer, M.R. (1985). A new method for studying cell growth in suspension, and its use to show that indomethacin enhances cell killing by methotrexate.   J. Pharm, Pharmacol., 37, 261-263.

Gaffen, J.D., Tsang, R. and Bennett, A. (1986).   Increased killing of malignant cells by giving indomethacin with methotrexate. Prog. Lipid. Res., 25, 543-545.

Henderson, G.B., Zevely, E.M. and Huennekens, F.M. (1978).   Cylic adenosine 3':5'-monophosphate and methotrexate transport in L1210 cells. Cancer Res., 38, 859-861.

Hewitt, H.B., Blake, E.R. and Walder, A.S. (1976).   A critique of the evidence for active host defence against cancer, based on personal studies of 27 murine tumours of spontaneous origin. Br. J. Cancer, 33, 241-259.

Langlois, A.J., Holder Jr., W.D., Iglehart, J.D., Nelson-Rees, W.A., Wells Jr, S.A. and Bolognesi, D.P. (1979).   Morpholigical and biochemical properties of a new human breast cancer cell line. Cancer Res., 39, 2604-2613.

Zor, U., Her, E., Talmon, J., Kohen, F., Harell, T., Moshonov, S. and Rivnay, B. (1987).   Hydrocortisone inhibits antigen-induced rise in intracellular free calcium concentration and abolishes leukotriene C4 production in leukemic basophils. Prostaglandins 34, 29-40.

INDEX

Biliary excretion, 39
Bleeding time, 130
  blood analysis, 20
Bradykinin, 145
Bronchoalveolar lavage, 20
Bronchoconstriction, 57-58,
    89, 196
  and leukotriene antagonists,
      57-58, 89, 198-199,
      200, 204, 205
  and 5-lipoxygenase
      inhibitors, 199, 200
      222
  and platelet activating
      factor antagonists, 95
Brotizolam, 95

Calcium ionophore A23187
  and eicosapentaenoic acid,
      186-187, 188
  and leukotriene metabolism,
      33-35, 37, 55, 56, 57,
      228-231, 232
  and lipoxins, 47-48, 49, 50,
      51-52
Calibration curve, 11-12, 13
Cancer chemotherapy
  breast cancer, 243, 244,
      245-247
  interactions between drugs,
      243-248
  see also Tumor cells
Carbenoxolone, 153, 155
  ISF 2715, 155-156
Cardiac anaphylaxis, 58-60
Cardiac transplantation, 72
Cardiomyocytes, and ischaemia,
    72, 73
Cardiovascular disease
  arterial thrombosis, 113-119
  and aspirin, 65-69
    primary prevention, 67-68
    secondary prevention, 66
    whith streptokinase, 67
  and prostacyclin/analogues,
      71-81
    cardioprotective
      mechanisms,
      74-76
    in clinical myocardial
      infarction, 76-77
  and renal prostaglandins,
      127-128
Cardiovascular system
  and leukotrienes, 55-56, 58-
      60
    biological activities, 58-
      60
    cardiac activities, 58
    generation, 55-56

CBFV, cyclical variations in
    blood flow, 113-119
Cell-to-cell contact, 236,
    239, 240
Cell types, and biosynthesis,
    31-36, 84, 183
Cerebrovascular disease, and
    aspirin, 66, 67, 68
Chemical ionization, 7-8
Cloning, see Molecular cloning
Collateral blood flow, 72-73,
    74
Coumadin, 131, 132
Crohn's disease, 145, 146, 201
  role of leukotrienes, 145,
      146, 147, 199
  and anti-inflammatory
      drugs, 146, 148, 149
Cutaneous inflammation, see
      Inflammation, cutaneous
Cyclical variation of blood
    flow, CBFV, 113-119
Cyclooxygenase, 23, 25, 31, 32,
    66, 227-228, 229-231
  localization, 35
  and transcellular
      metabolism, 31, 32, 35
Cyclooxygenase inhibitors
  and arterial thrombosis, 114
  BW755C, 166, 197, 200, 244,
      245, 246, 247
  in cancer chemotherapy, 244,
      245, 246, 247
  and gastric mucosa, 164, 166
  and macrophage eicosanoids,
      228-229
  and NSAIDs, 231-232, 233
  quantitative analysis, 19-20
  and renal disease, 125-126,
      127-128, 130, 131
Cyclophosphamide, 131
Cysteamine, 138, 139, 156
Cytochrome P-450, 23, 24
Cytokines, 187-188
Cytoprotection, cardiac, see
      Cardiovascular
      disease: aspirin,
      prostacyclins
Cytoprotection, gastric, 138,
    139, 140, 153-160
  "adaptive", 153-154
  cytoprotective drugs, 138,
      139, 155-156
  experimental models, 137-
      144, 153-155
  and prostaglandins, 138,
      142, 161-167
    exogenous, 139, 140, 156-
      157

and gastrointestinal mucosa,
137, 138, 139, 140,
154-155, 157, 162,
165-166
and cytoprotective drugs,
155-156, 157
and inflammation, 173, 174,
175-176, 177, 223
and inflammatory bowel disease, 146, 148
and interleukin-1, 239-240
and macrophage activation,
227, 228, 229, 235-236
and cytostasis, 236-239
microvascular effects, 173,
174, 175-176, 177
and NSAIDs, 162, 164, 165-
166, 229-230, 231,
232, 233
in renal disease, 124, 126
synthetase, 148
Prostaglandin endoperoxides,
31, 32-33, 34, 35,
115, 123
$9\alpha,11\beta$-Prostaglandin F2, 9α,
11β-PGF$_2$, 105-112
biological activities, 108,
109, 110
metabolism, 105, 108, 110
structure, 105, 108
Prostaglandins, PG
analogues, 139, 140, 153,
157
biological actions, 122, 146
biosynthesis, 65-66, 121-
122, 146
and cancer chemotherapy,
243-248
and cytoprotective drugs,
155-156
exogenous, 139, 140, 156-157
and gastrointestinal mucosa,
153-157, 161-167
gastroprotective properties,
137, 138, 139, 140,
142, 153, 157
in inflammation, 174-177,
178
in inflammatory bowel disease, 145-146, 148,
149
inhibition, 125-126, 243-248
metabolism, 31, 32
transcellular, 31, 32-33,
34, 35
microvascular effects, 174-
177, 178
and NSAIDs, 65-66, 156-157,
174, 175-176, 177
quantitative analysis, 19-20

renal, 121-122, 123-124,
125-128, 130
in chronic glomerular disease, 123-133
excretion, in disease,
123-124
vasodilative, 174-177, 178
see also 6-Keto-prostagladin
F$_2$
Psoriasis, 206, 208
Pyrexia, 224

Qualitative analysis, 6-7
Quantitative analysis
arachidonic acid, 11
clinical application, 19-20
derivatization, 18
immunoassays, 15-16
see also Gas chromatography-
mass
spectrometry; Mass
spectrometry
Quercetin, 197
Quinolines, 85, 86, 88, 89, 90

Radiochromatography, 106-108
Radioimmunoassay, 15-16
macrophage cytostasis, 237
Red blood cells, 33-34
Reductases
6,7-dihydroreductase, 47,
49, 51, 52
11-ketoreductase, 105, 108,
110
Renal eicosanoids, 24, 26,
108, 110, 121-136
biosynthesis, 121-123
glomerular, assessment,
123
localization, 121-122
cyclooxygenase, inhibitors
and renal function, 126-
127
glomerular disease, chronic,
121-136
eicosanoid inhibition,
129-133
thromboxane B$_2$ excretion,
123-125
urinary prostaglandin
excretion, 123-125
hypertension, renal, 26
prostaglandin inhibition,
125-126
and renal function, 127-
128
and renal failure, 124, 131
Reperfusion injury, 72-73, 74,
76

and gastric mucosal leuko-
    trienes, 137-141
  leukotriene C_4, 142
  platelet activating factor,
    141-142

Vascular studies, <u>see</u> Cardio-
    vascular disease; Car-
    dioascular system
Vasoconstriction, 74, 170-171
Vasoconstrictor hormones, 127-
    128
Vasodilating agents, 115
Vasodilation, 174-176, 178
Vasopressin, 127, 128
Verapamil, 244

Wheal reaction, 207